Large Gymnasium (

323 [illegible]

WI 1016, Wilson Hall, New College

The Neurobiology of Motivation and Reward

James R. Stellar
Eliot Stellar

The Neurobiology of Motivation and Reward

With 66 Figures

Springer-Verlag
New York Berlin Heidelberg Tokyo

James R. Stellar
Department of Psychology and
Social Relations
Harvard University
Cambridge, Massachusetts 02138
U.S.A.

Eliot Stellar
Department of Anatomy
and Institute of Neurological Sciences
University of Pennsylvania
Philadelphia, Pennsylvania 19104
U.S.A.

Library of Congress Cataloging in Publication Data
Stellar, James.
The neurobiology of motivation and reward.
Bibliography: p.
Includes index.
1. Motivation (Psychology)—Physiological aspects.
2. Reward (Psychology) I. Stellar, Eliot, 1919- .
II. Title. [DNLM: 1. Motivation—physiology. 2. Nervous
System—physiology. 3. Reward. WL 102 S8235n]
BF503.S82 1985 153.8 84-26729

Typeset by David E. Seham Associates Inc., Metuchen, New Jersey.
Printed and bound by R.R. Donnelley & Sons, Harrisonburg, Virginia.
Printed in the United States of America.

9 8 7 6 5 4 3 2 1

ISBN 0-387-96092-9 Springer-Verlag New York Berlin Heidelberg Tokyo
ISBN 3-540-96092-9 Springer-Verlag Berlin Heidelberg New York Tokyo

To Betty, Teresa, Jennifer, Liz, Chip, and Katie

Preface

This book was conceived many years ago as an abstract goal for a father–son team when the father was working in university administration and the son was just getting into the academic business. Eventually, the father returned to the laboratory, the son began to get his feet on the ground, and the goal became concrete. Now the work is finished, and our book enters the literature as, we hope, a valuable contribution to understanding the terribly complex and subtle problem of the neurobiology of motivated behaviors.

We would also like the book to stand as a personal mark of a cooperative relationship between father and son. This special relationship between the authors gave us an extra dimension of pleasure in writing the book, and it would delight us if it gave anyone else an extra dimension of enjoyment from reading it. One thing we hope happens is that anyone considering a similar partnership, or simply considering entering similar fields, will take the existence of this book as encouragement. Such relationships are highly satisfying if both parties take care to protect the partnership.

When we actually sat down to write the book, we were humbled by the immense literature and the smallness of both our conceived space for putting it down and of our brains for processing all the information. In some places, we consciously did not discuss a particular study or area of literature. Certainly, there are also papers we have forgotten to cite or of which we are unaware. Therefore, we invite you to write to us with your suggestions if you feel some important work or a body of literature is neglected.

We would like to acknowledge the many people who helped us with the preparation of this work. First, we would like to thank the other members of our family, who allowed this book to occupy much of our time together, and who actively supported us in its writing. Richard Solomon, Alan Epstein, Dale Corbett, and Meg Waraczynski all gave us their professional opinions on some of the chapters. Janet Gulotta, Mary Jack, Aimee Hamilton, and Kristin Quinlan provided valuable assistance on the word processors and in production aspects. Teresa Stellar helped us with the bibliography and with proofreading. Finally, the staff of Springer-Verlag gave us the encouragement and support we needed to work through the vagaries of production of a finished manuscript.

March, 1985

James R. Stellar
Eliot Stellar

Contents

1
Introduction

The Scope and Use of This Book

This book is intended for the reader who already has some familiarity with psychobiology. It is for researchers, graduate students, and upper level undergraduates who are interested in the topic of motivated behavior in animals and people. Our hope is that it will not only serve as a text for graduate and advanced undergraduate courses, but also that it will be enjoyed by those doing research on motivation and/or reward processes.

We did not, however, intend the book to be a handbook that completely surveys the field and includes all relevant references. Instead, we have tried to construct a conceptual map that will serve as a guide to the reader and be a useful source of ideas. Therefore, we focused on what we felt were key issues. For example, in the chapters dealing with brain-stimulation reward, we focused on behavioral measurement of the reward (chapter 5) and the implications of measures that separate reward and motoric consequences of drug administration (chapter 7). In the chapters on motivated behavior, we were selective in choosing examples so as to illustrate the principles and concepts of motivation and its underlying physiology.

Extensive reviews and studies of motivation are already available. Hoebel and Novin (1982) present a symposium on the topic of feeding behavior and reward. Feeding behavior itself is reviewed in a number of places (Stunkard & Stellar, 1984; Novin, Wyrwicka, & Bray, 1976); so is thirst (Epstein, Kissileff, & Stellar, 1973; Weijnen & Mendelson, 1977). The general topic of motivation has recently been treated in a series of contributions edited by Pfaff (1982b) and Morrison and Strick (1982) and in a handbook by Satinoff and Teitelbaum (1983). Reward from electrical stimulation of the brain is discussed in a volume deriving from an international symposium (Wauquier & Rolls, 1976) and in recent reviews (Gallistel, 1983; Routtenberg, 1980; Hall, Bloom, & Olds, 1977). Drug effects on reward or motivational processes are reviewed in many places (e.g., Iversen & Iversen, 1981; Cooper, Bloom, & Roth, 1982). The hypothalamus is discussed comprehensively in a three-volume handbook (Morgane & Panksepp, 1979 and 1981; see particularly the two parts of Vol. III on behavioral studies of the hypothalamus).

We consciously tried to make the book somewhat personal, and in light of the many reviews in this area of research, we feel that this is a strength rather than a weakness. The personal tone should *not* convince the reader that the book is simply idiosyncratic, however. Over 500 references were reviewed in its preparation, and strong emphasis was placed on the most current materials. We believe this gives the book a depth that will make it a useful source of references for anyone reviewing the neurobiology of motivation and reward.

The Book's Structure

Chapter 2 begins with a brief history of motivation and reward, the older notions of hedonism and temperament converge with more modern notions of regulatory physiology and the neurobiology of motivation. In chapters 3 and 4, the topic of motivated behavior is addressed in its modern conception, first as a behavioral problem, and second, as a problem of physiology and neurobiology. Chapter 3 deals with such behavioral concepts as incentive, competition among drives, acquired motivation, and affect. Chapter 4 considers the brain states that underlie these behavioral processes. It emphasizes the concept of a hierarchy of neurological control mechanisms and of peripheral/central-neural interactions in the generation of motivated behavior.

Reward is treated along with motivation in chapters 2, 3, and 4, but receives special attention through the study of brain stimulation in the next three chapters. Again, the progression from behavior to physiology is followed, with the exception that the physiology is divided into two chapters. Chapter 5, which deals with behavior, treats the important, and often underestimated, issue of how to make clear and specific measurements of the rewarding effects of electrical stimulation of the brain. Chapter 6 addresses the question of the tissue that is directly excited by the rewarding brain stimulation from electrodes located in one key place, the lateral hypothalamus. Chapter 7 presents the major hypothesis for the role of an important neurotransmitter, dopamine, and this discussion takes us well beyond brain stimulation.

Finally, in chapter 8, we deal with more synthetic issues of brain stimulation's interaction with motivation and offer some ways to bring the concept of reward and motivation together. Chapter 8 concludes the book by attempting to provide a broad overview of the field, noting the pendulum-like swings in our thinking, and setting out what the problems might be for the future.

The Book's Direction

The direction of the book and its many conclusions are difficult to summarize. It is especially difficult to identify concepts that will stand the test of time. When researchers 100 years in the future look back on the present, they will have many new concepts, born of advances in technology and new discoveries. We are not at all confident, however, that presently meaningful terms such as reward and motivation will have much scientific significance to those future psychobiologists, although the terms will probably always have a general use and meaning in common language.

We are sure, nevertheless, that behavioral concepts will remain central. Despite all the precision and rich diversity of presently understood and yet-to-be-discovered facts of molecular and cellular neurobiology and the anatomy and physiology of brain systems, it is well to remember that *the primary business of the brain is behavior.* The brain is organized so that its structure generates behavior, and it is only through a psychobiological approach that we will ever understand how the brain performs such a prodigious feat. The separate disciplines of neurobiology will never solve the problem alone. It is only in the combination of behavioral analysis with the rest of neurobiology that progress ultimately will be made.

In its conclusions, the book emphasizes seven major points. First and foremost is the common biological and behavioral basis of motivation and reward. In the vertebrates, at least, all motivated behaviors involve stimuli that function as rewards, and thus, direct and modify behavior. Activation of neurons in the lateral hypothalamus and anatomically related structures (ventral tegmental area and nucleus accumbens) make up a major component of the arousal of motivated behavior and reward. In addition, dopamine appears to be a neurotransmitter that plays a major role in both.

Second, peripheral and central-neural interaction is the rule in the biological control of motivated behavior and reward. The brain is sensitive to the internal environment and monitors metabolic and visceral events in the periphery, integrating this information with sensory information from the external environment as well as with information from past experience. All of these inputs control the brain, and in turn, the brain's output controls the periphery, including both the internal and external environment. Many of the pathways involved in motivation and reward have been traced, and we are beginning to develop concepts of how the motor control of motivation and reward is generated.

Third, the brain is organized in a hierarchical fashion, and so is behavior. While major integrators lie in the hypothalamus, they are under the influence of more rostral structures and exert their effects through a number of other integrators lying caudally in the neuraxis. What we are learning is that important components in the hierarchy of behavioral control also lie in the brainstem, even the caudal medulla. What may be even more important for our thinking is that the basic units of motivated behavior may be revealed here, including the specific responses of acceptance and rejection and approach and withdrawal.

Fourth, the study of brain-stimulation reward shows us that the psychophysical methods practiced by sensory psychobiologists are fruitful in the investigation of motivation and reward. Clearer behavioral measures, with emphasis on the quantitative rather than the qualitative, are important to the development of the field. Recent progress in quantitative psychobiology and structure–function relations in the field of vision is very encouraging and is being frankly emulated in self-stimulation studies.

Fifth, at the other end of the spectrum is the need for psychobiologists to include more data from human experience in our inquiry. In the attempt to be scientific in the past, we may have confused behaviorism with materialism and the avoidance of philosophical dualism. To the psychobiologist, subjective human experience comes from the physical brain, and is as much a function to be measured as overt behavior. The measurement may be difficult, but that does not mean that the function of reportable experience should be ruled out. Therefore, we have included human subjective reports, given on an analogue rating scale or in a magnitude estimation, along with accompanying behavioral data on the same subjects. Taken together with animal data, the human data add a new dimension to the inquiry.

Sixth, in one area, that of brain-stimulation reward, we may be close to identifying the brain substrate in a way that has never been done for a behavioral phenomenon as "psychological" as reward. We have two major clues: a rapidly growing, fine-grained psychophysical characterization of the behaviorally relevant axons that are directly excited by an electrode in the lateral hypothalamus (Gallistel, Shizgal, & Yeomans, 1981), and a strong implication of dopamine as an important neurotransmitter (Wise, 1982). What makes the field even more exciting is the possibility of forming a link between these two clues. That is, the behaviorally relevant axonal characterization suggests a connection between the axons excited by the electrode and the brain area containing dopamine cells.

Finally, we see the study of motivation and reward as moving in two directions. One direction is yielding a better and more powerful biological reductionism, which is coming about because of the development of powerful cellular and neurochemical techniques. Such techniques let us trace anatomic pathways in great detail and specify neurotransmitters and peptide neuromodulators, their agonists and antagonists, and their specific cellular receptor sites and channels. The other direction is our greater ability to use concepts and principles to synthesize and see function as a whole. The principles of hierarchical organization and peripheral/central-neural interaction are fundamental insights. Perhaps broader and of even greater impact is the recognition that motivated behavior is generated by the neurobiological mechanisms responsible for homeostasis and physiological regulation on the one hand, yielding reward and reinforcement/and producing affect and human hedonic experience on the other.

2

A Brief History of Motivation and Reward Concepts

The modern concept of motivation derives from the historical need to account for the arousal and direction of behavior. Human and animal activity occurs in peaks and troughs and it shifts its direction from one goal to another many times throughout a day. Even the ancients knew that these shifts in levels of activity and direction were the result of some combination of changes in external stimuli and internal state. What they did not know, however, was that the brain was the organ that integrated these inputs and was responsible for both behavior and conscious experience. Plato (428–348 B.C.), for example, thought that reason was in the head, but that courage was in the chest and appetite in the abdomen. The temptation to think in terms of separate central-neural and peripheral physiological controls of motivated behavior is still with us today. The lesson of history, however, is that there must be a biologically coherent mechanism integrating both peripheral and central controls. That mechanism is in the brain.

As we trace the roots of current thinking about motivated behavior (see Cofer & Appley, 1964; and Brown, 1979), we can see that it represents the convergence of different lines of inquiry in the history of both philosophy and science. One of the earliest and most relevant is the development of the concepts of *instincts and taxes* (tropisms), leading directly to the observations of naturalists and to the more recent work of ethologists. A second ancient line of inquiry is seen in the history of the concept of *hedonism* (pleasantness and unpleasantness). A third, related to hedonism in recent times, is one aspect of the history of *sensory psychology and physiology,* particularly beginning with Wilhelm Wundt's (1832–1920) concern with the nature of feeling. A fourth, related in a different way, is the emergence of the concepts of *temperament, emotion, and affect.* Fifth is the development of the concept of *reinforcement,* the role of rewards and punishments in learning new responses and in determining the vigor of existing responses. Sixth, and equally important, has been the idea of *regulatory physiology,* for many of the basic biological motivations are in the service of homeostasis and the survival of the individual and the species. Seventh, perhaps most important of all, have been developments in *neurobiology,* for it is the brain that is the organ of all behavioral functions, and we are now learning much about the organization, localization, and chemistry of brain circuits that form this common substrate for motivated behavior. Finally, from all of these converging lines, there emerges a very specific history of the development of the *concept of motivation,* including the concepts of drive and satiation, goal-directed behavior, and incentive.

All of these lines of inquiry and investigation also overlap and converge among themselves, particularly in the work of individual scholars. As we discuss the ideas and the people involved, keep in mind the overall hypothesis of this book: that a core neurological substrate serves the functions of physiological regulation, all motivated behaviors, reinforcement and reward, affect, and human hedonic experience. The view that these functions are anatomically, physiologically, and behaviorally related provides us with the opportunity for a broader theoretical synthesis. Furthermore, both the concepts and the techniques we use to investigate any one of these functions should help in the investigation of the others. Consequently, the headway we make in understanding the simpler functions like regulation and basic, biological motivation should stand us in good stead in the investigation of more complex functions like reinforcement and hedonic experience.

Before reviewing these eight historical lines, it should be pointed out that much of the early thinking about them has been permeated by mind–body dualism. Certainly the ancient Greeks forced themselves into a dualistic viewpoint, for they made the distinction between rational and non-rational determinants of behavior. In their view, only man possessed a rational soul (reason). Animals had a lower soul (instinct), which man also shared and which could be thought of in mechanistic terms. Descartes (1596–1650) set the tone for modern thinking by adopting this dualism and by providing a mechanism in the nervous system posited to allow for mind–body interaction—the pineal gland. To some extent, the distinction between rational and irrational processes continues today in the division of behavior into cognitive and affective processes. The division is all right, but any vestige of dualism should be eliminated from our thinking. As Aristotle (384–322 B.C.) anticipated, the mind–body problem can be resolved into a matter of form and function. All behavior and all psychological processes (mind) are the functions of the nervous system and its internal environment (body or form) and the ways in which the external environment impinges on them.

Instincts and Taxes

The Stoics of ancient Greece (304–205 B.C.) are credited with the first use of the term *instinct,* but the concept permeated ancient thought about the roots of behavior. The two essential elements of the ancient concept are still with us today: the arousal and the direction of behavior. Arousal was thought to require some special energy or vital force, and direction was predetermined and even "pre-known," and thus, teleological. Both were thought to be innate. Only gradually did growing biological knowledge eliminate the appeal of the vitalistic and teleological forces thought to be at work, but much of the mystery and myth about instinct has persisted through the modern era. Descartes held a mechanistic view of instinct and thought of it as a complex of reflexes, made up of animal spirits flowing in hollow nerve tubes. Darwin (1809–1882) placed it in evolutionary perspective and described instinct as a major behavioral adaptation to the environment. Generations of naturalists before and after Darwin, moreover, did us the great service of describing and cataloguing myriad instinctive behaviors in a wide range of species, pointing out that they were both species-specific and adaptive.

One class of instincts included behaviors we would count as motivated behaviors today: hunger, thirst, mating, nest-building, maternal behavior, filial behavior, migration, homing, herding, schooling, aggression, territorial defense, and so on. In another class were complex behaviors believed to be innate, but not considered as distinctively motivated. These included walking, swimming, flying, vocalization, imitation, motor coordination, and sensory perceptual processes.

As psychology came of age during the last century, it relied heavily on the concept of instinct, as in the writings of William James (1842–1910) and later, William McDougall (1871–1938). Both extended the concept of instinct to human behavior, but it was McDougall (1908) who gave instinct a central place in his theory. He made two valuable contributions to our thinking: First, he thought of instincts as prime movers, and therefore, as motivated behavior. Second, he believed that instincts had both cognitive aspects (knowing the object or end-point of the instinct) and affective accompaniments (feelings of pleasure and pain) and represented a striving toward or away from some object (approach–avoidance). But McDougall made the unfortunate error of using instinct *only* as an explanatory concept. Humans fought, therefore they had an instinct of pugnacity; they gathered together in groups, and this called for an instinct of gregariousness. In this way, McDougall also listed the odd assortment of flight, repulsion, curiosity, self-abasement, self-assertion, reproduction, acquisition, and construction as major human instincts, or as he later called them, *propensities*. They were innate and they determined human behavior and purpose.

The term *instinct* fell into deep disrepute because McDougall used it as an explanatory concept and because it implicated innate processes at a time when learning and experience were being successfully put forward as explanatory concepts by Watson (1878–1958) and the behaviorists (Watson, 1919). At most, the Watsonian behaviorists admitted three basic emotions—fear, anger, and love—that might be innate. Thus, the notion of instinct was all but dropped (Beach, 1955) until modern experimental and physiological psychologists used the term *motivated behavior* in place of instinct, and most important, went on to investigate the behaviors involved and their biological basis.

At the same time that behaviorists and experimental psychologists were turning away from the concept of instinct, the ethologists in Europe brought the study of instinct under notable scientific scrutiny (Tinbergen, 1951). In their terms, instinctive behavior was species-specific behavior, innately determined, primed by the internal environment, and triggered by external stimuli. Dealing with the classic issues of arousal and direction of behavior, the early ethologists saw the internal state building up a hydrostatic-type pressure that could overflow its bounds and appear as displacement behavior and even as a "vacuum reaction"—that is, it could be released without the benefit of external stimulation. Generally, however, the instinctive behavior was viewed as inhibited until a sign stimulus released it so that it could be expressed. The sign stimulus is a highly specific configuration, such as the red belly of the fighting stickleback fish and its vertical threat posture, or the red dot that is precisely positioned on the anterior beak of the gull that elicits gaping behavior and feeding in the young.

In very general terms, Tinbergen thought of each phase of instinctive behavior as the expression of a succession of central neural mechanisms arranged in a hierarchy. Each mechanism was subject to arousal by the internal state and to release by external sign stimuli, and each exerted an influence on the mechanisms below it in the hierarchy. For example, Tinbergen describes the reproductive behavior of the stickleback fish. The highest level of neuronal organization serves in migration, triggered by increases in gonadal hormones that are caused by increases in the amount of daily light. In response to these conditions, the next level in the hierarchy is released, and the fish move into their territories, guided by water temperature and response to green vegetation. Nest-building is then released at the next level, and this provides the focus for both territorial defense against red-bellied males and the attraction of females to the nest by the male's increasingly red belly and his execution of a zig-zag dance. Finally, mating is released, and then, the male participates in the care of the eggs by fanning them with his fins. The theory is that migration, territory selection, nesting, territorial defense, attracting of the female, mating, and parental behavior represent a succession of steps in the hierarchy of instinctive behavior.

Thus instinct evolved, in the history of thought, into two modern lines of investigation. One is the field work of the European ethologists on mammals, birds, amphibia, fish, and invertebrates. The work consists of observing, describing, and experimentally analyzing species-specific behavior thought to be innate. The other is the laboratory work of the American physiological psychologists interested in motivated behavior, working mainly on mammals (rats, cats, monkeys), who see much that is "hard-wired" in the basic biological motivations of hunger, thirst, sex, aggression, and so on, and much that is species-typical. But they also see how modifiable in experience motivated behavior is, particularly in mammals, and how dependent upon experience its full expression may be. Both the ethologists and the psychologists recognize the common ground they are on, and one of the big challenges they both face is to understand the neurological basis of instinct and/or motivated behavior.

At a simpler level, the same issues arose in the work of Jacques Loeb (1859–1924) and H. S. Jennings (1868–1947). Reduction of behavior to its underlying biological mechanism, indeed its physical and chemical basis, was the lofty goal of Jacques Loeb (1918). He chose for study simple organisms (invertebrates) and simple behaviors he called *tropisms*—essentially "forced" movements toward or away from some source of stimulation, such as the phototropism of protozoa or the rheotropism of fish (swimming directly into the current). The orientation depended on the innate tendency of the animal to equalize stimulation on both sides of the body. Moreover, the more intense the stimulation, the stronger the behavior. The sign (toward or away) was also innate. The scientific task, as Loeb saw it, was to learn the physical and chemical basis of these two innate mechanisms.

As a mechanistic biologist, Loeb was a direct descendant of Descartes. It is a matter of some historical interest that, unlike the students of instinct or motivation, he never ascribed much of a role to the internal state of the organism nor to the expression of affect. Neither did he allow much room for biological variability or modification of behavior through experience, although he thought there could be "psychic life" in animals capable of associative memory. It remained for H. S. Jennings (1906) to recognize the importance of the variability of the organism and the trial and error nature of its behavior, even among protozoa. At the same time, he searched for the biological basis of behavior, placing importance on the organism's internal physiological state.

The experimental psychologists were much influenced by Jennings. The ethologists derived many of their ideas from Loeb, but they replaced the term tropism with *taxis,* reserving tropism for the orientation of plants by growth. Furthermore, they saw the orientations they called taxes as components of instinctive patterns of behavior, part of *fixed action patterns* that allowed the organism to approach or avoid some object (appetitive behavior) and to perform specific acts upon it (consummatory behavior). Distinguishing the appetitive and consummatory aspects of instinct and motivation was an important advance in thinking, originated by Craig (1918), and it had great impact on the work of both ethologists and psychologists.

Hedonism

Almost at the other end of the spectrum from instinct were the thoughts of the ancient Greek philosophers about *hedonism*—human experiences of pleasantness and unpleasantness. Aristippus of Cyrene (ca. 435–356 B.C.), a contemporary of Socrates, made a philosophy of life of hedonism, emphasizing the happiness and good in striving for pleasure. Epicurus (341–270 B.C.) and his followers continued the cult, and when the cult died, hedonism diminished in philosophical importance. It was the British associationists and empiricists and their French counterparts who emphasized the utilitarian role of good and happiness in the determination of behavior, including the concept of "the greatest good for the greatest number." Hobbes (1588–1679), John Stuart Mill (1806–1873), and especially Jeremy Bentham (1748–1832) and the Utilitarians, were most influential in developing and perpetuating this special role of hedonic experience.

None of these philosophers, however, raised the question of the biological basis of hedonism nor its role in animal behavior. It was Herbert Spencer (1820–1903), a Darwinian concerned with the study of instinct, who did both. He saw pleasure and pain as guiding principles in evolution and adaptive behavior, and he wrote (1872) that "pains are the correlatives of actions injurious to the organism, while pleasures are the correlatives of actions conducive to its welfare." Spencer (1872) foretold Thorndike's law of effect by stating: "every animal habitually persists in each act which gives pleasure—and desists from each act which gives pain," thus describing the effect of positive and negative reinforcement on behavior. For humans, he felt that pleasure was "a feeling which we seek to bring into consciousness" and pain "a feeling which we seek to get out of consciousness and to keep out."

Troland (1928), dealt with pleasure and pain as essential parts of human motivation. Borrowing from Sherrington, he classified stimuli as nociceptive, neutroceptive, and beneceptive, thus emphasizing the sensory basis of hedonic experience. In his theory, thalamic relay nuclei were thought to play facilitative and inhibitory roles (cf. Head & Holmes, 1911, *syndrome thalamique*).

Coming from the tradition of Wundt (1832–1920) via Titchener (1867–1927) and Boring (1886–1968), Beebe-Center (1932) also discussed pleasantness and unpleasantness in sensory terms. Starting with the Wundtian concept that weak stimuli were pleasant and strong stimuli unpleasant, he thought of pleasantness–unpleasantness as an intensity continuum passing through some neutral zone. He wrote a book on the subject and tried to make the study of these affective states as scientific and objective as psychophysical methods would allow. Although Beebe-Center studied saccharine preference in rats later in his life (Beebe-Center, et al., 1948), true to his historical tradition in sensory psychology, he focused on human hedonic experience, and concerned himself very little with the motivational or reinforcement aspects of hedonism or the question of its biological basis beyond the role of sensory reception.

It remained for P. T. Young (1936, 1941) to attempt a direct and objective study of hedonic processes in animals. He also focused on sensory processes, however, and he used the study of food preference and food choice in animals as his main vehicle of investigation. Because of this, he was, of necessity, also interested in motivation and emotional expression. In studies of rats, he used both the measure of relative amount of food and fluid intake (consummatory response) and the measures of approach and choice without substantial ingestion as in his brief-exposure preference tester or with a T-maze (appetitive response). Preference was indicated by greater intake of a substance, more frequent choice of a small taste of the substance, or more rapid running to the substance. Since some non-nutritive substances like saccharine were preferred, Young, unlike his contemporary, C.P. Richter, emphasized the role of palatability rather than biological need or internal state in determining preference and motivation. Furthermore, because of the intensity and persistence of preference behavior, he also assumed that it was accompanied by the expression of some affective process that contributed to the arousal of the motivated behavior (incentive) and also served as a reinforcement or reward in the acquisition of new behavior.

Building on the food preference work of Young as well as of Richter, Pfaffmann (1960, 1965, 1980, 1982) sought to understand directly the neural basis of food preferences, and as he called them, "the pleasures of sensation." In this way, he brought together the traditions of animal motivated behavior, sensory psychology, and sensory neurophysiology. His work focused on two aspects of the role of the nervous system. First and foremost, he described the relation of peripheral afferent nerve discharges to the generation of preference, reinforcement, and hedonic effect, particularly in the gustatory system. Secondly, he concerned himself with the central nervous system, the central terminations of the sensory pathways, and he and his students showed how the gustatory pathways led to the hypothalamus and limbic system as well as to the thalamocortical system (see Figure 4.5). In addition, he showed the relationships among the afferent neural discharges in animals, the preference behavior of rats, and affective or hedonic ratings of tastes by humans.

While Pfaffmann clearly recognized the role of post-ingestional events and the internal environment in food preferences and palatability, it was Cabanac (1971, 1979) who showed how human ratings of concentrated sugar solutions changed from pleasant to unpleasant as a function of ingestion or gastric preloading with the sugar (see Figure 3.12). This is a phenomenon Cabanac calls "alliesthesia"; it also shows up in the evaluation of the pleasantness and unpleasantness of odors, and as a function of core body temperature in the hedonic evaluation of warm and cold stimuli. As the temperature example makes clear, the gustatory and olfactory systems are not alone in generating pleasant and unpleasant effects. Butler (1953), for example, demonstrated the importance of visual stimulation as a reinforcer of learning in visually deprived monkeys. In addition, Harlow has made eminently clear in his study of infant rhesus monkeys how important "tactile comfort" is in normal emotional and social development, what motivation tactile deprivation can engender, and how much attachment depends on early experience with this form of sensory stimulation (Harlow and Zimmerman, 1959).

To bring the history of hedonism up to date, we should mention Solomon's opponent process theory of affect (Solomon, 1982). In a nutshell, this theory holds that the negative after-effect of pleasure is pain, and of pain is pleasure (see Figure 3.3). Thus the abstinence agony of the drug addict, the grief of the recently widowed, and the separation-distress of the imprinted duckling are all negative after-effects of highly positive experiences. So, according to the theory, are the highs of sport parachute jumping and long-distance running, as well as the elation of the dog released from a shock box or from social isolation the after-effects of highly negative experiences.

History shows that hedonic responses can be induced experimentally and studied objectively in humans by use of rating scales. They can also be studied in animals by use of operant conditioning technology and by observing affective display behavior. It is our hypothesis that these hedonic responses use the same neurological mechanisms operative in motivated behavior and reinforcement.

Sensory Psychology and Physiology

It is remarkable to realize that the mainstream of the history of experimental psychology, starting with Wilhelm Wundt (1873), borrowing heavily from the early great sensory physiologists (Johannes Müller, 1801–1858, and Hermann von Helmholtz, 1821–1894), never addressed the question of motivation. Wundt acknowledged feeling as one of the attributes of sensation, and Boring (1929), in his *A History of Experimental*

Psychology, discusses hunger and thirst along with urination and defecation as some of the organic sensations. But motivation is mentioned only briefly in the discussion of the dynamic psychology of Freud and McDougall; neither is affect nor pleasantness and unpleasantness discussed. Nor does motivation fare much better in Boring's book, *Sensation and Perception in the History of Experimental Psychology* (1942), although the concept of drive is mentioned.

It remained for Beebe-Center, in *The Psychology of Pleasantness and Unpleasantness* (1932), to summarize the contributions of experimental psychology to the question of hedonic experience. However, he did not deal with the question of motivation. Rather, his contribution was to show that psychophysical methods could be used to scale the pleasantness and unpleasantness of stimuli as well as the sensations they produced. He also suggested use of the term *hedonic-tone,* ranging from positive (pleasantness) to negative (unpleasantness) through some neutral zone, to take the place of *affective-tone* and *feeling-tone,* terms used by earlier writers. Finally, he summarized, and discussed as unverifiable, extant theories of the physiological and neurological basis of hedonic-tone: Herrick (1918) wrote that "Normal discharge . . . of definitely elaborated nervous circuits resulting in free, unrestrained activity is pleasurable. . . . Conversely the impediment to such discharge . . . results in a stasis of nerve centers . . . and the development of a situation of unrelieved nervous tension which is unpleasant. . . ."; F. H. Allport (1924) thought pleasantness was associated with peripheral parasympathetic nervous system activity and unpleasantness with sympathetic; Troland (1928) speculated that "hedonic tone depends on the average conductance of cortical synapses . . .", pleasantness (and learning) resulting from increased conductance.

As pointed out previously, it wasn't until Pfaffmann took direct steps to investigate the hedonic aspects of afferent neural input that sensory psychology and sensory physiology began to make contributions to our understanding of the basis of motivation and reinforcement. More recently, Berridge and Grill (1983), have challenged the concept of a single continuum from pleasantness to unpleasantness through a neutral point. On the basis of their observation of rapid alternation between ingestive and aversive responses in rats given taste solutions by mouth cannula, they suggest instead that the nervous system may organize hedonic-tone in two separate mechanisms, one positive and one negative.

Temperament, Emotion, and Affect

Attempts to understand the biological basis of temperament date back to Hippocrates (460–370 B.C.). Based on Empedocles' (490–435 B.C.) list of the four cosmic elements (air, earth, fire, and water), Hippocrates believed that there were four corresponding bodily fluids or "humors" that determined temperament (Figure 2.1). *Black bile* was responsible for the *melancholic* temperament, (the sad, the love-sick); *yellow bile,* for the *choleric* temperament, (the angry, the irascible, the fighter); *phlegm,* for the *phlegmatic* temperament, (the apathetic, the sleepy, the flaccid); and *blood,* for the *sanguine* temperament (optimism, hopefulness, expectancy). As with all typologies, it was thought that people had different amounts of the four humors and that temperament was determined largely by which one was dominant. However fanciful, Hippocrates' notion began the search for the internal states that determined temperament, mood, affect. The search still goes on today with the focus on the internal environment of the nervous system and concern about the role of hormones, neurotransmitters, and peptide neuromodulators, especially the endogenous opiates.

The history of investigation of the biology of emotion can be divided

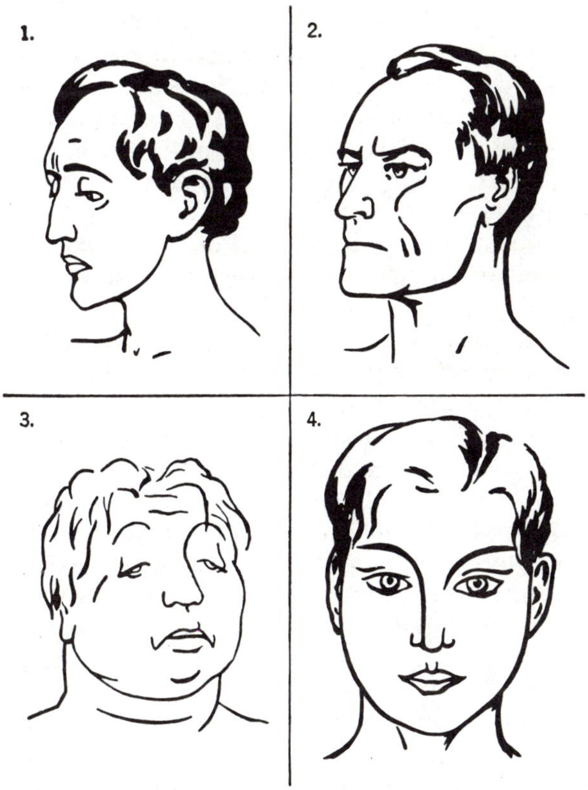

Figure 2.1 Representations of the four temperaments: (1) melancholic, (2) choleric, (3) phlegmatic, (4) sanguine (G.W. Allport, 1937.) Reprinted by permission.

into three phases: (a) emotional expression and its adaptive value, (b) peripheral autonomic manifestations of emotion, and (c) central neural mechanisms controlling emotion. Emotional expression was thought of as the accompaniment of instinct, and as Darwin said in *Expression of the Emotions in Man and Animals* (1873), emotional expressions were remnants of adaptive behaviors, innately given (see Figures 3.6, 3.7, and 3.8). Some expressions could be enhanced or strengthened by habit, and a few were learned, cultural gestures. As the ethologists later pointed out, many served as sign stimuli, releasing instinctive behavior in other animals, especially conspecifics.

Peripheral autonomic nervous system activity was proposed in the James–Lange theory (Lange, 1885; James, 1894) to be the cause of emotional experience. Thus the peripheral expression of emotion was actually thought to precede the conscious experience of emotion and provide the afferent neural basis for it. A generation of psychophysiologists, armed with the means of recording autonomic activity (galvanic skin response, blood pressure change, heart rate change, local temperature change, etc.) failed to find specific patterns of response for each of the emotions that could provide the specific afferent neural input needed. What they found instead was general arousal during all emotions, reflected in the EEG as well. More recently, however, Ekman (1982; Ekman, Levenson, & Friesen, 1983) has found specific autonomic patterns associated with different facial expressions of emotion. So the pendulum swings, and feedback from the periphery may prove to be more specific than previously thought.

It was Cannon (1927) and Bard (1928) who proposed, contrary to the James–Lange theory, that emotion involved the arousal of the central nervous system, which simultaneously caused the peripheral expression of emotion, both skeletal and visceral, and the conscious experience of emotion through activation of the cerebral cortex. In keeping with Head and Holmes' (1911) report on the striking changes in emotion following thalamic lesions *(syndrome thalamique)*, they thought the focus of the central neural mechanism was in the thalamus.

Bard and his coworkers later went on to show other foci in the hypothalamus (Wheatley, 1944) and the cortex and amygdala (Bard & Mountcastle, 1947). By that time, Bard already knew of Papez's (1937) proposed circuit for emotion in the rhinencephalon: hippocampus, fornix, mammillary bodies, mammillo-thalamic tract, anterior thalamus, cingulate cortex, cingulum, and hippocampus again. These structures were major portions of what Broca (1878) had called the grand limbic lobe, forming a ring or limbus around the thalamus and brainstem.

Also during this period, Moruzzi and Magoun (1949) discovered the arousal function of the reticular formation of the brainstem. Receiving collaterals from all the main sensory pathways, the reticular formation through the non-specific nuclei of the thalamus activated or aroused all of the cerebral cortex, the hypothalamus, and the spinal cord. In keeping with the arousal theory of emotion, which argued that emotional arousal was non-specific behaviorally as well as physiologically, Lindsley (1951) proposed the reticular formation as the central neural mechanism of emotion.

Although general arousal is important, emotion has its specific behavioral forms—as in anger, fear, aggression, love—and it shows up in radically different manifestations in psychopathology: depression, mania, anxiety, compulsion, and the pathological changes in affect seen in schizophrenia. We have no clear understanding of the detailed neural mechanisms involved in these disorders, but we do know that different neurotransmitters, endocrines, and peptide neuromodulators are involved and that great changes in affect can be produced by pharmacological agents that are antagonistic and agonistic to these neurochemicals.

Reinforcement

The idea that behavior is controlled by its hedonic consequences is as old as philosophy. It was not until the English associationists, however, that the utility of behavior became a formal part of the theory of associative learning. Studying trial and error learning in animals in 1898, E. L. Thorndike (1874–1949) formulated the *law of effect,* which stated that the reward of success stamped in stimulus–response associations; punishment or other negative consequences stamped them out (Thorndike, 1898, 1911). Thus was born the modern concept of reinforcement of learning and performance, adopted by the major learning theorists of the 1930s (cf. Hull, 1943) and made an integral part of the empirical work of B. F. Skinner (1938) in shaping the operant behavior of animals and humans.

Pavlov (1927), it should be remembered, originated the concept of reinforcement in his classical conditioning studies. He conceived of it as the activation of the cerebral cortex by the unconditioned stimulus, irradiating in close temporal contiguity to a neighboring cortical area activated by the conditioned stimulus. Although it is now known that the cortex is not essential for Pavlovian conditioning, some special form of neural activation by the reinforcing event is probably common in all kinds of learning.

Kety (1970) has suggested that the reinforcement of learning depends on the neurosecretion of biogenic amines widely in the brain and into the cerebrospinal fluid. He pointed out that neurons, using catecholamines as their neurotransmitters, have many-branched axons that arise from cell bodies in the brainstem and extend monosynaptically to the forebrain as well as the cerebellum. The axons secrete neurotransmitters at varicosities along their way, as well as at their terminals. His theory is that these central-neural biogenic amine secretions are induced in the brain by biologically significant events, just as they are in the peripheral autonomic nervous system, and may form the basis for reinforcement of learning by inducing changes at synapses that were active at the time. Epinephrine, norepinephrine, and dopamine have been suggested as candidate neurotransmitters.

Whether such activation of biogenic amines takes place in all cases of associative conditioning is not known, however. What is known is that in many instances of classical conditioning, human and animal subjects are aroused by salient stimuli (USCs) and often they are motivated (e.g., aroused by food stimuli in the salivation experiments and by pain from or fear of electric shock in reflex-withdrawal experiments). Furthermore, food or shock termination (rewards) often appear following the conditioned response. Thus, even if motivation and reward are not necessary conditions for all classical conditioning, they often accompany it. In operant conditioning, of course, motivation and reward are clearly two conditions that must prevail if the law of effect is to apply. Otherwise, the organism will not work (when not motivated) or will undergo extinction (when not reinforced).

Despite this speculation, we still do not know what the actual reinforcing state of affairs is. For now, history will be served by reference to the classical experiment of Olds and Milner (1954) in which they demonstrated that electrical stimulation of parts of the limbic system (septal area and diencephalic regions) of the rat had a powerful reinforcing effect in that it shaped the rat's lever-pressing behavior and made it respond at an extremely high rate. Olds and others then went on to show that stimulation in some loci in the brain was aversive, in that it diminished and eliminated operant behavior (Olds & Olds, 1963; Valenstein & Valenstein, 1964; Hoebel, 1976).

It was as though the stimulating electrode had artificially activated parts of the brain that natural positive and negative reinforcers activate. But there were differences. For one thing, the rat extinguished almost immediately when the brain stimulation was omitted. This led Deutsch and Howarth (1963), and later Gallistel (1973), to postulate that the electrical brain stimulation produced both motivation (drive) and reinforcement at the same time. The validity of their concept became clear when it was shown that the behavior diminished as a function of the length of time since the last brain stimulation and could be restored by "priming" the brain with a "free" brain stimulation. It was as though the priming stimulus set up the motivational brain state so that the next brain stimulation could serve as a reinforcement or reward.

Thus, a way was opened up for the study of the neural basis of hedonic processes in animals, including both drive and reward. Parallel experiments in humans (Sem-Jacobsen & Torkildsen, 1960; Bishop, Elder, & Heath, 1964; Heath, 1964a) who had electrodes implanted in the same regions of the brain for treatment and investigation of intractable pain, epilepsy, and schizophrenia confirmed the reinforcing properties of such brain stimulation in humans and demonstrated that the effects could be highly pleasurable even though not always specifiable as to quality.

Regulatory Physiology

When physiology came of age and put aside vitalism and teleology in favor of empirical, scientific principles of function based on experimental work, it was Claude Bernard (1813–1878) who was at the forefront. Describing his own work in *An Introduction to the Study of Experimental Medicine* (1865), Bernard continued in the mechanistic tradition of Descartes. His many contributions to experimental physiology all led to his conception of the constancy of the internal environment, the *milieu interieur*. This concept implied physiological regulation of the internal environment. It was Andre Mayer (1900) who recognized in the study of thirst that behavior was also involved in the regulation of the internal environment.

Later, W. B. Cannon (1932) extended Bernard's conception and introduced the term *homeostasis* to signify maintenance of the constancy of the internal environment. His *Wisdom of the Body* also made it clear, moreover, that behavior was an essential part of physiological regulation. He and his student, Philip Bard (1934a), recognized the arousal function of emotion and established the role of the autonomic nervous system in it. As mentioned earlier, they made the important proposal that it was the central nervous system (thalamus) that integrated the emotional behavior and yielded both the expression and the conscious experience of emotion. Extending the concept further, Bard (1940) went on to apply the same thinking and same type of investigation to the study of sexual behavior and thus laid the modern foundations for the neurology of motivated behavior.

It was C. P. Richter (1942–43), however, who was most explicit about the role of behavior in physiological regulations. He used the term *self-regulatory behavior* and specifically identified these behaviors as drives in the sense that Woodworth (1918) defined them. Thus, thirst, hunger, specific hungers, behavioral temperature regulation (nest-building), and so on, all fell into place for Richter, bringing together motivation and physiological regulation.

In an independent line, stemming from Bernard, E. F. Adolph (1943) focused directly on the processes and the laws of physiological regulation. He too recognized the importance of the behavioral contribution to regulation and was followed by Brobeck (1946), who carried the problem of regulation and control systems into direct investigations of the central nervous system.

Neurobiology

How the brain mediates physiological regulation, motivation, reinforcement, emotion, and hedonic experience has long been a mystery. Flourens (1794–1867) had observed that birds and other animals with ablated cerebrums did not initiate behavior. Later, Goltz (1892) reported that decortication of dogs produced what Bard (1934b) subsequently called "sham rage": they gave an angry response to even mild tactile stimuli, the response did not outlast the stimulus, and it was not directed toward the stimulus. Still later, Head and Holmes (1911), in describing the *syndrome thalamique,* gave the first insight into specific brain loci that might be involved in the experiences of pleasantness and unpleasantness. They reported clinical cases with thalamic lesions in which stimuli were either excruciatingly painful or exquisitely pleasant, and these included as diverse sources as light tactile stimulation (pain) and music (pleasure). They speculated that the thalamus is normally inhibited by the cortex in the expression of hedonic experience. Inhibitory cortico-thalamic connections are severed by the lesions, leaving the thalamus released to act alone in these affective responses. Bard and Mountcastle (1947) later identified both excitatory and inhibitory roles for neocortex and old cortex, respectively (see below).

In 1938, Lashley wrote an article, "An Experimental Analysis of Instinctive Behavior," in which he expressed the belief that motivated behavior was directly proportional to some excitatory process in the brain. Morgan, in 1943, labeled this process the *central motive state,* but neither man had any idea of where in the brain that process or state was represented. Their speculations were based mainly on studies of Beach (1942) who, at that time, had gotten only as far as exploring the role of the cerebral cortex in maternal and sexual behavior.

Actually, it was earlier, in the mid-1930s, that W. R. Hess (1957) identified the diencephalon as a region of the brain important in regulative processes and associated behaviors. He implanted electrodes in the brains of cats and was able to stimulate different loci in the hypothalamus and thalamus while the animals were awake and behaving. In this way, he demonstrated the elicitation of eating or bulimia, drinking, aggression, sleeping, and so on, and mapped the diencephalon in its autonomic as well as behavioral function. In general terms, he found that the posterior diencephalon was concerned with sympathetic functions, which he called *ergotropic* or energy-expending functions, and the anterior diencephalon, with *trophotropic* or energy-conserving, parasympathetic functions.

During this same period, as mentioned above, Papez (1937) identified the limbic circuit concerned with emotional behavior. Also in the late 1930s, Ranson (1939) and his colleagues (Hetherington & Ranson, 1942) at Northwestern adapted the Horsely-Clarke stereotaxic instrument, originally developed for human neurosurgery, to the experimental study of the effects of sub-cortical lesions in animals. During this fruitful period, they made bilateral hypothalamic lesions that greatly increased or decreased such motivated behaviors as eating, drinking, copulation, sleeping, waking, and temperature regulation (see Windle, 1981).

Nearby, at the University of Chicago, Klüver and Bucy (1939) were investigating the temporal lobes, including the amygdala and hippocampus within them. They did bilateral surgical ablations in monkeys and found great changes in aggression, visual exploration, and both oral and sexual behavior. The normally aggressive rhesus monkey became tame, it compulsively inspected all small visual objects, and if the objects could be picked up, brought them to its eyes and then put them in its mouth in a pattern reminiscent of primate grooming behavior. Almost everything went into the mouth: nuts, bolts, wooden blocks, small pieces of meat even though the rhesus is not carnivorous. The monkeys masturbated frequently and often engaged in indiscriminate mounting behavior and copulation.

This work was followed up by the investigations of Bard and Mountcastle (1947) who found that amygdala lesions produced ferocity in cats; so did lesions of the old cortex, whereas lesions of the neocortex resulted in placidity. The conflict in findings with amygdala lesions were originally ascribed to species differences, but Schreiner and Kling (1956) later found that stereotaxic lesions of the amygdala in cats produced placidity. This conflict within one species was probably due to differences in what parts of the amygdala were damaged, although no careful comparison of the anatomy in the two experiments was ever done. However, more recent findings of Flynn and his associates, evoking rage and attack behavior in cats by perifornical stimulation, show that such aggression can be either facilitated or inhibited by prior stimulation of two different sites in the amygdala (Flynn, Vanegas, Foote, & Edwards, 1970). It is possible that lesions in these two different sites would yield opposite effects on aggressive behavior.

During this same period, Moruzzi and Magoun (1949) made their discovery of the activating role of the reticular formation, and Lindsley (1951) identified the reticular formation as an important structure in emotional behavior. In the 1940s and 1950s, there were a great number of investigations of the consequences of hypothalamic lesions by both physiologists and psychologists. By 1954, E. Stellar was able to write a paper on the "Physiology of Motivation," in which he suggested the hypothalamus as the focus of extensive limbic systems involved in motivated behavior (Stellar, 1954). He envisaged excitatory and inhibitory mechanisms for all motivated behaviors, subject to the influence of both the internal environment and external sensory stimulation. Support for the extensive anatomical substrate involved came from Pribram and Kruger's

(1954) paper, "Functions of the Olfactory Brain," and support for the motivational and affective role of these structures came from MacLean's (1949) paper, "Psychosomatic Disease and the 'visceral brain.' "

It was also in 1954 that Olds and Milner demonstrated the reinforcing value of electrical brain stimulation in the septal area and the lateral hypothalamus (medial forebrain bundle) as well. Heath (1964b) and his colleagues, furthermore, extended these findings to humans and were able to elicit reports of hedonic experience upon brain stimulation in the same regions.

Thus, the outlines of a neurobiology of motivation were established. Many details have now been worked out and are reported later in this book. Much more remains to be learned, particularly about the neurochemistry of motivated behavior, but also about the detailed circuitry involved.

The Concept of Motivation

Much of the meaning of the foregoing discussion depends upon the value of the concept of motivation. However crudely they may be defined, no one questions the validity of affect, emotion, or pleasure and pain, and no one questions the validity of hunger, thirst, sleep, or aggression. But the concept of motivation has had a stormy history.

Morgane (1979), for example, attacked the concept as mystical and without representation in the nervous system. Yet motivation is a definable property of behavior, and behavior is the outcome of activity in the brain. It seems to us that it serves no purpose to dismiss it with a wave of the hand. The issue, as this book demonstrates, is to investigate motivation as one of the complex functions of the brain, showing its behavioral validity and uncovering its neurological basis. Caution is needed, however, because motivation—and for that matter, reinforcement—is the result of the operation of *many* brain mechanisms. Thus, these terms may be very difficult to relate to specific brain mechanisms (see the beginning of chapter 6 for further discussion of this point).

As mentioned earlier, motivation refers to the arousal and new direction of specific behaviors and their satiation, and the new arousal and direction of other behaviors, representing shifts in motivation. Historically, much of this conception has been included in the term instinct, and the motivational aspects of instinct were emphasized by William James (1890) and William McDougall (1908). But as "instinct" fell into disrepute, the question of the arousal and direction of behavior was neglected. Experimental psychology focused on cognitive processes, particularly sensory and perceptual processes, as studied by Wundt (1873–74), Titchener (1896), Boring (1929, 1942), and the structuralists. It also emphasized the role of learning and experience in the determination of behavior, exemplified by Watson (1919) and the behaviorists. It was the functional psychologists (John Dewey, 1886) who took a Darwinian and evolutionary view toward behavior and who saw the need for the concept of motivation. As psychology matured, the concept re-entered. Woodworth (1918) introduced the term *drive* to replace instinct and to represent some urge or impulse, based upon bodily need, that impelled the organism to action. In the 1930s, Clark Hull (1943) adopted a drive theory of reinforcement and learning in which bodily need led to drive, which then led to new learned behavior to correct the need and reduce the drive, thus reinforcing the learning. Miller (1959) recognized that the bodily need often was not corrected when reinforcement took place, and therefore, he proposed a drive-reduction rather than a need-reduction theory of learning.

Tolman (1932) had earlier recognized that behavior was purposive and directed toward goals and places where goals could be obtained. He developed an expectancy concept of motivation in which an animal that had already learned, developed an expectation of a specific goal (e.g., food, sexual partners), and this goal functioned as an *incentive,* increasing the arousal of motivated behavior. Skinner (1938), on his part, refused to speculate about what went on inside the organism and took the view that he could account for reinforcement and learning in terms of external stimuli and responses.

It was the internal state of the organism, however, and particularly what went on in the central nervous system, that was the concern of the physiological psychologists. They studied biological motivation, essential for the survival of the individual and the species: eating, drinking, fighting, fleeing, sleep, mating, parental and filial behavior, migration, homing, territoriality, aggression, pain avoidance. All of these behaviors had been called instinctive by an earlier generation of psychologists and are currently called instinctive by the ethologists. Many, but not all, of the behaviors contribute to homeostasis and physiological regulation, but all involve the same kind of neurological mechanism and have the same properties of arousal and satiation, and under appropriate conditions, reinforcement. Furthermore, all these processes that can be identified in humans are also accompanied by positive or negative hedonic states or affect.

Finally, it should be said that motivation is a behavioral property that emerged in evolution and became more complex and richer as it evolved. The blowfly, for example, can be aroused to exploratory activity and ingestion upon external stimulation of its taste receptors, but its eating behavior is unaffected by its internal metabolic state (Dethier, 1976). Eating is terminated (satiation?) by the development of pressure in the foregut, which stimulates the recurrent nerve. Food, however, is not a ready reinforcer of new learning. Thus, the blowfly may have only a rudimentary form of motivated behavior or a precursor of what we see in vertebrates. Yet other invertebrates, like the ant, the bee, and the octopus, can learn on the basis of food reward. And negative reinforcement works well in the octopus and the sea slug, aplysia; the emergence of motivated behavior must have begun early in phylogeny.

That these changes continue later in phylogeny is illustrated by the example of sexual behavior in vertebrates (Beach, 1947). The female rat, for example, is heavily dependent on estrogen levels, as its 4–5-day estrous cycle shows and gonadectomy and replacement therapy verify. Sensory deprivation and decortication have little effect on the female rat. Female cats and dogs, on the other hand, are more dependent on sensory stimulation and more affected by decortication, though still dependent on hormones. It is in the primates, particularly apes and humans, that the female's relative independence of the hormones becomes possible, with a greater dependence on sensory and cerebral processes.

Finally, it is only with humans that we have a way of knowing about hedonic experience, for we can measure pleasantness and unpleasantness with suitable rating scales or magnitude estimation techniques. Animals have the hedonic processes of motivated behavior, approach and avoidance, and positive and negative reinforcement, and they express emotional states autonomically and somatically. But we can only speculate about their hedonic experience.

History tells us that the concept of motivation derived from many different lines of inquiry. As we trace its historical roots, we also see that it evolved in ontogeny and emerged in phylogeny through a process of encephalization in which more and more complex function is added as more levels in the neural hierarchy are added. At the simpler levels, approach or avoidance and innate consummatory acts are possible. As the nervous system becomes more complex, sensory and internal environment controls are added, and learning and the process of reinforcement become possible. Motivated behavior is now more variable and modifiable and serves much more than homeostasis. Affect and affective display become an important accompaniment, and in humans, hedonic experience. How the evolving and developing brain generates these related psychological and behavioral states is the task of this book to elucidate.

3

Behavioral Aspects of Motivation and Reward

History makes it clear that the concept of motivation has great heuristic value, for it brings a diverse range of behaviors into one theoretical framework. We begin with the fact that motivation is inferred from behavior, particularly to account for the many shifts in the arousal and direction of behavior throughout the day and the seasons of the year (as well as in intermediate-range rhythms such as the 4–5-day estrous cycle of the rat). Stimuli that are not particularly arousing at one point in time become so at another point in time when the internal environment or the state of the animal's brain is changed. The arousal may have a general component, especially evident in the searching behavior that occurs when appropriate stimuli are not encountered in the environment. But arousal is not *only* a general response. It is very specific and selective in both the pattern of stimuli (e.g., sign stimuli or releasing stimuli) that do the arousing and in the patterns of appetitive and consummatory responses that follow. Arousal leads to specific consummatory behaviors such as eating or mating that lead to satiation or refractoriness, which itself may be quite specific. All motivated behaviors obey this general rule of specific arousal, appetitive and consummatory responses, quiescence (Craig, 1918).

Some of the basic, biological motivated behaviors are what Richter (1942–43) called self-regulatory behaviors; these serve in homeostasis and thus the survival of the organism (e.g. thirst, hunger, thermoregulatory behavior). They parallel the purely physiological regulations concerned with fluid balance and energy homeostasis, for example, and are heavily dependent on the state of the internal environment. Others, like sex, maternal behavior, and defense of territory and the young, are critical for the survival of the species, but they do not serve in homeostasis. They are, however, also heavily dependent on a predisposing state of the internal environment produced by gonadal and pituitary hormones. A third class of motivated behaviors do not depend on a predisposing state of the internal environment to any degree (pain avoidance, some cases of aggression, and other emotions) although they may be influenced by it. All of these motivated behaviors have in common, however, a dependence on the same general neurological mechanism in the limbic system of the brain. Sensory, neuroendocrine, and neuroanatomical details are different and response patterns are different, but the principles of operation, as discussed below, are the same in all motivations, even, we speculate, in acquired motivations of the most complex sort.

All motivated behaviors also have the property that they lead to reward and reinforcement. Arousing stimuli may be positively reinforcing (e.g., sweet tastes, sexual stimulation), and the organism approaches them and seeks more of them. In some cases, removal or avoidance of the arousing stimuli is what is reinforcing (e.g., with pain stimuli and extreme ambient heat or cold), and this is called negative reinforcement. Change in the internal environment following consummatory behavior may contribute to reward and reinforcement (e.g., restoring fluid balance by drinking). Or it may be that simply carrying out the consummatory behavior itself is reinforcing (e.g., drinking, mating, attacking). Most probably, reinforcement consists of some combination of all of these factors, facilitated by learning or expectancy that comes with experience, such as finding food regularly at the end of a runway in the laboratory or returning to a "salt lick" in the wild.

In vertebrates, particularly birds and mammals, all of these motivated behaviors are accompanied by affective displays, both somatic and visceral. It helps to list some obvious examples: tail-drooping, yelping, and cardiovascular changes in the dog escaping shock; growling, spitting, hissing, pilo-erection, pupillary dilation, and arched back in the attacking cat; bowing and cooing in the mating male ring-dove; treading, rubbing, and calling in the sexually aroused female cat, and the rolling, licking, and vocalizing afterreaction following copulation.

For humans, the reinforcement and affect accompanying all motivated behaviors are reported as hedonic experiences, registering as positive or negative, pleasant or unpleasant. The case of thermoregulatory behavior in humans illustrates how all these facets of motivation fit together, for it contributes to temperature homeostasis and is an example of highly motivated behavior. Behavioral thermoregulation is also rewarding or reinforcing in that it can provide the basis for new learning and the control of performance. In addition, it may be accompanied by major autonomic and somatic changes and affective expressions, and it registers as a highly pleasant hedonic experience, marked on an analogue rating scale or verbally reported.

All of this means that the scope of our effort is much greater than it was in 1954, when the focus was mainly on the consummatory aspect of motivated behavior and the recently discovered role of the hypothalamus (Stellar, 1954). Now we wish to include appetitive behavior, the role of incentives, reward and reinforcement, affect, and reports of hedonic experience in humans because we believe they are all organized according to the same neurological and physiological principles. If this is true, what we learn about one kind of motivated behavior will tell us something not only about how other kinds of motivated behavior may be organized, but also about what constitutes reward and reinforcement. In addition, knowing something about the neurological mechanisms underlying motivation and reward will give us some insight into what underlies affect and hedonic experience.

The general scheme envisaged in 1954 still applies today, although we know, more clearly than before, that the hypothalamus is only one part of a larger central-neural control system. As the original diagram showed (Figure 3.1), all motivated behaviors are under *multifactor* control. A variety of internal and external stimuli contribute to central-neural states, leading to both the arousal and quiescence of behavior. There may be learned as well as unlearned sensory influences. Where chemical and physical changes in the internal environment play a role, they contribute to the same arousal and quiescence. The implication of this convergence of sensory and internal environment influences is that there are central-neural mechanisms or systems that integrate a variety of sources of information.

Both excitatory and inhibitory central-neural mechanisms control the arousal and satiation of motivated behavior in some instances (e.g., hunger, rage and aggression, sleep). In other instances (e.g., thirst and sex), the main evidence is for only excitatory mechanisms, although septal lesions cause hyperdipsia (Harvey & Hunt, 1965) and amygdalectomy leads to hypersexuality (Klüver & Bucy, 1939). Certainly the hypothalamus is involved in these central-neural mechanisms, and in many cases, may be the major integrator in a hierarchy of integrators along the neuraxis (Gallistel, 1980a, 1980b). But it must be remembered that the hypothalamus is only part of an extensive limbic system involving the brainstem, diencephalon, and forebrain, with both ascending and descending pathways running through it (see Figure 6.1).

How central and peripheral mechanisms interact is certainly more complex than previously envisaged. Peripheral sensory and metabolic mechanisms play an important role in processing information reaching the central-neural mechanism, and may in turn mediate some of the effects of experimental manipulation of the brain mechanism. Thus, the gut and the liver generate satiety signals that control food intake, and

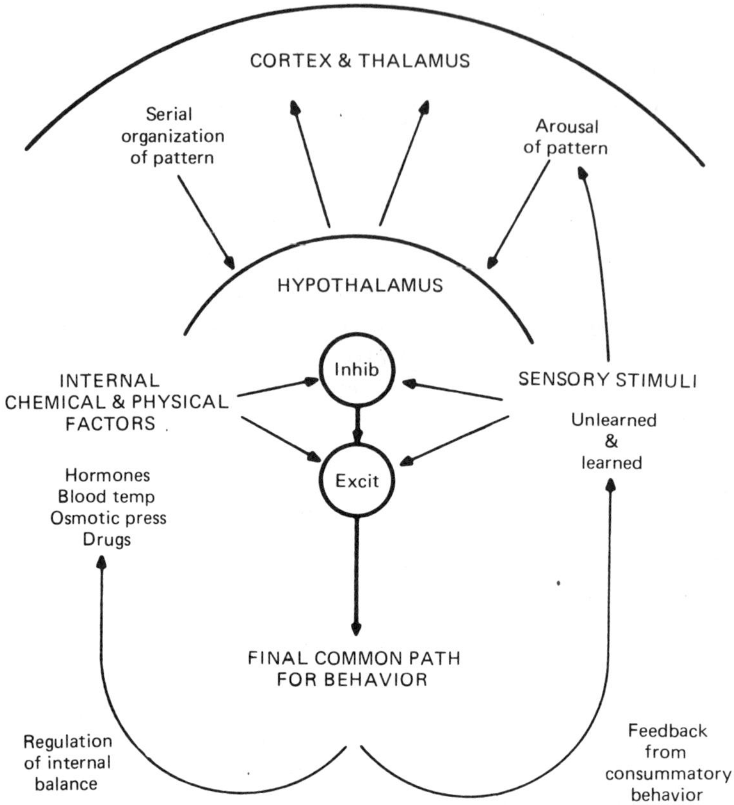

Figure 3.1 The physiological control of motivated behavior envisaged in 1954, in which internal environmental and internal and external sensory factors and learned as well as unlearned influences converge on a central neural mechanism with its major integrators in the hypothalamus (Stellar, 1954).

these are conveyed to the brainstem over afferent vagal pathways and thence to the hypothalamus (Friedman & Stricker, 1976; Hyde & Miselis, 1983; Novin & VanderWeele, 1977). Similarly, the medial hypothalamus plays part of its role in feeding by controlling insulin levels by means of vagal output (Powley & Opsahl, 1974; Inoue & Bray, 1980). In the end, however, it is obvious that the brain has to be the source of the final common path to behavior. How it gets the information it acts on and how it controls the pathways over which it acts are complex, but important, questions to investigate.

In order to deal with these questions about the brain mechanisms of motivation, and of reinforcement, affect, and hedonic experience as well, we need better definitions of both the behavioral and psychological and the physiological and neurological substrates. Behavioral definitions must be operational and must apply to both the laboratory and the natural environment. Specifying the physiological substrate requires defining both peripheral and central-neural physiological processes, including afferent neural input, metabolic and endocrine signals, and efferent control mechanisms that make up the final common path to behavior. We need, on the one hand, to be able to specify the organizing behavioral principles and concepts such as motivation (drive and satiation), reinforcement, affect, and hedonic experience. Just as much, we need, on the other hand, to define physiological and neurological principles and concepts such as homeostasis, excitation and inhibition, central-neural integration, hierarchical neurological organization, biological rhythms and neuronal oscillators, and motor subsystems. In this chapter, we review the behavioral specifications, and in the next chapter, we discuss the physiological and neurological mechanisms.

Behavioral Concepts and Definitions

Motivated Behavior

Motivated behavior is goal-directed behavior and is thought by most theorists to be dependent upon specific arousal or *drive* of the organism. The drive may be due to a specific state of the organism's internal environment, it may be the result of arousing sensory stimulation, or it may be learned (acquired drive). It may also be some combination of these. The *goal* may be an object or another organism on which a specific consummatory act is performed (e.g., eating food, copulating with a mate), the goal may be a change in the external environment of the organism (e.g., a move from cold to warm, withdrawal from a specific noxious stimulus), or the goal may be the consummatory behavior itself (e.g., sham drinking, executing threatening postures in defense of territory). All of these behaviors are *consummatory behaviors*. Typically, they lead to *satiation* or quiescence when they are completed (Craig, 1918; Antin, Gibbs, Holt, Young, & Smith, 1975; Smith & Gibbs, 1979). The organism is then unresponsive to the previously arousing stimuli, but still responsive to stimuli for other motivations.

Distinguished from consummatory behaviors are *appetitive behaviors* (Craig, 1918), the arousal of the organism and the approach to or avoidance of the goal. Appetitive behavior may be restlessness, increased locomotor activity, foraging. It may be courtship in the natural environment or an approach to a mate or to water in the laboratory. Or it may be a learned instrumentality that leads to the goal object, such as bar-pressing for food, or that leads away from it, such as moving, on signal, from one end of a compartment to another in order to escape or avoid electric shock.

Reinforcement and Reward

The ability to promote learning of new instrumental acts is dependent upon the reinforcing or reward value of goals or goal objects. Reinforcement, as used by students of operant conditioning, is defined by the establishment of operant (instrumental) behavior as well as by the maintenance of the vigor of performance (Skinner, 1938). Reward is a term used interchangeably with reinforcement by many psychobiologists, and we have followed that tradition here. In our observation, if there is any small difference in the use of these terms, reward is more often used to represent the stimulus, whereas reinforcement is used to refer to the process of strengthening specific responses of the organism. The removal of reward or reinforcement leads to performance decrement and extinction. Reinforcements may be positive rewards (e.g., food, a mate, warmth) or the reward of escape or avoidance of negative or aversive consequences (e.g., pain, shock, fear), but both promote learning and both control performance. Rewards and reinforcers may also be learned (e.g., secondary rewards such as money or tokens).

Incentive

Once learning takes place, either with secondary rewards or natural rewards, then the rewards themselves can become incentives and arouse motivated behavior (Bindra, 1968). Thus, the hungry rat runs faster to a high concentration of sucrose reward that it regularly receives at the end of a runway than to a low concentration reward (Figure 3.2). For a given concentration, it runs faster when deprived of food overnight than when deprived for only a few hours (Figure 3.2), showing the interaction of the incentive stimulus and the state of the internal environment (Stellar, 1982). Some stimuli (e.g., sweet taste, sexual) are naturally arousing and rewarding. Others become so only after associations are formed to them (e.g., a whiff of a particular perfume). In both cases, both incentive and reward value are greatly enhanced by learning to "expect" them in the same way the rat learns to "expect" a strong sugar solution at the end of the runway.

Preference, Aversion, and Choice

Motivation and reward value are also indicated by preference, aversion, and choice. Animals, including humans, develop preferences and aversions and choose some substances or goals over others when given the opportunity. Choice is affected by both the nature of the stimulus (e.g.,

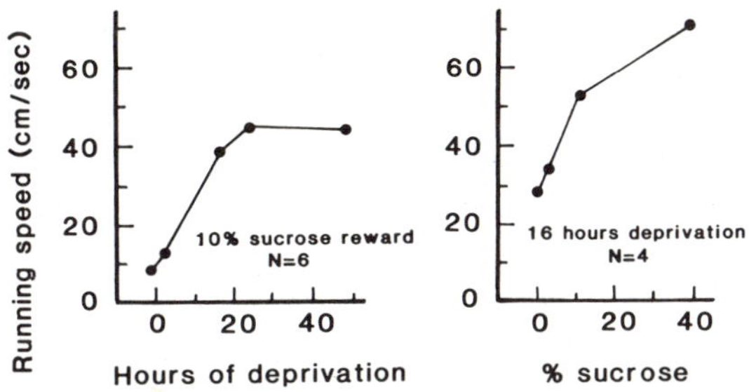

Figure 3.2 (Left) Food intake and running speed for 0.1 ml 10% sucrose rewards as a function of hours of deprivation (Stellar, 1982). (Right) Running speed to small (0.1 ml) sucrose rewards in a meter-long runway as a monotonic increasing function of concentration (Stellar, 1982).

saline concentration, a female rat in heat) and the internal state (e.g., loss of salt from the internal environment or hormonal changes). If the choice test allows the animal to perform the consummatory act, then the choice is altered by the feedback from consummatory behavior. In the case of food preferences, for example, behavior is greatly influenced by post-ingestional factors such as gastric distension, osmotic or dehydrational effects, intestinal hormonal secretion, or post-absorptive effects. Thus a rat will choose a 30% sucrose solution over a 10% solution, but because of post-ingestive effects, it can only drink a small amount of the hypertonic 30% solution compared to the 10% solution (Stellar & McCleary, 1952; Young & Greene, 1953). So if amount ingested is the measure, 10% is preferred; if choice is the measure, 30% is preferred. Thus, how preference is measured matters a great deal.

Competition Among Drives

A classical method of assessing motivation is the obstruction box, which requires a rat to run across an electrified grid to reach a goal (Warden, 1931). The faster the animal runs, or the more frequently it crosses, in the face of a given current level, the more motivated the animal is said to be. The method has been used as a standard way to assess the effects of deprivation and to compare the strength of different drives. In Warden's studies, it was reported that maternal drive was strongest by this measure, then came thirst, hunger, sex, and exploration. Later, the obstruction box was used to demonstrate that electrical self-stimulation of the brain was a very strong motivated behavior, for rats took very strong foot shock in order to stimulate their own brains (Olds, 1958c). The basic principle involved here is to measure a motivation in competition with another motivation (shock avoidance). In less dramatic form, this is what running speed in a runway measures, for the unmotivated animal yields to the motivation to explore, sniff, and groom, and thus gets to the goal only slowly, whereas the highly motivated animal runs avidly to the goal without time for sniffing, exploring, or grooming.

Motivation

In behavioristic terms, then, motivation is goal-directed behavior that may be determined by one or more of the following variables: *some specific internal state* that contributes to drive; *specific patterns of sensory stimulation,* such as innate sign stimuli or learned discriminative stimuli, that may function as incentives and arouse drives or may function as goals or rewards, and direct and shape behavior; and *learning or experience,* which may provide the basis for acquired drive and conditioned satiation (Booth, 1972) as well as new appetitive and even new consummatory behaviors such as voluntary feeding by gastric tube (Teitelbaum & Epstein, 1963; Jordan, Stellar, & Duggan, 1968).

To illustrate how complicated the interactions among all these variables can be, the sensory stimulation provided by the bowing and cooing of the male ringdove not only arouses the female dove behaviorally, but also causes her ovary to grow, thus altering her internal hormonal environment so that she becomes more sensitive to the male's behavior (Lehrman, Wortis, & Brody, 1961). In the male dog or rat, it has been shown that previous mating experience makes the animal less dependent on sensory input. Thus, its sexual behavior survives peripheral surgical ablation of as many as two sensory modalities, whereas the inexperienced rat shows no sexual behavior after such treatment (Beach, 1942a). Similarly, in the male cat, previous sexual experience makes a great deal of difference in how long sexual behavior survives after castration (Beach, 1942b).

Measurement of Motivation

The measurement of motivation is the measurement of the intensity (latency, magnitude, frequency, or probability) of behavior and its duration and persistence. These dimensions apply to both the appetitive and consummatory aspects of the behavior, observed in the natural or semi-natural environment or in the laboratory. Intensity and duration measures apply to the expression of behavior that is largely unlearned, such as copulation in the female rat; to those behaviors that are modified by learning, like following behavior in the imprinted duckling; to those in which the animal makes a choice, such as drinking from either a water or sugar solution bottle. Intensity and duration dimensions also make valuable measures in those situations in which some arbitrary act or behavioral sequence is learned and performed, such as pressing a lever to avoid shock or to turn on a heat lamp, running down an alley and pressing a lever for food or for electrical stimulation of the brain. The same intensity and persistence variables are also used in the measurement of affective displays, like the courtship behavior of a sage grouse or peacock, or the threatening posture of a stickleback fish or an attacking cat. These variables are also used in the measurement of autonomic responses and other neurophysiological indices of arousal or quiescence (EEG during waking and sleep). Finally, measurement of intensity also applies to human subjective reports of hedonic experience, especially when magnitude estimation techniques or analogue rating scales are used to express the degree of pleasantness–unpleasantness, liking–disliking, satisfaction–dissatisfaction, comfort–discomfort, pleasure–pain.

Not all measures of motivation agree, however, and this presents both problems for measurement and opportunities for analysis. For example, appetitive measures (where there may be little or no ingestion or other feedback from consummatory behavior) may differ from consummatory measures. The best example, already mentioned, is the response to different concentrations of sugar solutions. Where rats press a lever or run down an alley for very small rewards, response is a monotonic, increasing function of concentration (Gutman, 1953; Stellar, 1982). Where they ingest, it is an inverted-U-function that peaks near isotonic concentration because of negative post-ingestive consequences of hypertonic solutions in the stomach (McCleary, 1953). If the hypertonic sugar does not reach the stomach, as in the rat with an esophageal fistula, but water does instead, then drinking yields an increasing function of concentration (Mook, 1963). The same is true when choices between the tastes of two concentrations are measured, as in the brief exposure method of P. T. Young (1945).

Another reason for disagreement among measures is that in some instances, performance (skill, work capacity) may be at stake, as in high-ratio schedules of bar-pressing. This is seen dramatically in the hypothalamic hyperphagic rat's unwillingness to work to obtain food at the same time that it overeats from an open dish (Miller et al., 1950). Also, experimental manipulations (e.g., drugs) may interfere with motor performance as much as with motivation. A different example is the effect of food deprivation, which reaches its peak (but not a motoric limit) after 24 hours, with ingestion or running speed to food as the measure (see Figure 3.2) but is still increasing after 5 days with running wheel activity as the measure (Wald & Jackson, 1944). The remarkable thing, however, is how often and how well the different measures of motivation we have discussed agree with each other under comparable experimental conditions.

Biological rhythms make a difference in the magnitude of motivated behavior. Activity level and consummatory responses vary markedly in these rhythms, as seen in the night–day cycle of activity, eating, and drinking in the rat, the 4–5-day cycle of activity and sexual behavior in the female rat, or seasonal migration and premigratory hyperactivity and hyperphagia in birds.

Deprivation and Drive

Deprivation is a common manipulation, used in the laboratory to change the magnitude of motivation, but it does not work in the same way in all types of motivated behaviors. It works well in hunger and thirst, although water intake is a monotonic, increasing function of deprivation (Stellar & Hill, 1952) and food intake is not. Prolonged deprivation of food produces anorexia, probably related to the inactivity of the gut, for it can be avoided in rats, as Hamilton showed, by letting them eat a non-nutritive vaseline–cellulose mixture during the period of starvation (Hamilton, 1969). Humans have the same problem after long starvation, and even if they think they want to eat, they can eat only small amounts. This also happens in patients who are fed solely by intravenous hyperalimentation. They are often anorexic and require time to reinstate oral ingestion, probably because of their inactive gastric tracts (Jordan, Moses, MacFayden, & Dudrick, 1974).

Deprivation works well in increasing the motivation for sleep. However, it operates over only a few hours in the maternal behavior of the rat before it becomes negative and leads to reduced maternal interest (Rosenblatt, 1965). It may play a minimal role in increasing drive in temperature regulation and other motivated behaviors.

Drive and the magnitude of motivation may also be raised by the intensity and duration of sensory stimulation such as a sweet taste, cold temperature on the skin, sexual stimulation, the prolonged presence of infant rat pups, eliciting maternal behavior in the virgin female rat (Wiesner & Shepard, 1933). In the laboratory, direct manipulation of the internal environment or the brain may also be used to arouse motivated behavior, such as the systemic injection of insulin to elicit eating, introduction of estrogen into the hypothalamus of the ovariectomized rat to elicit lordosis, or hypertonic solutions in the preoptic area to elicit drinking.

Satiation and Satiety

Drive may also be manipulated in the negative direction by increasing satiation or satiety. In LeMagnen's terms (1971), *satiation* is measured by how soon the consummatory act terminates and thus how long the duration of a meal is, for example. *Satiety* is the measure of how long it is before the terminated consummatory act returns—for example, how long the intermeal interval is. Preloading food by gastric intubation will shorten a meal without affecting its onset and thus produces satiation. Varying the size of a prior meal determines satiety in the rat, for the larger the meal, the longer it is until the next meal. This is also true in the "free running" human in a sleep laboratory where there are no external signs to tell when a meal should occur, for long intermeal intervals follow large meals (Bernstein, Zimmerman, Czeisler, & Weitzman, 1981).

Satiation and the onset of satiety are marked, in the rat, by a regular behavioral sequence that includes sniffing, exploring, grooming, drinking, lying down, and sleeping after a meal (Antin et al., 1975). The sequence is seen in many animals and in humans, and it shows up after the satiation of thirst in the rat in much the same pattern (Stellar & Hill, 1952). In some ways, this may be a special case of competition among motivations, in which grooming, exploring, and sleep may come into ascendancy after hunger and thirst are satisfied.

It has been only recently that attention has focused on satiation and satiety in the study of food intake. Even in recent work, the distinction between them has not always been made. But it is a useful one and should be applied more widely in the measurement of motivation.

Acquired Motivation

Taste-Aversion Learning

Organisms that learn readily can develop acquired motivation under a variety of conditions, leading to acquired drive, conditioned satiety, and secondary reinforcement. One of the most potent examples is the conditioned aversion to foods, developed as a result of poisoning. This is an associative learning paradigm in which a novel taste is paired with a negative gastrointestinal consequence such as that produced by lithium chloride poisoning. These studies, done mainly in the rat, show that if rats are allowed to drink a preferred saccharine solution and then are poisoned with lithium, one trial is sufficient to make them avoid saccharine on the next test (Nachman, 1970). The time between the original saccharine drinking and the poisoning can be as long as an hour or more and the association is still made. An aversion can even be developed to water if rats are reared with saccharine solutions to drink and are given water as the novel stimulus before poisoning (Garcia & Koelling, 1967). Pairing saccharine with electric shock does not work, indicating that the effect is specific to gastrointestinal distress. The original experiments in this field were on the rat and dealt with the aversive effects of x-radiation (Garcia, Kimmeldorf, & Koelling, 1955; Smith, 1971), which can produce the aversion to saccharine and other tastes. More recently, it has been shown that strong taste aversions are also produced in human adults and children undergoing radiation therapy (Bernstein & Webster, 1980; Bernstein, 1978).

Opponent Process Theory

Although motivation may be acquired through various processes of associative learning, Solomon (1982) has pointed out that non-associative experience can make an important difference in the generation of drive, reward, affect, and hedonic experience. In his opponent process theory, he describes the induction of powerful new motivational states by the repeated arousal of affect of the opposite sign. Thus, the pain and fear induced initially in a dog by electric shock in an avoidance conditioning situation, yield an opponent process of excitement and euphoria, which is clearly evident after the animal is released from the apparatus. Similarly, the distress and distress-calling of an imprinted young duckling is an opponent process state of motivation induced by the termination of the positive state, marked by following of the mother duck (i.e., attachment). The more experience the duckling has with the following response, the more intense the distress-calling upon separation of the duckling from its mother.

Solomon and Corbit (1974) describe the two opponent processes and their relationship as follows (see Figure 3.3). An initial motivational state (a-process) is aroused by electric shock, for example in dogs. This is attenuated by an opposite motivational state or opponent process (b-process), which follows the a-process with a short latency (Panel A, middle row, Figure 3.3). Solomon and Corbit show that with repeated presentations of the shock, the b-process strengthens and occurs with shorter latency, to the point where the dog's affective response to the shock is minimal (habituation, Panel B, top row, Figure 3.3). A second phenomenon is apparent when, after repeated experiences, the dog is released from the apparatus and goes through an excited, euphoric response of tail-wagging, licking, and yelping. This is the positive b-process unopposed by the negative a-process now that shock stimulation has ceased (Panel B, top). The general rule is that, if the a-process is positive, the b-process is negative, as in the distress-calling of the duckling; if the a-process is negative, the b-process is positive, as in the shock-avoidance

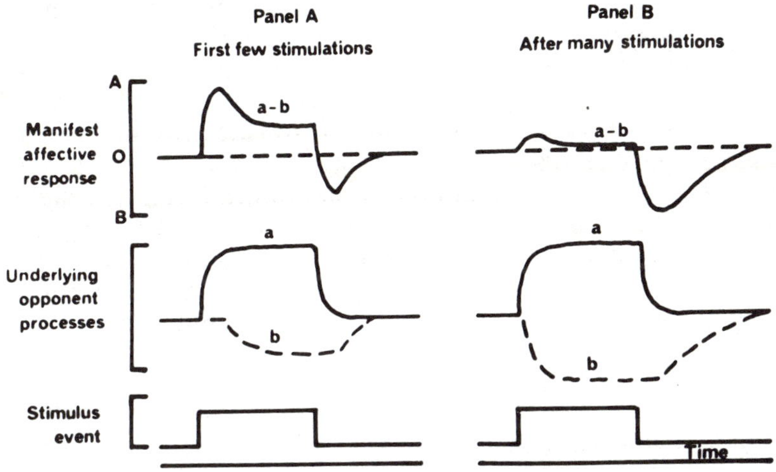

Figure 3.3 Affective response to arousing stimulation (top row) during and after stimulus (bottom row), showing the relations of opponent process (a and b in middle row) and the growth of the opponent process (b) manifested in shorter latency, greater magnitude, and longer duration after many stimulus repetitions (Panel B, middle). This results in a minimal affective response (a–b) to the stimulus (habituation), with a big after-response or opposing affective response (Panel B, top) that is the acquired motivation (Solomon, 1982.) Reprinted by permission.

situation. The new idea is that the b-process is an acquired affective and motivational state, generated, through a *non-associative* experience, by another emotional state of opposite sign. The implication is that the opponent process mechanism is a basic property of the nervous system.

Opiate addiction is a striking example, for opiates produce a highly positive a-process (rush and euphoria in humans), and only with repeated use do they set up a highly aversive, opponent b-process, evident in the absence of the opiate (withdrawal). As is well-known, the best way to eliminate the aversive b-process is to counteract and cancel it by arousing the a-process by taking opiates. Now the motivation is to get rid of the withdrawal symptoms rather than just to gain the euphoria. Solomon (1977, 1980) draws similar conclusions about taste-pleasure and taste-craving in hunger as opponent processes; love and grief; fear and risk (as in sport parachuting) and the consequent thrill (that develops slowly with experience); and jogging or running and the subsequent high.

We have no firm idea of what the neurological basis is for the opponent process mechanism. There may, in fact, be many different bases. Studies with opiates suggest that opponent process may be related to the development of excess opiate receptors that remain unactivated during withdrawal (Snyder, 1977). Naloxone, which blocks opiate receptors but does not activate them, induces withdrawal symptoms in addicts and thereby supports this interpretation. Even more suggestive evidence is that rats become more tolerant to the pain of radiant heat after they have habituated to repeated electric shocks, but naloxone blocks the tolerance (Grau, Hyson, Maier, Madden, & Barchas, 1981). Other possible neural mechanisms may involve reciprocal excitation and inhibition, the positive and negative systems revealed in self-stimulation studies (Olds & Olds, 1963; Hoebel, 1975), and approach and withdrawal systems revealed by brain stimulation (Stellar, Brooks, & Mills, 1979). At this point, we can only speculate, but we should recognize the important properties of the nervous system implicated by the potent, and perhaps very general, opponent process systems revealed by behavioral studies of motivation and affect.

Non-Homeostatic Motivation

Some motivated behaviors, like sexual behavior, aggression, and acquired motivations, do not serve homeostasis. Some actually work against homeostasis and are maladaptive. Two examples are illustrative. One is *schedule-induced polydipsia* sometimes called psychogenic polydipsia (Falk, 1971). If a hungry rat is given a small (45 mg) pellet of food every 60 seconds or is allowed to press a lever to get food on that schedule, it will begin to drink from its water spout immediately after each pellet, while waiting for the next food pellet. In the course of an hour, the water-satiated rat may drink 5 to 10 times the amount of water it would ordinarily drink while eating dry pellets from a dish. Quite clearly, its behavior toward the water is highly motivated, but no one knows why it comes about. The drinking has been called "adjunctive behavior," implying that the rat uses it to fill the time while waiting for the next pellet.

It has also been suggested that the rat drinks to wash down the dry pellets, but in fact, it drinks much more than it needs to for that. Solomon (1982) has suggested that the drinking may be the expression of an opponent process. That is, the drinking is the only response available to the rat to oppose the taste-craving that develops when the pellet is eaten and gone. Ordinarily another pellet (taste-pleasure) would be eaten to cancel the taste-craving, but since it is unavailable for one minute, the water is drunk. Supporting this interpretation is the finding that, when stronger taste-cravings are induced by more highly preferred pellets (sucrose-flavored), the schedule-induced drinking is even greater (Rosellini & Lashley, 1982).

More readily understandable is the highly motivated behavior animals express toward sweet solutions. If the satiated rat is given a saccharine or sucrose solution to drink at the same time every day, it will begin to drink more and more each day until it becomes polydipsic and may take

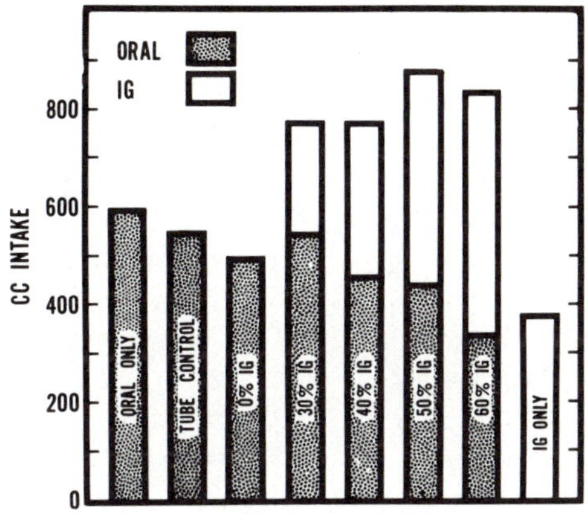

Figure 3.4 Total food intake in a human subject during a meal when liquid diet is voluntarily pumped simultaneously into the mouth and into the stomach via nasogastric tube (IG). Oral intake is reduced as a function of the increasing percent of the total going into the stomach (%IG), but not enough to prevent overeating (Stellar and Jordan, 1970).

excessive calories from the sugar solutions (Ernits & Corbit, 1973). Still more dramatic is the polydipsia seen with mixtures of 3% glucose and 0.125% saccharine. These are intensely sweet solutions with little osmotic or caloric post-ingestional consequences. As a result, the rat will *drink its body weight* of the glucose-saccharine mixture overnight and be forced to secrete vast amounts of fluids (Valenstein, Cox, & Kakolewski, 1967; Smith, Williams, & Jue, 1976). Quite clearly, taste drives ingestion and may do so way out of proportion to what is required by homeostasis. For example, rats overeat and become obese on the so-called "supermarket" diet, which consists of a variety of cookies, candies, luncheon meats, and so on, in addition to their laboratory chow (Sclafani & Springer, 1976). They also overeat and become obese when fed a highly palatable high fat diet (Corbit & Stellar, 1964).

In human studies, taste and other oral factors also drive intake. For example, although Jordan (1969) found that human subjects are quite capable of regulating the size of a liquid diet meal when taste is eliminated by pressing a button to pump the diet directly into their stomachs via a nasogastric tube, taste can also play an overriding role. If they are given two pumps that simultaneously deliver equal volumes to the mouth and to the stomach, they eat in accordance with their oral stimulation and ignore the extra amount going into the stomach by nasogastric tube, virtually doubling their intake (Figure 3.4). The oral stimulation is described as pleasant and satisfying, and without it, subjects report their hunger is less satisfied, even though they eat the same volume by stomach alone as they do by mouth alone (Figure 3.5). Some insight into this dissociation of the regulation of food intake and subjective satiation is given by the anecdote of the subject who tried to drink a milkshake and eat a hamburger after an intragastric meal because he felt so unsatisfied. After one bite of the hamburger and a taste of the milkshake, he said "my mouth wants it but my stomach doesn't."

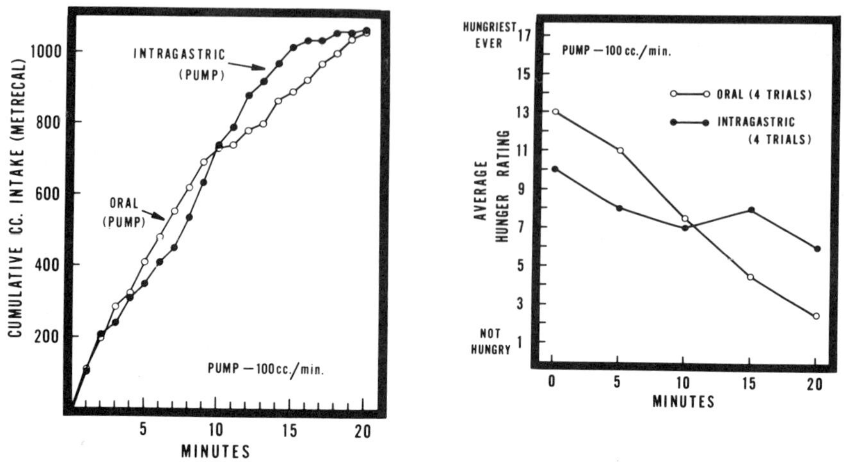

Figure 3.5 Voluntary ingestion of liquid diet by stomach tube is the same as oral ingestion (left panel), but hunger ratings are not reduced as much by the intragastric meal (right panel). (Stellar, 1967).

Emergence of Motivated Behavior and Hedonic Responses in Phylogeny

Most of what we have said about motivation to this point is based on experimental work with rats, humans, and a few other representative vertebrates. We know from the work of both ethologists and psychologists that fish, amphibia, and reptiles as well as mammals exhibit the properties of drive, goal-directed behavior, and satiation, and they display autonomic and somatic signs of affect. Most important, they all are able to learn operant responses on the basis of both positive and negative reinforcement that demonstrate their appetitive as well as consummatory behavior.

What about invertebrates? They eat, mate, and defend territory. Does this behavior qualify as motivated behavior? We think it does, although not all the components that we see in vertebrates are always present. The blowfly, for example, lowers its proboscis and ingests food in response to chemical stimulation of taste receptors on its legs (Dethier, 1976). The stronger a sugar solution, the more the blowfly ingests, up to the point where negative post-ingestive effects enter. While sensory adaptation may cause ingestion to slow, the main mechanism that turns eating off is the post-ingestive filling of the foregut. This response can be eliminated by sectioning the recurrent nerve from the foregut. As a result, the blowfly doesn't stop eating and may literally burst. There seem, however, to be no post-absorptive effects in the blowfly's internal environment that turn eating off, for nutrients infused into the lower gut have no effect on ingestion. Is foregut distension satiation? We think it is, but it is based on a very limited, single factor as compared to mammals, in which stomach distension, intestinal hormones like cholecystokinin, metabolic signals from the liver over the vagus, and possibly, metabolic signals directly affecting the brain play important roles.

So the blowfly fits a simple stimulus-response model, with the taste of sugar turning ingestion on and distension of the foregut turning it off. But it is somewhat more complicated than that. Salt turns ingestion off, so there is an aversion mechanism. Female blowflies develop a protein appetite preceding egg-laying, indicating that, under the right conditions, there can be specific hunger other than for carbohydrates. The nutritionally depleted fly is more active in flight than a satiated one. Also, taste can arouse the blowfly to increased locomotor activity as well as ingestion. For example, if the wings are clipped and a blowfly is allowed to encounter a drop of sugar solution on a flat surface, it will burst into a zig-zag pattern of running, the speed and extent of which is a function of the concentration of the sugar (Dethier, 1957). To date, however, it has not been shown that the blowfly can learn an operant response on the basis of food reward; it may lack that aspect of motivated behavior.

Dethier, who is responsible for this work on the blowfly, argues that the concept of motivation is superfluous in accounting for the blowfly's ingestive behavior because the main variables controlling food ingestion can be specified (Dethier, 1982). We would argue that the blowfly exhibits a rudimentary form of motivated behavior, limited by the level of development of its nervous system in phylogeny, but also limited by its specialization as a non-social animal. The bee, by contrast, readily learns to use arbitrary discriminative cues that signal the location of food, and it is aroused to make its waggle-dance (cf. the blowfly's zig-zag pattern of running) in response to the intensity of food stimulation as well as its location (von Frisch, 1967).

The seaslug, *aplysia,* is another invertebrate that shows many of the characteristics of motivated behavior (Weiss, Koch, Koester, Rosen, & Kupfermann, 1982). Its feeding has a diurnal rhythm and exhibits both appetitive and consummatory aspects of motivation. Presentation of seaweed near a food-deprived aplysia elicits appetitive locomotion and headwaving. Contact with the seaweed evokes the consummatory response of biting and ingestion. Satiation is exhibited after a large meal by failure of response to food, probably due largely to distension of the gut. Both heart-rate and blood pressure parallel hunger and satiation behavior with increases and decreases. Food stimuli elicit these increased cardiovascular responses, and so do arousal by tail pinch and handling, which decrease the latency to bite the food. On the other hand, strong electric shock or stretch of the gut decrease all the somatic and cardiovascular signs of food arousal. As shown by Weiss et al. (1982), paralleling these behavioral and physiological effects, and undoubtedly at the root of them, is the activity of the metacerebral cells of the cerebral ganglion,

A

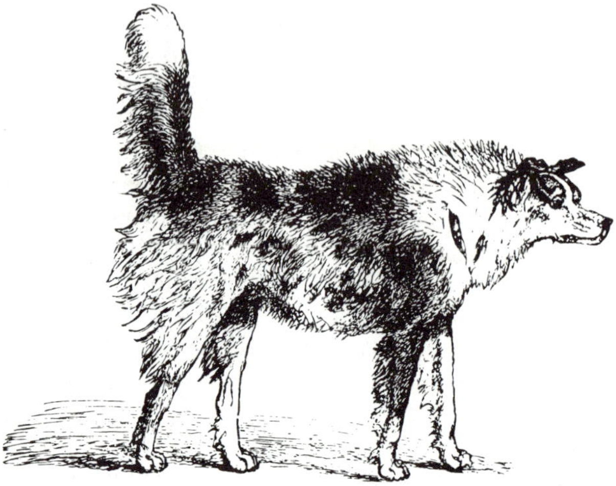

B

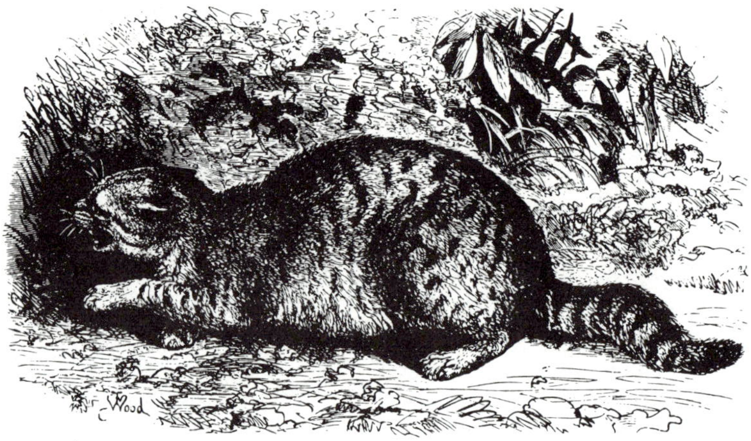

Figure 3.6 Affective display. (A) From Darwin's original legend: "dog approaching another dog with hostile intentions" (B) From Darwin's legend: "cat, savage and prepared to fight" (Darwin, 1873).

which use serotonin as their neurotransmitter. Silent during behavioral quiescence, these cells fire (1–10 spikes per second) when food touches the tentacles or lips. Furthermore, the responses of the metacerebral cells persist after the food stimulus is withdrawn, as long as the animal is hungry. When *aplysia* is fed or given strong shock, there is no longer any response of the metacerebral cells to food.

While *aplysia* learns associations based on shock to the mantle, and thus has the property of negative reinforcement, there is no evidence as yet that it learns appetitive, operant responses to food rewards. Thus, as Weiss et al. point out, it is evident that *aplysia* exhibits many, but not all, of the characteristics of motivated behavior. Whether these behaviors

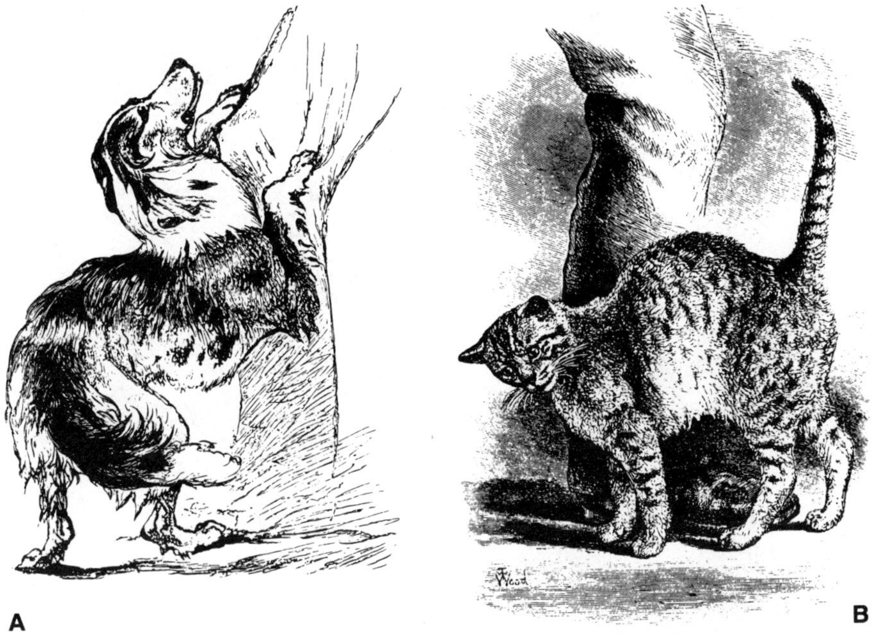

Figure 3.7 Affective display. (A) From Darwin's legend: dog in a "humble and affectionate frame of mind" (B) From Darwin's legend: "cat in affectionate frame of mind" (Darwin, 1873).

are called instincts as Epstein suggests (1982a), precursors of motivated behavior, or limited and rudimentary motivated behavior, it is fruitful to take them into account in trying to understand the behavioral and physiological basis of motivation.

Affect and Hedonic Response

As we study motivation, we see many instances of affective display and hear many reports of hedonic experience from human subjects. Neither of these two aspects of behavior has received adequate investigation, nor do we know much about their physiological and neural basis. Somatic and autonomic expressions of emotion and affect have been recognized back to the beginning of humanity and they are what we now call non-verbal communication, so necessary to human interactions. Darwin (1873) recognized them for their adaptive value. By analogy to human experience, he labeled animal expressions as showing "hostile intentions" (Figure 3.6A) or "savage" (Figure 3.6B), "affectionate frame of mind" (Figure 3.7A and B), and "terrified" (Figure 3.8). Darwin saw these expressions as part of the animal's adaptive response to challenges in

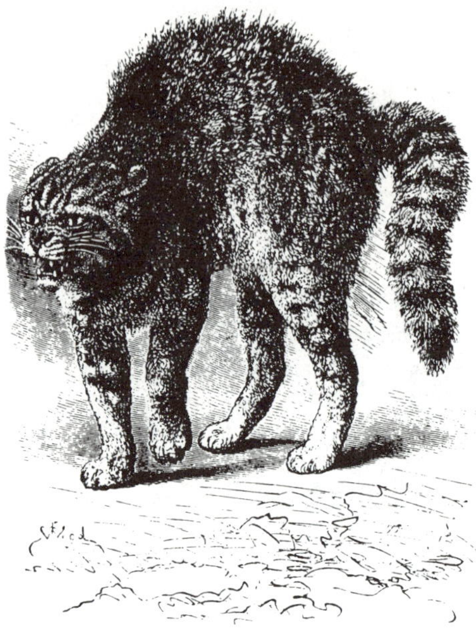

Figure 3.8 Affective display. From Darwin's legend: "cat terrified at dog" (Darwin, 1873).

the environment, and he extended his thinking to human facial expressions, which he believed were remnants of adaptive actions such as the baring of teeth in human anger and rage. It was the ethologists who later made it clear that affective displays were also sign stimuli that signaled other animals about the affective state of the displaying animal (Tinbergen, 1951).

In the study of food intake, we have learned that ingestion of food with tastes that human infants prefer (Desor et al., 1973) namely, sugar solutions, evoke very positive facial expressions in the newborn (Steiner, 1977), whereas quinine produces a negative facial expression of rejection (Figure 3.9). Even the anencephalic infant, without most of its forebrain, shows these positive and negative facial expressions. It is interesting, moreover, to note that similar acceptance and rejection expressions are also possible in the decerebrate rat (Norgren & Grill, 1982). Accompanying the human infant's positive facial responses to sugar solutions, furthermore, are immediate changes in the pattern of sucking and increased heart rate, even when the effort of sucking is controlled (Crook & Lipsitt, 1976; Ashmead, Reilly, & Lipsitt, 1980). Adult humans also reflect different emotions in facial expression, and these are accompanied by specific patterns of autonomic changes (Ekman et al., 1983).

While affective expression is readily observed and recorded, hedonic experience is indirectly revealed only in human subjective reports or by psychological scaling methods. Using a simple rating scale, ranging from pleasant (+2 and +1) to unpleasant (−1 and −2), Cabanac (1971) has studied the hedonic experience of human subjects under different tem-

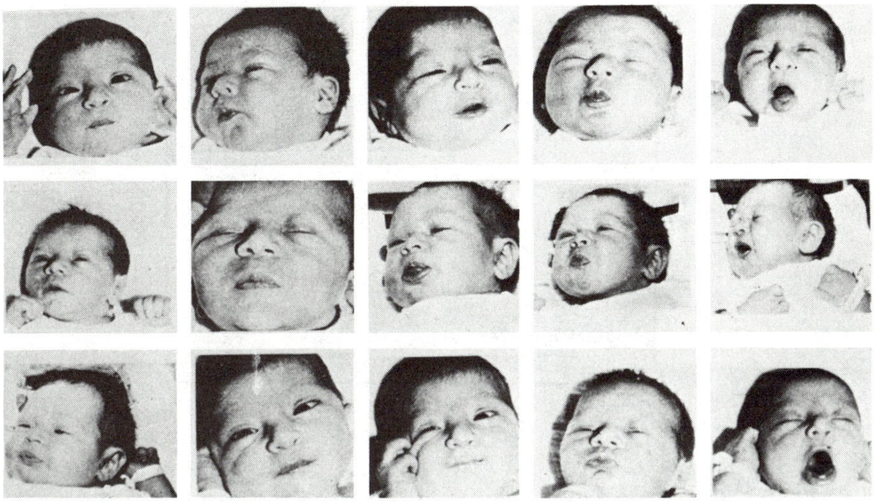

Figure 3.9 Affective facial expressions in infants right after birth: (1) resting, and responses to (2) distilled water, (3) sweet, (4) sour, (5) bitter (Steiner, 1977.) Reprinted by permission.

perature conditions. When they are made hyperthermic by immersion in a warm bath, they judge cold temperatures on their hands as most pleasant and warm temperatures as unpleasant. With hypothermia, cool hand temperatures were unpleasant and warm ones very pleasant (Cabanac, 1971; Cabanac, Massonet, & Belaiche, 1972). These findings illustrate Cabanac's (1971, 1979) concept of *alliesthesia,* whereby the pleasantness of sensory stimuli is determined by the state of the internal environment. The findings also fit with the more general concept in the study of motivated behavior whereby sensory responsiveness is determined by the state of the internal environment. For example, salt hunger in the rat is determined by salt depletion, and even humans on low-sodium diets report salty soup as more pleasant than when they were on a regular diet (Bertino, Beauchamp, Riskey, & Engelman, 1981).

Hawkins (1975) replicated Cabanac's finding by heating and cooling subjects in a constant temperature bath. He then asked them to judge the pleasantness of buckets of water, ranging from very cold (20°C) to very hot (48°C), by dipping one hand in each bucket after adapting the hand to a neutral 35°C. The results are shown in Figure 3.10. Even more striking was the second part of Hawkins' study, in which he asked subjects to stand up out of the tub and adjust a shower to the most pleasant temperature when the shower came on at tub temperature. Figure 3.11 shows the result. When body temperature was elevated or lowered 0.5°C–

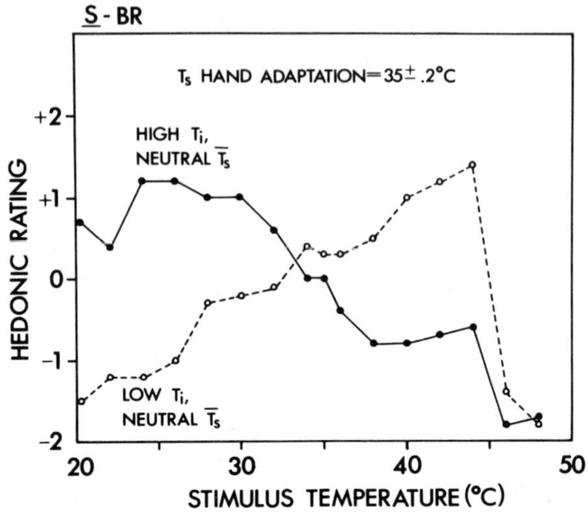

Figure 3.10 Ratings of pleasantness and unpleasantness of hand baths (from 20–48°C) when core temperature (Ti) was raised or lowered by immersing the subject in a warm (40°C) or a cold (30°C) constant temperature bath (Hawkins, 1975).

1.0°C, subjects were very uncomfortable and promptly adjusted the shower temperature to the opposite extreme (a high of 40°C and a low of 30°C). These extreme shower temperatures were experienced as very pleasant, and subjects maintained them for as long as 10 minutes, a behavior reminiscent of the proverbial roll in the snow after a sauna. On the other hand, if the subjects were asked to take the showers before rectal temperature changed, the same bath temperatures (and therefore skin temperatures of 30 and 40°C) were only moderately unpleasant, and the subjects took only moderately warm (35°C) and moderately cool (33°C) showers, which they rated as moderately pleasant.

Cabanac has reported similar alliesthesia with olfactory and taste stimuli with hungry and fed or gastrically loaded human subjects (Cabanac, Minaire, & Adair, 1968). A successful experiment is shown in Figure 3.12, in which the subject judges the pleasantness of hypertonic (20%) sucrose solutions that he samples in 50-ml mouthfuls every 3 minutes. In one case, he tastes and spits, and the pleasantness rating does not change in its positive value over a 90-minute period. In the other case, each 50-ml mouthful is swallowed after its pleasantness is rated. Within about 30 minutes, after the subject has ingested 500 ml of 20% sucrose, the pleasantness ratings drop and become quite negative. The same effect can be obtained by intubating 500 ml of 20% sucrose into the stomach, but intravenous infusion is without effect. Cabanac (1979) believes that the ingested sugar must reach the small intestine to have the alliesthesia

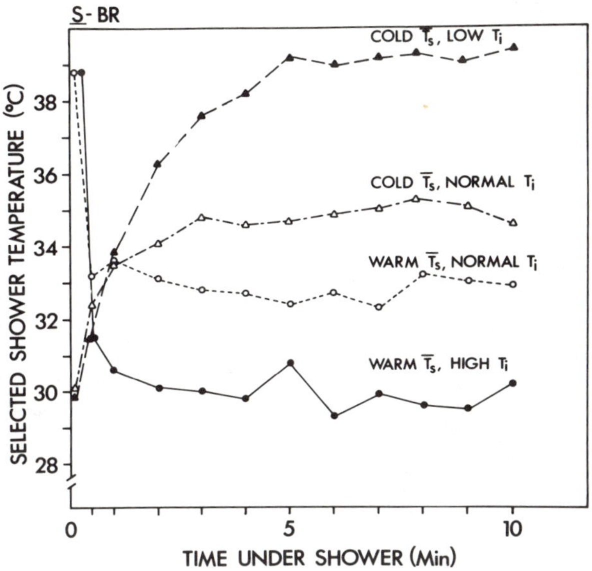

Figure 3.11 Shower temperature selected as most pleasant by a human subject after skin temperature (Ts) was raised or lowered and after core temperature (Ti) was also raised or lowered (Hawkins, 1975).

effect. He finds, however, that obese subjects and undernourished subjects do not show this alliesthesia. He also reports the same results in judgments of the pleasantness of olfactory stimuli that are relevant to food (Cabanac, 1979).

Food-related alliesthesia does not appear to be as robust a phenomenon as temperature-related alliesthesia, however, for other investigators have reported difficulty in obtaining the food effects (Grinker, 1977). In our laboratory, using experienced subjects, we found the decreased ratings of pleasantness with ingestion, but they seemed to be related to gastric distress, slight nausea, and the reluctance to swallow any more hypertonic sucrose. Gastric distress upon over-ingestion, of course, may itself be only one step beyond ordinary fullness and satiation, and these post-ingestive effects may be reflected in judgments of oral pleasantness.

On the other hand, in her work on sensory-specific satiety, Rolls has found support for the alliesthesia concept (Rolls, Rolls, & Rave, 1982). Her subjects gave lower hedonic ratings to a food they had just eaten a few minutes before, compared to a similar food they had not yet eaten. Furthermore, they ate less of the food previously eaten than they did of the new food. Because this effect took place within minutes after eating, she called it *sensory-specific satiety*. She found similar specific satiety with the shape and color of foods as with the taste. These findings indicate that post-ingestive effects are important in both the hedonic rating of

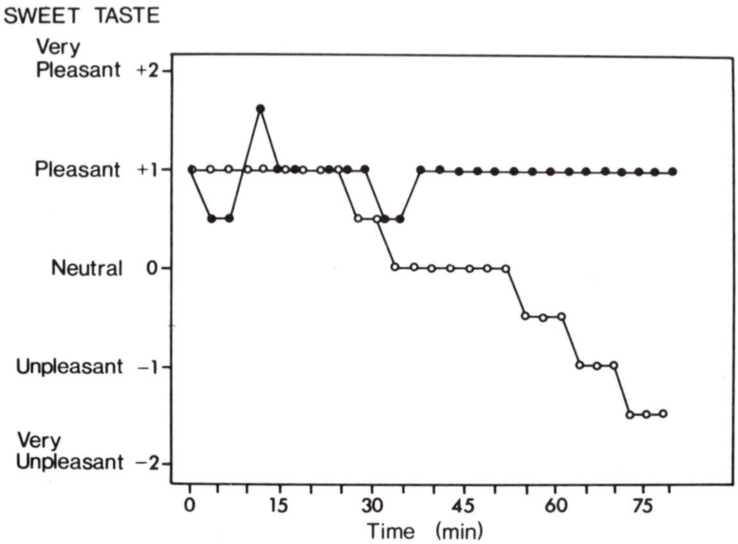

Figure 3.12 Change in the hedonic rating of 50 ml of 20% sucrose solutions, depending on whether the solution was spit out (closed circles) or swallowed (open circles) (Cabanac, 1971.) Reprinted by permission.

foods and how much subjects eat. These observations fit very well with McCleary's (1953) finding that rats intubated with hypertonic sucrose solutions do not drink very much hypertonic sucrose, compared to rats not tubed or intubated with plain water.

Studies of taste hedonic ratings, where there is no ingestion, show that, for many human subjects, there is an enhancement of hedonic ratings when sugars and fats are mixed (Drewnowski and Greenwood, 1983). Adding 10% sucrose to unsweetened heavy cream (37.6% fat) or heavy cream with 15% safflower oil (52.6% fat) greatly increased the hedonic rating of those relatively unpalatable concentrations of fat. By the same token, addition of the fat increased the relative acceptability of the higher concentrations of sucrose. Overnight food deprivation, interestingly enough, did not make a change in these functions. However, when obese and normal-weight subjects were compared, there was a difference. The obese clearly preferred the highest fat content (52.6%), mixed with a relatively low concentration of sucrose (5%). Normal-weight subjects preferred mixtures of less fat (30%) and more sucrose (8%). The pleasantness of food stimuli, therefore, varies not only with taste and texture, but also with immediate post-ingestive effects, and with chronic internal conditions such as those associated with obesity.

Summary

The process of motivation is inferred from behavior to account for the shifts in arousal and direction of behavior throughout the day and the season. Motivated behavior may be aroused (drive) by a change in the internal environment, by naturally arousing stimuli (incentives, sign stimuli), and by previously neutral stimuli that come to arouse because of learning and experience. The first phase of motivation is appetitive behavior, the arousal and approach or avoidance, leading to the second phase, the consummatory act. Satiation is produced by the consequences of the consummatory behavior. For example, satiation can be produced by: ingestion and consequent change in the internal environment; a change produced in the external environment; simply the execution of the consummatory act itself; or some combination of these. The result is quiescence and reduction of the specific behavior. The object or end-point of the consummatory act (food, mate, and perhaps even the execution of threatening posture) is the goal toward which motivated behavior is directed and may function as both incentive and reward.

Motivated behavior thus leads to reward or reinforcement, which operate in the promotion of new learning and the maintenance of performance. In birds and mammals, at least, motivated behavior and reward, in turn, yield expressions of affect, both visceral and somatic. In humans, all of these processes yield hedonic experience that can be reported or measured on a psychophysical scale.

Motivation can be measured by preferences, aversions, choice, and willingness to overcome barriers to achieve the goal (cf., obstruction box) or to work and perform (e.g., operant responses). Some preferences and aversions may be learned, and thus acquired motivation, such as food aversion, is developed through associative processes. Motivation and affect may also develop non-associatively in experience, for example, through the operation of opponent process mechanisms. Some motivated behaviors do not serve homeostasis, but are adaptive; others may be maladaptive—for example, schedule-induced polydipsia.

Motivation emerges in phylogeny from simpler reflexes and taxes that lead to approach and withdrawal and to various fairly stereotyped consummatory acts such as eating, mating, or attacking. Among representatives of the invertebrates, fewer factors may control arousal and satiation than in the vertebrates. There may be little expression of affect, and learning may play little or no role. So motivation here may be in rudimentary form, a limited precursor of what is seen among the vertebrates. In vertebrates, the full complement of motivated behaviors appears where multiple internal environmental, internal and external sensory, and learned factors operate and where affect is fully expressed and reinforcement occurs. In the vertebrate series, from fish to primate, sensory factors and learning become more important and internal environmental and humoral controls relatively less important, as Beach (1947) has described for sexual behavior. In humans, hedonic experience emerges that can be reported or marked on a rating scale, and it may have its precursors in animals in the hedonic processes of motivation, reward, and affect.

As the next chapter describes, we believe that all motivated behaviors and associated hedonic processes share similar neurological mechanisms in the limbic systems and that all operate according to the same basic physiological and behavioral principles.

4

Physiological Aspects of Motivation and Reward

What are the properties of a biological mechanism that could underlie the general characteristics of motivation and reward? What properties do we need in order to satisfy the requirements of the related concepts of arousal, drive and satiation, approach and withdrawal, positive and negative reinforcement, affective display, and pleasant and unpleasant hedonic experience? We need to envisage a central-neural mechanism that is readily influenced by changes in the internal environment, that receives visceral, endocrine, and somatic afferent inputs from all modalities, and that has visceral, endocrine, and somatic efferent outputs to control or prime response mechanisms in the brainstem and spinal cord. At the same time, the mechanism must have an influence on forebrain structures to yield the more complex hedonic processes and hedonic experience itself, which we presume to occur at the highest levels of the neural hierarchy. In turn, the central-neural mechanism must itself be controlled by these structures at a higher point in the neural hierarchy.

So we envisage a hierarchical organization in which the major controlling mechanism is capable of integrating varied neural and humoral influences of an excitatory and also of an inhibitory nature, so that both the arousal and satiation of motivated behavior can be controlled in a graded fashion. The behavioral facts tell us that this mechanism must be highly discriminative in what arouses it (specific releasing sign stimuli), and at the same time, capable of discrete behavioral control, so fine that a hungry animal eats rather than drinks and the maternal rat cleans its newborn pups, but does not eat them. Yet these systems are activated by general arousal (e.g., tail pinch leading to eating or copulation) and part of their output contributes to the general activity or quiescence of the organism as well as to the arousal and satiation of specific responses. Furthermore, all motivated behavior yields the conditions for positive or negative reinforcement, approach and withdrawal, and positive and negative affect, so they have those in common, too. The challenging question is the identification of the common mechanism and how the different motivations find their way into it. To address this challenge, we must first identify the specific mechanisms of each kind of motivated behavior, and then, show how they participate in the general mechanism.

Complicating the task is the fact that the neural mechanisms involved are anatomically intertwined and overlapping, so that our crude experimental interventions with lesions, stimulations, drugs, and even recording almost always involve more than one system at a time. For example, it is reasonable to assume that in the hypothalamus, as in the visual system, adjacent neurons may have different functions: some may be concerned with metabolic and hormonal events and others with autonomic display and behavioral control; some may be concerned with hunger and others with thirst; some may be involved in general arousal and others with specific functions. The remarkable thing is that we get as much separation and isolation of behavioral function as we do. Some of this may be due to the fact that we often focus on just one behavior and may ignore others that are also affected. But some may well be due to the fact that our recording, stimulation, and lesion techniques are manipulated until we do succeed in isolating, to a sufficient degree, neurons with quite specific functions. Most of the investigations described in this chapter are designed to analyze and separate functions. Part of our task, however, is also to synthesize and generalize so as to include, in one rubric, not only the various motivated behaviors, but also reward, affect, and the hedonic experience reported by humans.

Brain States

We begin the analysis with a central-neural mechanism, an enduring brain state, brought about by some combination of influences produced by a pattern or sequence of sensory stimulation, and in some cases, a state of the internal environment. To illustrate how this works, we can take the case of Flynn's experiments (Flynn et al., 1970) in which the brain state is the central-neural activation produced by lateral hypothalamic, perifornical stimulation through an elecrode implanted in the cat's brain. In that state, the pattern of sensory stimulation provided by a prey animal (e.g., a rat) is sufficient to evoke a predatory attack culminating in a lethal bite in the back of the neck, even on the part of tame laboratory cats that would not otherwise kill rats. If the rat is anesthetized or dead or a toy rat, it is less adequate to provoke attack, or it takes more brain stimulating current to elicit the attack. The peripheral input and the central arousal must, then, be additive in some way.

If the cat is in an empty arena and there is no prey stimulus, the brain stimulation produces only general arousal, circling, and searching behavior, but no attack. The central arousal, then, looks very general, but closer examination shows that it has some highly specific components. For example, if the lip of the cat, contralateral to the electrode, is touched around the mouth, it will elicit head orienting and a biting response (MacDonnell & Flynn, 1966). If the brain stimulation is weak, then the region is small, but if stimulation is increased, the receptive field to elicit the head orienting and bite increases in area (Figure 4.1). If there is no brain stimulation, the cat either gives a face-rubbing response to stimulation of the lip or else withdraws its head, but there is no bite. The same thing is seen in the rooting response of the hungry human infant. The hungrier the baby, the larger is the area around the mouth that will elicit head turning, mouth opening, and initiation of sucking.

The second question is how the specific brain state comes about naturally, so as to produce an animal responsive to specific stimuli and with specific motor patterns. One way is through specific changes in the internal environment, due to the presence of circulating hormones. As Pfaff (1980) has pointed out, the evocation of the lordosis response (back arching, tail deflection) in the female rat is an excellent illustration, for it is dependent upon the presence of naturally occurring or artificially

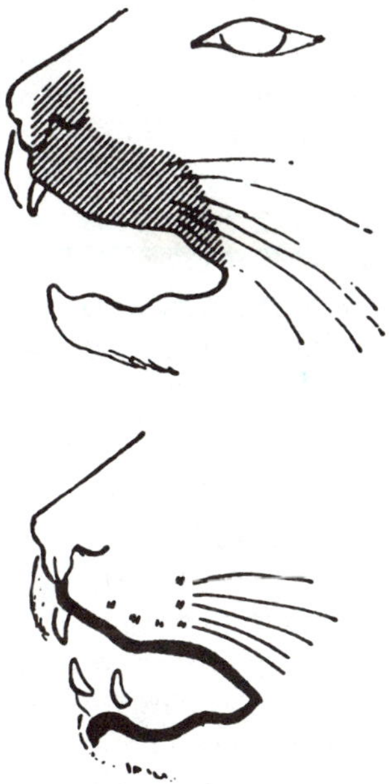

Figure 4.1 (Top) Maximum sensory field for head-orienting response during intense contralateral perifornical stimulation. (Bottom) Maximum sensory field for jaw opening, leading to bite; with weak brain stimulation, only the region of the lip close to the midline is effective (MacDonnell and Flynn, 1966.) Reprinted by permission.

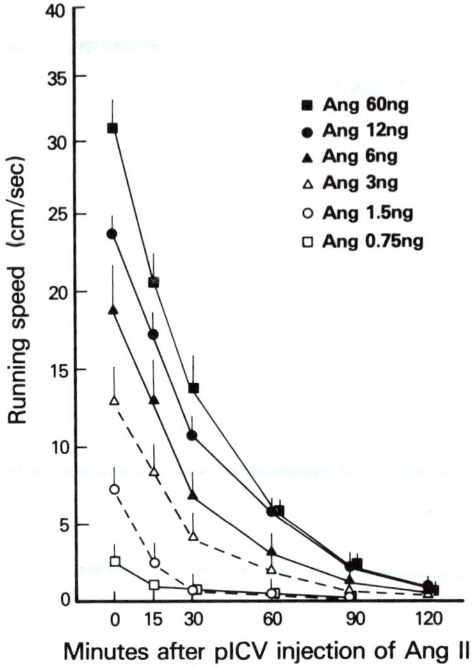

Figure 4.2 Running speed to water reward as a function of the dose of angiotensin II at different times after pulse intracerebroventricular (pICV) injection in the rat (Zhang et. al., 1984.) Reprinted by permission.

administered estrogen. Only then will cutaneous pressure on the flanks, rump, and perineal area arouse lordosis. If there is no estrogen, the female rat avoids such stimulation with aggressive kicks and withdrawals. Binding studies show that estrogen is taken up rather specifically by the ventromedial and anterior hypothalamic areas and the medial preoptic area. Implantation of estrogen in these areas is most effective in the elicitation of the lordosis response, and so is electrical stimulation.

In the control of thirst, very similar evidence implicates the subfornical organ (SFO) in the anterior wall of the third ventricle as a major site of action of angiotensin II in the elicitation of hypovolemia-induced drinking (Epstein, 1982b). Angiotensin binds here. Introduced through a cannula directly on the SFO, the lowest concentrations of angiotensin, in physiological amounts (femtomoles), evoke drinking. Lesions here block the hormonal effect of blood-borne angiotensin. What makes the angiotensin example even more interesting is the fact that it not only elicits the consummatory response of drinking upon pulse injection into the anterior cerebral ventricles, but it also produces dose-dependent appetitive response in which the water-replete rat avidly runs down a familiar runway for a 0.1-ml reward of water (Figure 4.2, Zhang et al., 1984).

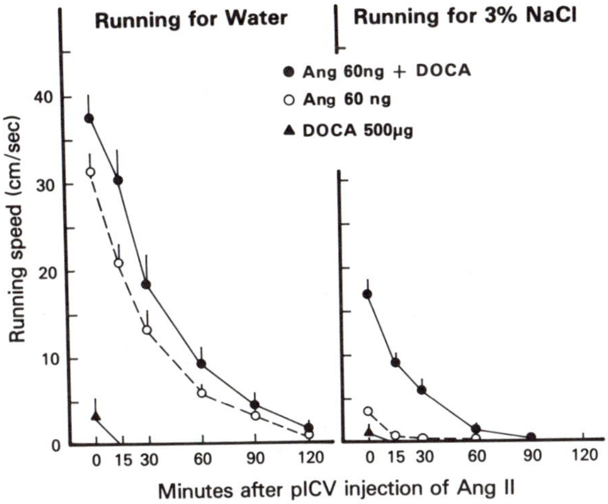

Figure 4.3 (Right) Running speed to 3% NaCl reward, initiated by the synergistic effects of intracerebral angiotensin and systemic DOCA (to raise aldosterone levels). (Left) DOCA adds little or nothing to angiotensin's effect on running to water (Zhang et. al., 1984.) Reprinted by permission.

These mechanisms are not simple. Intracerebroventricular injection of angiotensin also elicits avid salt appetite in both consummatory and appetitive responses if the animal is previously treated with subcutaneous DOCA to raise its aldosterone levels (Fluharty & Epstein, 1983; Epstein, Zhang, Schultz, Rosenberg, Kupsha, & Stellar, 1984; Figure 4.3). Of course, both water drinking and salt ingestion are important behavioral facets of fluid balance and maintenance of the integrity of vascular volume, as are the direct vascular effects of angiotensin, leading to increased blood pressure. So the direct physiological effect and the two types of motivated behavior that are produced by angiotensin are consonant in their homeostatic results. Furthermore as Epstein (1982b) points out, angiotensin may also act on the organum vasculosum of the lamina terminalis (OVLT) in thirst and produces its vascular effects through midbrain sites and the area postrema.

The origin of the central-neural state in the case of thirst is even more complicated, for there are two consequences of water depletion that are signaled separately and that have two different central-neural mechanisms (Epstein, Kissileff and Stellar, 1973). One cause of thirst is hypovolemia, signaled by the level of circulating angiotensin II and also by the response of baroreceptors in the great veins and the left atrium of the heart. As we have pointed out, the subfornical organ is a receptor area for blood-borne angiotensin. A second cause of thirst is osmotic, and there are osmoreceptors in the lateral preoptic area that respond to cellular dehydration (Blass & Epstein, 1971; Peck & Novin, 1971).

Both kinds of depletions are involved in the thirst of water deprivation, and the two combine quantitatively in an additive way when they are separately manipulated in experiments (Blass & Fitzsimons, 1970). How their central-neural effects, through the lateral preoptic osmoreceptors and the subfornical organ, are integrated into regulatory drinking responses is not known. However, neurons in the preoptic area (Nicolaidis, 1968, 1980) and the subfornical organ (Miselis, Shapiro, & Hand, 1979; Miselis, 1981) send their axons into the medial forebrain bundle of the lateral hypothalamus. These relationships are not simple or exclusive, however, as is shown by the anatomical tracing of neurons of the subfornical organ with autoradiographic transport methods (Figure 4.4, Miselis, 1981).

In hunger and the regulation of food intake, we still do not know what changes in the internal environment provide signals for the arousal and satiation of behavior. Blundell (1984) describes 19 endogenous and exogenous substances that are known to increase food intake and 27 that decrease it. Glucostatic, lipostatic, protein, and temperature mechanisms have been suggested, and Nicolaidis (1981) believes that all are combined into a single metabolic or "ischymetric" signal to which neurons in the lateral hypothalamus are sensitive. We also know that afferent neural impulses from the liver and the gut coming into the brain, particularly through the vagus nerve, provide the brain with information about the metabolic state of the animal (Friedman, 1980; Novin & VanderWeele, 1977; Stricker, 1983). Undoubtedly, there are both peripheral metabolic signals that reach the brain over afferent neural paths and metabolic signals that reach the brain directly, crossing the blood-brain or cerebroventricular-brain barriers or perhaps arising in the brain's own metabolic and neurosecretory activity.

Exteroceptive afferent neural activities also contribute directly to the arousal of the central brain state in hunger. These activities may be learned as well as unlearned sensory inputs, arousing appetitive and consummatory behaviors and functioning as incentives. Rolls has traced some of these afferent inputs electrophysiologically to the lateral hypothalamus, substantia innominata, anterior hypothalamus, lateral preoptic area, and the region below the anterior commissure (Rolls, 1982; Rolls & Rolls, 1982). Recording from single neurons in the brain of the waking monkey, he and his associates have found units that are selectively responsive to the taste and/or the sight of food. In one study, 13.6% of the 764 hypothalamic units sampled were responsive. But they responded only when the animal was food-deprived and hungry, showing their dependence on the state of the internal environment. Furthermore, they did not respond to general arousal by aversive stimuli or thirst or by drinking water. Rolls also found that these hypothalamic units increase their firing in the same way to the sight of the syringe he habitually uses to deliver the taste stimuli to the mouth. Other visual stimuli, not as-

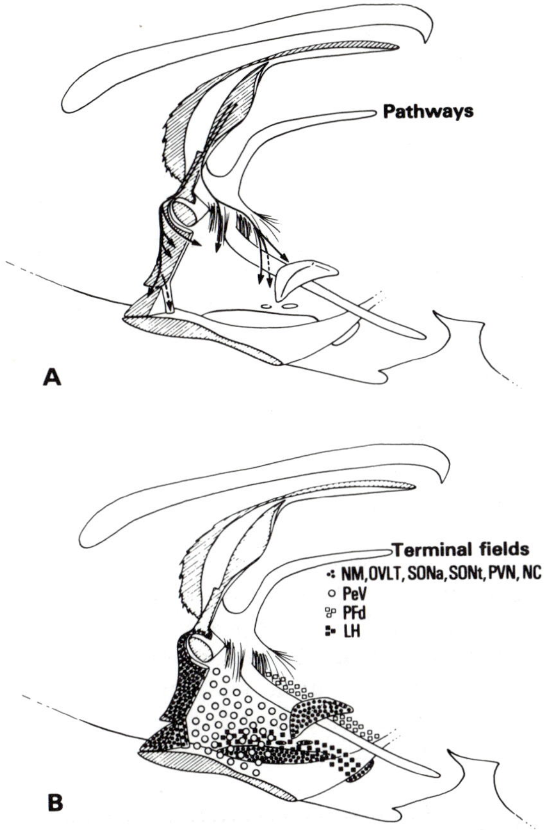

Figure 4.4 Connections of the subfornical organ (SFO). (A) Pathways. (B) Terminal fields. NM, nucleus medianus of medial preoptic area; OVLT, organum vasculosum of the lamina terminalis; PVN, paraventricular nucleus; NC, nucleus circularis; PeV, periventricular nucleus; PFd, dorsal perifornical area; LH, lateral hypothalamus. (Miselis, 1981.) Reprinted by permission.

sociated with feeding, are ineffective in arousing these neurons. Furthermore, visual stimuli become ineffective in arousing these units if subjected to extinction procedures. Thus, it is clear that it is only through associative learning that visual stimuli become effective in increasing the firing rate of these hypothalamic units. Finally, since these units can be driven antidromically from the cerebral cortex, especially prefrontal cortex and supplementary motor cortex, they must have important input to the forebrain.

Similar units have been found in the preoptic and anterior hypothalamic areas in temperature regulation (Guieu & Hardy, 1971; Hardy & Guieu, 1971). These neurons are responsive to the arousal of warm and cold receptors in the skin, they change their firing rate to local heating and cooling of the brain, and they are responsive to input from other regions of the nervous system that are also temperature-sensitive.

Neural Hierarchies

All of this evidence points to a major central integrating role of the hypothalamus, but it also shows quite clearly that the hypothalamus does not act alone. It is but one integrator in a hierarchy of integrators at different levels of the neuraxis. In temperature regulation, for example, Satinoff (1983) has pointed out that there are regions of the nervous system sensitive to temperature changes in the spinal cord, medulla, and midbrain as well as in the preoptic-anterior hypothalamic area and the septal area.

Decerebration experiments in the study of temperature regulation reveal some of the details of the hierarchical organization. The spinal, medullary, and midbrain preparations (cat and monkey) are capable of temperature regulatory reflexes below the transection, but these are relatively fragmentary and ineffective. Without the hypothalamus, Satinoff points out that there are three deficits in temperature regulation: (a) thermoregulatory responses occur only at abnormally high and low body temperatures, (b) they usually do not succeed in maintaining normal body temperature, and (c) inappropriate thermoregulatory responses can sometimes occur.

Furthermore, not all regions of the neuraxis play an excitatory role in temperature regulation. Some are inhibitory. For example, Chambers, Siegel, Liu, and Liu (1974) have shown that, in the cat, although midbrain decerebration abolishes shivering and vasoconstriction in the forelimbs when the body is cooled, subsequent pontine and medullary decerebration reinstates these responses. Thus, there is an area between the midbrain and the pons that inhibits forelimb thermoregulatory responses. The same result has been described in the monkey (Liu, 1979).

Studying sexual behavior in the ovariectomized female cat and guinea pig, Bard (1940) and Dempsey and Rioch (1939) also made it clear that control of motivated behavior is through a hierarchy of integrators. In both species, transections at the spinal, medullary, and midbrain levels yield animals capable of more and more complicated patterns of sexual reflexes upon genital stimulation. But in none of these preparations did systemic administration of estrogen make any difference. Only when the hypothalamus was left in did the full pattern of sexual response occur, and then only when estrogen was administered. The hypothalamus, then, is a major integrator of sexual responses that are mediated by other integrators lower in the neuraxis, and as we know, it is the site of action of the sex hormones in their facilitation of sexual responses.

The importance of the integrators below the hypothalamus should not be underestimated. In the study of the feeding behavior of the thalamic and decerebrate rat, Norgren and Grill (1982) have shown remarkable integrative functions. Their ingenious innovation was to provide the rat with a mouth cannula so that food stimuli could be delivered directly into the mouth. The normal rat accepts and swallows sucrose solutions through the cannula until it is satiated. Then it lets them dribble out of the mouth. If quinine is infused, it is rejected immediately, and the animal rubs its face on the floor, shakes its head, and washes its face with its paws. Video monitoring of the orofacial responses of the rat during these stimulations reveals an ingestive sequence of mouth movements, tongue protrusions, and lateral tongue movements when sucrose is infused. With quinine, the orafacial response is gaping in repeated (2–6) bursts.

In the decerebrate rat, transected just rostral to the superior colliculus and posterior to the mammillary bodies, sucrose solutions are accepted with normal orofacial ingestion expression. Quinine is rejected with gaping responses and chin rubbing, head shaking, and face washing at high concentrations, although the complete rejection pattern may not always be present. The decerebrate rat is also sensitive to its own internal state, for it does not ingest when it has just been fed, although it does so when deprived. The decerebrate also shows cephalic-phase, or pre-absorptive insulin release when glucose is infused into the mouth, and it responds to subcutaneous insulin injections by ingesting more sucrose when its blood sugar drops (Flynn & Grill, 1983). In contrast, the decerebrate rat does not learn taste aversion and fails to reject a previously preferred saccharine solution on which it has been poisoned with lithium chloride. Finally, it should be pointed out that the decerebrate does not increase its acceptance of water when it is dehydrated and does not accept salt solutions when it is salt-deprived. Its ingestive abilities are specific to food.

Thus the behavior of the decerebrate is limited. It does not have the appetitive responses involved in the search for food and the approach to it, and it does not develop learned taste aversions. Yet it responds differently to its own state of repletion and to positive and negative tastes. One can ask whether it is hungry and has motivation for food. The answer may be "yes," but to a limited degree, consonant with the limited neuraxis available to the response mechanism.

In contrast, the thalamic rat, with all forebrain above the thalamus removed, rejects all stimuli, gaping to water and weak sucrose solutions, chin-rubbing and face-washing. It is aphagic and adipsic and does not accept or ingest any liquid stimuli introduced into the mouth through the cannula. Since many of the components of food acceptance and rejection are organized and integrated below the level of the hypothalamus, this rejection behavior means that, between the thalamus and the decerebration transection, there may be an inhibitory or aversive mechanism for food acceptance that keeps the thalamic animal from ingesting sucrose solutions the decerebrate will accept. On the other hand, the rejection of food might be produced by a functional lateral hypothalamic lesion, owing to the loss of forebrain-lateral hypothalamic connections. For example, it has been shown that a unilateral thalamic rat will be seriously impaired in its food intake by a contralateral lateral hypothalamic lesion, but not by an ipsilateral lesion (Pon & Stellar, 1981). This contralateral lesion impairment is equivalent to that seen in an intact rat given bilateral lateral hypothalamic lesions, and is much greater than that seen when an intact rat is given a unilateral hypothalamic lesion. All of this suggests that lateral hypothalamic tissue may be functionally impaired by the forebrain lesions done in the thalamic rat, even though the hypothalamic tissue remains surgically intact.

We still don't know all the capabilities of the brainstem mechanisms in the control of feeding behavior, but much of the relevant sensory input enters the brain here. The taste afferents (facial, hypoglossal, vagal; Norgren and Leonard, 1973), and the vagal innervation from the abdominal viscera (Hyde & Miselis, 1983) all have their inputs here. The taste afferents send axons into the rostral region of the nucleus of the solitary tract (NTS), and via the parabrachial nucleus of the dorsal pons, send afferents rostrally. The rostral taste afferents divide into (a) a dorsal branch that goes to the ventrobasal thalamus and then to the cortex, and (b) a ventral branch that goes to limbic structures (lateral hypo-

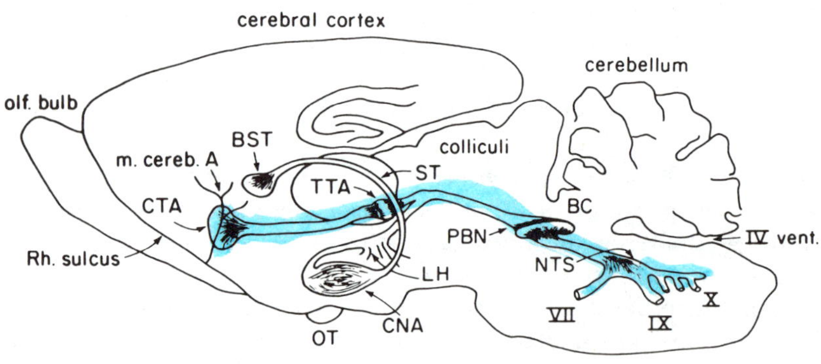

Figure 4.5 Lateral view of the rat's brain, schematically showing two taste pathways. (1) The classic thalamo-cortical pathway, arising from cranial nerves VII, IX, and X, synapsing in the rostral nucleus tractus solitarius (NTS) and proceeding to the parabrachial nucleus (PBN) of the pons, the thalamic taste area (TTA), and cortical taste area (CTA). (2) A ventral pathway from PBN to the lateral hypothalamus (LH), the central nucleus of the amygdala (CNA) and the stria terminalis (ST), and its bed nucleus (BST). Other abbreviations: BC, brachium conjunctivum; OT, optic tract; Rh, rhinal sulcus (Norgren, 1977.) Reprinted by permission.

thalamus, central nucleus of the amygdala, and the bed nucleus of the stria terminalis), concerned with motivational and affective functions (Figure 4.5, Norgren, 1977).

The input from the abdominal vagus terminates in the area postrema (AP), the caudomedial nucleus of the solitary tract (cmNTS), and the dorsal motor nucleus of the vagus (Figure 4.6). These structures are interconnected and send second- and third-order neurons directly—and synaptically through the parabrachial nucleus—to limbic structures (lateral hypothalamus, paraventricular nucleus, dorsomedial and arcuate nuclei, substantia innominata, and the bed nucleus of the stria terminalis). Descending fibers have also been traced from the paraventricular nucleus, the ventromedial nucleus, and lateral hypothalamus to the caudal medial NTS, the area postrema, and the dorsal motor nucleus of the vagus.

In addition to having this sensory input from the abdominal vagus, the area postrema is one of the seven circumventricular organs that lie outside the blood-brain barrier (Figure 4.7, Phillips, 1978). The AP also lacks the tight cerebrospinal fluid (CSF)-brain barrier of the other circumventricular organs and thus is in an excellent position to monitor the internal chemical environment directly as well as through its vagal input. This region of the brain, for example, must contain glucoreceptors, because glucoprivation restricted to the fourth ventricle by injection there of the glucose analog, 5-thioglucose, causes feeding and hyperglycemia in rats (Ritter, Slusser, & Stone, 1981). Lesions here cause a transient (12-day) hypophagia and a long-term lowering of body weight (27% loss) that the animals defend (Hyde & Miselis, 1983). Thus the caudal medulla may have a food intake control and a body weight set-point mechanism as well.

In addition to a hierarchy of integrators below the hypothalamus in the neuraxis, there are also integrators rostral to it. The case of aggressive behavior is illustrative of both rostral and caudal integrators. Classical studies by Bard and Mountcastle (1947) demonstrated the excitatory role of the neocortex (removal made cats placid) and the inhibitory role of the old cortex (removal made cats fierce). In keeping with this finding, they also reported ferocity after bilateral amygdalectomy similar to the ferocity previously reported in that laboratory by Wheatley (1944) after ventromedial hypothalamic lesions in the cat. However, Klüver and Bucy (1939), in the monkey, and Schreiner and Kling (1956) in the cat reported placidity following amygdalectomy, in contrast to Bard and Mountcastle. This conflict has never been resolved, but through Flynn's stimulation studies, the suggestion arises that the difference may be in what part of the amygdala was damaged. Flynn, for example, found that concomitant stimulation of the lateral nucleus of the amygdala facilitated the attack evoked by perifornical stimulation, and that stimulation of the rest of the amygdala inhibited it (Flynn et al., 1970).

Flynn's exploration of the neuraxis also showed even more extensive

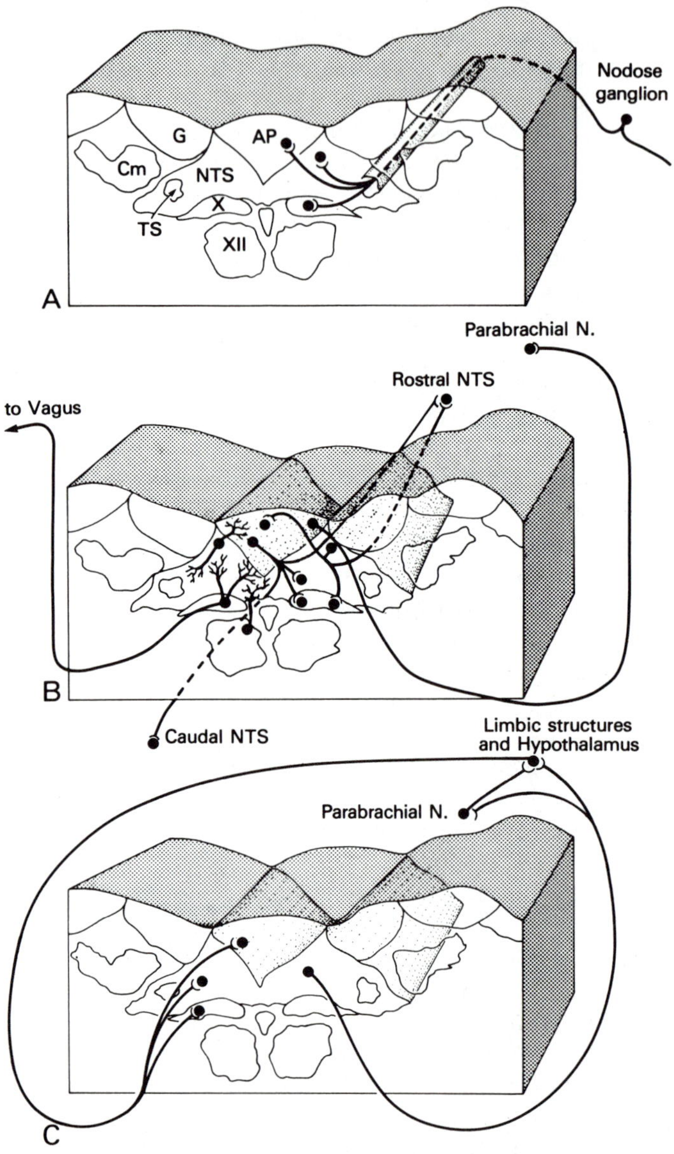

Figure 4.6 Central connections of the afferent input of the vagus to the caudal medulla. (A) Synapses in the area postrema (AP), caudal medial nucleus tractus solitarius (NTS), and the dorsal motor nucleus of the vagus (X); XII, hypoglossal nucleus; TS, tractus solitarius; CM, medial cuneate nucleus; G, gracile nucleus. (B) Connections between AP, caudal medial NTS, rostral and caudal NTS, X, and parabrachial nucleus. (C) Ascending connections directly to hypothalamus and via parabrachial nucleus. Descending connections from hypothalamus to AP, NTS, and X. (Hyde and Miselis, 1983.) Reprinted by permission.

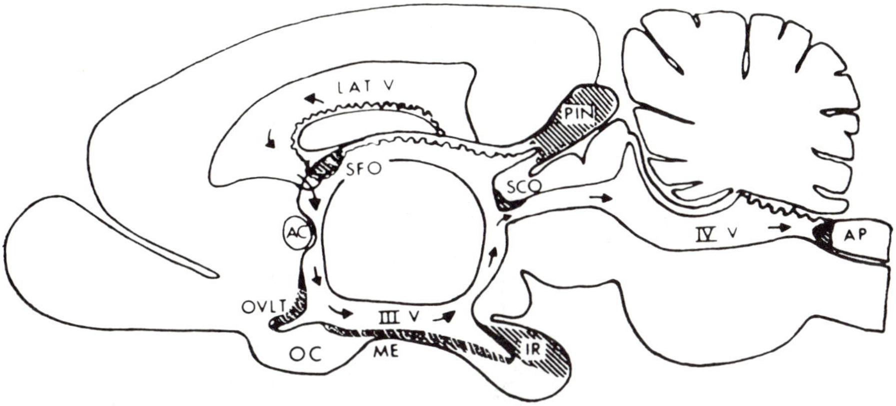

Figure 4.7 Lateral view of the rat's brain, schhematically showing the seven circumventricular organs that have little or no blood-brain barrier. SFO, subfornical organ; OVLT, organum vasculosum of the lamina terminalis; ME, median eminence; IR, infundibular recess and neurohypophysis; SCO, subcommissural organ; PIN, pineal; AP, area postrema. (Phillips, 1978.) Reprinted by permission.

roles of structures rostral and caudal to the hypothalamus, for he could evoke attack from the stria terminalis, the thalamus, and midbrain central gray and reticular formation as well as the perifornical area. Moreover, perifornical stimulation can be facilitated or inhibited by these and other structures in the brain. For example, attack is facilitated and the threshold for perifornical stimulation is lowered when there is prior and concomitant stimulation of the ventral hippocampus, the lateral nucleus of the amygdala, the midbrain central gray and reticular formation, or mediodorsal and midline thalamus. Attack is inhibited and the perifornical current must be increased if the dorsal hippocampus, the amygdala outside the lateral nucleus, and the thalamic structures (these only after prolonged stimulation) are also stimulated at the same time as perifornical stimulation. In a similar fashion, the preoptic area facilitates and the diagonal band, prefrontal cortex, and anterior cingulate cortex inhibit attack when they are stimulated concomitantly with perifornical arousal. Thus, there appear to be excitatory (summating) mechanisms and inhibitory (suppressor) mechanisms in control of aggressive behavior.

Some of these relationships are shown in Flynn's diagram (Figure 4.8), which also portrays the hypothalamus in the pathway that facilitates brainstem and spinal cord response mechanisms. One response is the general arousal and "searching" behavior (appetitive). The other is the specific response directed by the pattern of stimulation provided by the target animal (consummatory). This picture is further complicated by the fact that medial perifornical stimulation produces an affective attack

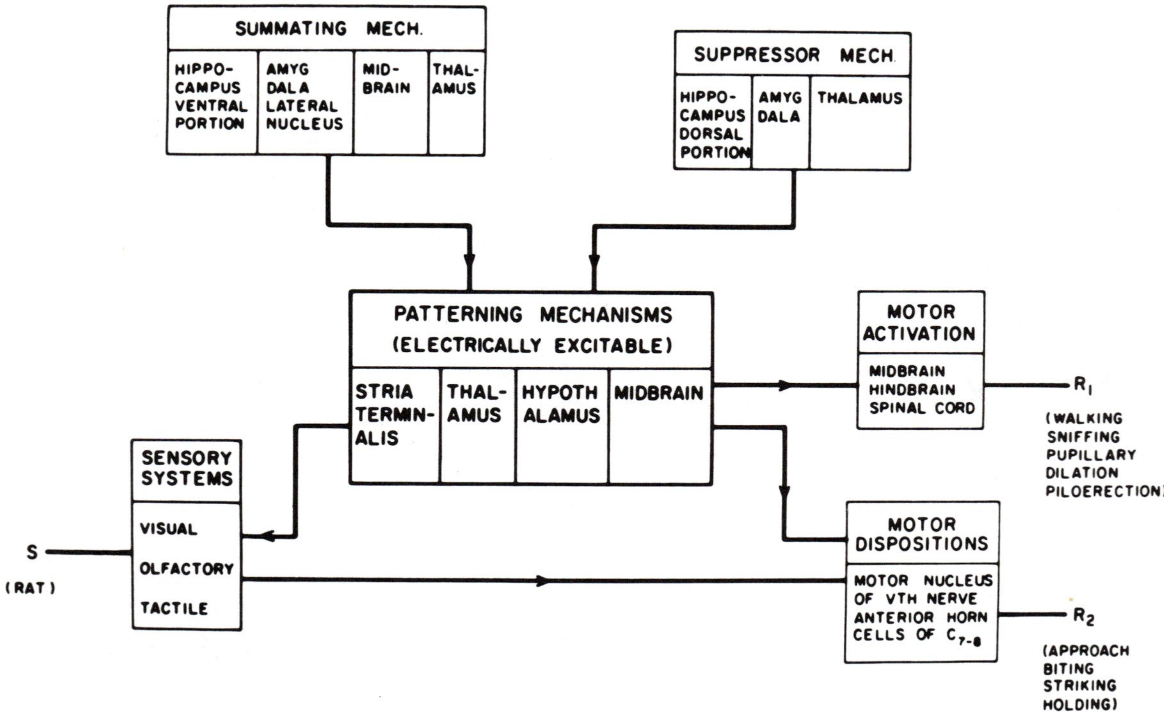

Figure 4.8 Flynn's diagram of the central-neural mechanism involved in the arousal of attack behavior by diencephalic and midbrain electrical stimulation of the cat's brain via implanted electrodes. R_1 is the appetitive behavior—arousal and searching; R_2 is the consummatory behavior—specific attack on the prey stimulus. Rostral and caudal facilitating (summating) and inhibitory (suppressor) mechanisms are shown (Flynn et. al., 1970.) Reprinted by permission.

with full sympathetic display, characteristic of the rage response in the cat, while the lateral perifornical stimulation elicits a predatory attack, the quiet biting attack.

Peripheral and Central-Neural Interactions

It is clear from the foregoing discussion that peripheral afferent neural and humoral influences contribute significantly to the control of the brain mechanisms involved in the arousal and maintenance of motivated behavior, as well as its satiation and quiescence. These inputs can be at all levels of the neuraxis, but their major integration takes place in the hypothalamus, as we have seen in the examples of sexual behavior, temperature regulation, aggression, and thirst. At one time, it was believed that hunger and the regulation of food intake represented the clearest example of this kind of integration operating in control of motivated behavior (Stellar, 1954; Stellar & Jordan, 1970). The lateral hypothalamus was thought of as a hunger or feeding mechanism because lesions there produced aphagia, and stimulation produced eating in the satiated animal. The ventromedial hypothalamus was considered a satiation and satiety mechanism, for lesions there led to larger and more frequent meals, and stimulation inhibited eating in the hungry animal. Even transient changes produced by local anesthetic and excitatory hypertonic saline injections yielded the expected results. Taken together, all of these findings fit the conception of anatomically separate, excitatory and inhibitory neural mechanisms for hunger and satiety.

Medial Hypothalamic Interactions

We now know, however, that the mechanism is more complicated than this. The critical region in the medial hypothalamus is not the ventromedial nucleus (VMN) itself, but more likely the paraventricular nucleus (PVN), that lies just ahead of it. Ventromedial area lesions simply interrupt fibers passing through the region to the PVN, as knife-cut experiments that spare the VMN have shown (Gold, 1973; Kapatos & Gold, 1973). Furthermore, a good deal of evidence suggests that the medial hypothalamus and PVN may not be involved as much in short-term satiation and satiety as it is in long-term regulation of body weight through both metabolic and feeding effects (Panksepp, 1971a, 1971b). Furthermore, many of the effects of medial hypothalamic lesions are not simply direct behavioral effects, but rather are also the result of peripheral metabolic changes. For example, a good bit of the hyperphagia and obesity produced by medial hypothalamic lesions may be a secondary result of the hyperinsulinemia caused by the lesions (Han & Frohman, 1970; Hustvedt & Løvø, 1972; Powley, 1977).

The increased insulin levels, which may occur in the first hours after ventromedial hypothalamic (VMH) lesion (Rohner et al., 1977), lead not only to increased glucose utilization, but also to increased lipogenesis. The result is that, with energy stored and utilized at a high rate, the animal must eat to replenish its nutrient sources. Depriving rats of neurally released insulin by treating them with streptozotocin and maintaining them with transplanted fetal pancreatic islets eliminates the hyperinsulinemia and attenuates obesity caused by VMH lesions, but the animals do overeat moderately (20%) (Inoue & Bray, 1980). Subdiaphragmatic vagotomy can also abolish the hyperinsulism, hyperphagia, and obesity (Powley & Opsahl, 1974), but much of the effect on eating may be due to slowed gastric emptying (Inoue and Bray, 1980) or to the acute gastrointestinal distress caused by vagotomy. Bernstein and Goehler (1983), for example, using a conditioned taste-aversion paradigm with rats, have shown that vagotomy can lead to avoidance of novel foods. Concerned with the finickiness and hyperreactivity to negative stimuli of VMH-lesioned rats, King et al. did their vagotomies 70 days before the VMH lesions (King, Carpenter, Stamoutsos, Frohman, & Grossman, 1978). Recovered from the acute effects of vagotomy, their animals showed prompt and marked hyperphagia and obesity following VMH lesions, even though there was no increase in basal insulin levels. It has also been shown that VMH-lesioned rats will show hyperphagia after acute vagotomy if fed a high-fat diet (Powley & Opsahl, 1974) or a highly palatable supermarket diet (Sclafani, Aravich, & Landman, 1981).

Quite clearly, the peripheral metabolic and visceral functions of the medial hypothalamus are an important part of the pathway, leading to food-motivated behavior. Furthermore, while the afferent and the efferent fibers of the vagus are also an important part of this pathway, it is clear that the vagus is not the only route, for the vagotomized animal still eats and satiates, even if the processes are not entirely normal. Therefore, even in the vagotomized animal, there must be behavioral control mechanisms in the brain that the metabolic signals of depletion and repletion reach over afferent pathways or by means of some direct influence on the brain.

Thus, the question remains: where in the brain are such signals for hunger and satiety received? The brainstem and the lateral hypothalamus are obvious candidates, but the medial hypothalamus should not be overlooked as a mechanism for behavioral control simply because it also has metabolic and visceral functions. In addition to the fact that electrical and chemical stimulation of the medial hypothalamus and local anesthetization produce prompt, stimulus-bound feeding effects, local microinjection of norepinephrine into the PVN increases food intake (Leibowitz, 1978, 1982). These are specific, localized, and transient effects that should not be overlooked in investigating the central targets of peripheral metabolic and visceral signals of hunger and satiety.

Lateral Hypothalamic Interactions

The direct role of the lateral hypothalamus (LH) in feeding has also been called into question. First of all, lesions there produce a wide range of deficits in a variety of motivated behaviors: hunger, thirst, thermoregulatory behavior, sleep, self-stimulation. They also lead to sensory neglect, akinesis, and catalepsy. Some of these symptoms may be due to the fact that LH lesions destroy much of the nigostriatal pathway and deprive the caudate and putamen of dopamine terminals. They also destroy the mesolimbic pathway, depriving the accumbens and other limbic structures of dopamine, and they destroy a variety of norepinephrine and serotonin inputs as well.

By injection of the neurotoxin, 6-hydroxy-dopamine (6OHDA), into the medial forebrain bundle of the LH, very similar syndromes to those seen after LH lesions can be produced. But they are not identical. First of all, 6OHDA lesions must deplete striatal dopamine by 90–95% before they are effective (Stricker & Zigmond, 1976b), whereas LH lesions usually don't cause depletions of more than 40–60% (Oltmans & Harvey, 1972; Glick, Greenstein, & Waters, 1974) and sometimes are effective in producing the syndrome of aphagia and adipsia with as little as 20–25% dopamine depletion (Grossman, 1984). Marshall, Richardson, and Teitelbaum (1974) report that rats with 6OHDA lesions eat much earlier in recovery and are not as finicky to tastes as rats with electrolytic LH lesions. Furthermore, bilaterally injected kainic acid, which destroys the cell bodies in the LH and the zona incerta and subthalamus, but not the fibers of passage, can produce the LH syndrome of aphagia and adipsia, and—after recovery—the failure to respond to acute drinking and feeding challenges (Grossman, Dacey, Haloris, Collier, & Routenberg, 1978; Stricker, Swerdloff, & Zigmond, 1976). Dopamine and norepinephrine levels are not affected by the kainic acid.

However DA-NE depletion is not whole story

A number of things happen when the LH is lesioned or when it is stimulated. First, as Stricker (1983) pointed out, there is a big effect on the arousal of the animals. Lesions make them slow to respond, especially to stressful homeostatic challenges. Stimulation arouses the animal to explore and investigate. Secondly, there are metabolic and visceral effects. Stimulation leads to glucagon release, hyperglycemia, and increases in gastric motility and secretion, oxygen consumption, and body temperature. Lesions have pretty much the opposite effects (Nicolaidis, 1980; Grijalva, Lindholm, & Novin, 1980). As would be expected, vagotomy abolishes or reduces many of these effects, either by interrupting efferent vagal output or afferent feedback from the periphery or both. Third, there are specific effects. Eating and drinking patterns over the 24 hours are changed by lesion (Kissileff, 1970), and direct stimulation can evoke rapid stimulus-bound eating or drinking that stops dead-beat when the stimulation goes off.

Ball (1974) has reported that vagotomy can block or attenuate evoked eating and LH self-stimulation from the same electrodes, but not septal self-stimulation, so again a peripheral feedback loop may be involved. Powley and Opsahl (1976) report similar blockage of evoked eating by vagotomy, but evoked gnawing is not affected nor is self-stimulation, even in those placements where evoked eating was blocked. Thus, the effects are rather specific to feeding evoked by LH stimulation and may involve vagal efferent output via the caudal medulla and possibly also feedback through vagal afferent input from the liver and the gastrointestinal tract, as well as the cardiovascular system.

We also know that stimulation through an LH electrode that elicits eating in one situation may later elicit drinking in another, so there is not complete specificity in the face of variations in the internal environment, external stimulation patterns, and recent past experience (Valenstein et al., 1968). This is what happens, of course, in natural arousal of drives, but we should not overlook the importance of prompt evocation of highly specific patterns of behavior by LH stimulation. This is especially important since there are many different kinds of neurons in the LH, and not all placements in it are successful in eliciting eating and drinking even though only the successful loci are usually reported. As W. R. Hess (1954) showed in his pioneering work in the cat's diencephalon in the 1930s, a variety of ethologically significant, species-specific behaviors can be evoked by stimulation at different loci and with different stimulation parameters (Hess, 1954). The responses aroused are *both* autonomic and somatic and have the character of motivated behavior as we define it today.

A good illustration of the correlation of somatic and autonomic functions of the LH can be seen in the work of Misher and Brooks (1966). They measured gastric acid secretion in rats during both LH and VMH stimulation. If the LH stimulation increased eating, it also increased gastric acid secretion, and if VMH stimulation reduced eating, it also decreased gastric acid secretion. If the stimulations had no effect on eating behavior, they had no effect on gastric secretion. The two measures, then—the behavioral and physiological—are correlated, as one would expect from central-neural structures that have both somatic and autonomic functions. That the physiological effects may not be the cause, or at least the sole cause, of the behavioral effects, however, is suggested by the experiments of Schallert, Whishaw, and Flannigan (1977). Using LH lesions, they were able to separate the gastric and behavioral effects to some degree. They found that dorsolateral LH lesions led to aphagia and varying degrees of gastric pathology, whereas lesions medial and ventral to the LH produced gastric pathology and little or no aphagia. The most sensible hypothesis, at present, is to think of the autonomic (physiological) and somatic (behavioral) functions as parallel processes that may well interact and have significant effects on each other.

In evaluating the functions of the LH in feeding behavior, the great specificity that can be found in recording from single neurons in the LH of the waking monkey should be recalled (Rolls, 1982). As pointed out earlier, some units respond only to the taste and sight of food and only when the animal is hungry. So in addition to the taste pathways reaching the lateral hypothalamus through the ventral pathway from the parabrachial nucleus (see Figure 4.5), some additional and specific change in metabolism, associated with food deprivation, must reach the LH via the central connections of the vagus (see Figure 4.6), or directly as Nicolaidis (1981) has described in his ischymetric hypothesis.

Given the multiple inputs and outputs of the LH and the multiple ascending and descending pathways in it, we have already pointed out that it should be no surprise that lesions and stimulations yield multiple behavioral, visceral, and metabolic effects. Newer technologies may, however, permit better separation of functions. Recently, in their efforts to restore functions lost by 6OHDA lesions with transplantations of fetal substantia nigra tissue, Dunnett and Björklund (1983) reported remarkable separations of function in the rat (see also Dunnett, Björklund, & Stenevi, 1983). Transplantation in a cortical cavity dorsal to the caudate-putamen can compensate for amphetamine-induced ipsilateral rotation, following unilateral lesions of the nigrostriatal pathway. Contralateral sensory neglect, caused by unilateral 6OHDA lesions and akinesia caused by bilateral 6OHDA lesions are compensated for only by transplants that are placed in cortical cavities ventrolateral to the caudate-putamen. Additionally, only nucleus accumbens injections of nigral cell suspensions are able to compensate for apomorphine-induced hyperactivity. None of these loci for transplantation of nigral grafts, however, has been able to improve the regulatory deficits in eating and drinking, even though they can produce recovery from the akinesia following bilateral 6OHDA lesions of the nigrostriatal pathway. The deficits in feeding and drinking after LH electrolytic or 6OHDA lesions thus may not be dependent on the sensory, motor, or arousal deficits that accompany them.

Feeding, Satiation and Satiety

Given fuller delineation of the role of peripheral visceral and metabolic controls of feeding behavior, we can now describe the major features of the physiological and neural systems responsible for generating and sustaining hunger motivation, expressed as both feeding behavior and satiety (see Stricker, 1983; Friedman & Stricker, 1976; LeMagnen, 1983). Late in the postabsorptive state, when there are no nutrient sources from the intestines and stored fuels are being mobilized, the state of hunger is activated by peripheral metabolic input from the liver and by gastric activity over the vagus. This activation is reflected in the activity of catecholaminergic neurons that help to arouse the animal and bring it into contact with food. At the same time, cells in the LH are responsive to the change in energy available, what Nicolaidis called an ischymetric change, reflected in an abrupt drop in O_2 consumption, and what LeMagnen thinks of as decreased glucose utilization and availability. It is these conditions that make some of the LH neurons responsive to the taste and visual stimuli that Rolls used to activate them (see also Oomura, Shimaza, Miyahara, & Hattori, 1982), and it is what makes these sensory stimuli incentives and reinforcers. As food is tasted, there is a pre-absorptive or cephalic insulin release that can be mediated at the brainstem level, and this helps induce the organism to eat, utilize glucose, and store fat.

To complicate matters, insulin may also begin to induce satiation and satiety. For example, in experiments where insulin is infused into the lateral hypothalamus (rat), or into the cerebral ventricles (baboon), food intake is decreased (Nicolaidis, 1981; Woods, Lotter, McKay, & Porte, 1979). As the meal progresses, satiation approaches, abetted by these effects of insulin and possibly its effects in increasing cerebral serotonin release, by stomach distension and gastric chemoreception of nutrients, and by the duodenal effects of nutrients, including the release of CCK and other peptides from intestinal cells. In the early post-absorptive state, nutrients enter the liver through the hepatic portal vein and provide signals of satiation that are transmitted over vagal afferents (Russek, 1971; Novin and VanderWeele, 1977). What produces the longer term effects of satiety and postpones the onset of the next meal, we can only assume is the time it takes for the dissipation of the post-ingestional and post-absorptive effects of the mobilization of stored nutrients. But we do not know how this works in any detail, and more research is needed here.

These are the normal cycles of feeding and satiety that are determined, in part, by circadian rhythms. As LeMagnen (1981, 1983) has pointed out for the nocturnal rat, the night part of the circadian cycle is the period of positive energy balance when intake (5–8 meals at 1–6 gm/meal) exceeds energy expenditure, when glucose utilization is high, and when insulin is elevated—a period of lipogenesis. In the day, on the other hand, energy intake is below expenditure, for there is no eating for the first 4–5 light hours, then there are only a few meals, typically below 2 gm; this is a period of hypoinsulinism, glucose intolerance, and lipolysis. These circadian rhythms of feeding and satiety are also controlled by deprivation, the size of the last meal, and the palatability of foods available.

Thus, there is a complex interaction of peripheral- and central-neural events, both somatic and autonomic as well as metabolic. Conceptually, we have to think of reiterated peripheral–central–peripheral loops with both afferent and efferent components. Taste stimulation, for example, leads to cephalic insulin release via brainstem mechanisms and also arouses lateral hypothalamic units if the animal is food-deprived. Insulin release is also controlled by the medial hypothalamus, presumably over vagal efferent pathways. Vagal afferent pathways bring chemically specific information from the gut and liver as well as from the tongue to the brain. Synapsing in the NTS, these afferents reach the PVN, LH, and other hypothalamic structures directly or through synapses in the parabrachial nucleus of the pons. The hypothalamic structures, in turn, send efferents to the area postrema, cmNTS, and the dorsal motor nucleus of the vagus, thus exerting efferent control of the periphery.

Conceptual Schemes of Peripheral-Central Interactions

We don't know enough of the details yet to agree on how to put these peripheral and central-neural interactions together into a coherent scheme, but some significant attempts have been made. For example, in a schematic diagram (Figure 4.9), Stricker (1983) envisages the periphery providing metabolic (SE_1) and afferent neural (SE_2) activation of a general excitatory system in the brain. The metabolic signals (SE_1) are those arising in the post-absorptive state as the flux of calories from the intestine and liver decreases and energy stores are called upon (one in Figure 4.9). Encountering smell and taste stimuli in the environment sets up the afferent neural signals (SE_2) that act as arousers and incentives, pro-

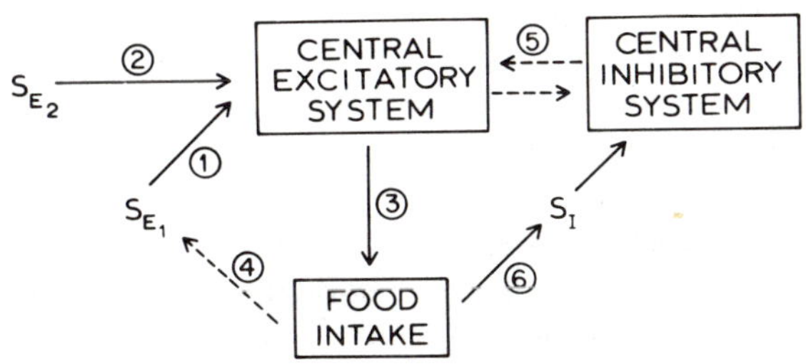

Figure 4.9 Schematic diagram of the central-neural control of food intake, emphasizing general arousal (excitatory) and inhibitory mechanisms that are controlled by peripheral sensory and metabolic input. Abbreviations and numbers explained in text (Stricker, 1983.) Reprinted by permission.

moting eating (two in Figure 4.9). Both kinds of excitatory input operate through activation of the reticular formation and particularly the catecholamines, NE and DA (three in Figure 4.9). Feeding eliminates SE_1 by restoring the flux of calories from the intestine and liver and also by increasing insulin activity (four in Figure 4.9). At the same time, the insulin favors the uptake of tryptophan, the precursor of serotonin in the brain. Serotonergic activity is thought to promote general inhibition (S_I) of behavior, and therefore, cessation of feeding and perhaps sleep (six in Figure 4.9). The central inhibitory system (serotonergic) and the central excitatory system (catecholaminergic) are thought to reciprocally inhibit each other (five in Figure 4.9). The focus here is on the elicitation of feeding by general activation and affect and not by metabolic influences, but there is no reason why the same brain mechanism could not serve both. They are not mutually exclusive functions.

Nicolaidis (1981) makes metabolism central to his conception, particularly the rate of cellular energy production, or what he calls the ischymetric control of food intake. He envisions brain cells in the LH that are sensitive to the availability of energy substrates and that are influenced by hormonal changes. These cells are involved in neurohormonal loops in which the chemoreceptors of smell and taste and those in the gastrointestinal tract project to the LH which, in turn, controls hormonal and metabolic events in the periphery. Thus, a basis is provided for preabsorptive or cephalic insulin and blood sugar changes as well as postabsorptive satiation long before cellular repletion and the restoration of the rate of cellular energy production. LH inhibition of glucagon and increase of insulin secretion are thought to be antagonistic to VMH inhibition of insulin and enhancement of glucagon. One very intriguing aspect of the neurohormonal loop that both Stricker and Nicolaidis stress is the satiating effect of insulin, seen experimentally when it is infused intrahypothalamically in rats (Nicolaidis, 1981) or intraventricularly in baboons (Woods et al., 1979).

We still need to learn more details of how the peripheral autonomic and metabolic and the central-neural mechanisms interact in the control of feeding, but the outlines of a complex mechanism are shaping up in a way that could provide an important model for other kinds of motivated behaviors as well. No longer can we envisage a simple lateral hypothalamic excitatory area and medial hypothalamic inhibitory area. As Hoebel (1984) points out, there is evidence for both excitatory and inhibitory controls in *both* the lateral and medial hypothalamus. Such a dual mechanism may still be the basis for potentiation and depotentiation of feeding behaviors and account for the behavioral facts of hunger and feeding on the one hand, and satiation and satiety, on the other. Many peripheral–central–peripheral loops may be involved. In the end, however, the brain has to control the response mechanisms that yield feeding and the various other kinds of motivated behaviors, not only in their consummatory, but also their appetitive aspects. We turn now to the question of how motivation controls the response mechanism.

Motor Control of Motivated Behavior

The most thoroughgoing investigation of the neural pathway involved in the execution of motivated behavior is the case of lordosis described by Pfaff (1980, 1982) (Figure 4.10). The pathway represents a convergence of hypothalamic influences on spinal cord reflexes via brainstem mechanisms. The output of ventromedial hypothalamic cells, excited by estradiol, converges on midbrain central gray neurons with afferent sensory input and on midbrain reticular formation neurons. From there, the descending influences are relayed through the reticular formation of the medulla and the lateral vestibular nuclei to ventral horn cells of the spinal cord via the lateral vestibulospinal and reticulospinal tracts. Here, between T-12 and S-1, the reflexes of vertebral dorsiflexion are executed in response to flank, rump, and perineal stimulation by the male rat. Thus lordosis and sexually receptive posture are executed by the female rat.

Taken as a model, this response system suggests that the motivational state serves to prime, facilitate, or potentiate a response mechanism that leads to the appetitive or consummatory behavior or some components of them. Furthermore, the hypothalamic structures are the major integrators of the motivational state under the direct influence of the sex hormones and sensory input, and they operate to facilitate integrators lower in the neuraxis that make up the response mechanisms. This conceptualization leads to the more general question of how such a model applies to other kinds of motivated behavior. How does the neural representation of the motivated state prime, facilitate, potentiate, and depontentiate the specific response mechanisms of each kind of motivated behavior? How do these mechanisms yield reward, reinforcement, affect, and hedonic experience, common to all motivated behaviors?

Gallistel (1980a, 1980b) is very specific in addressing the question of how motivation influences the motor response mechanisms. He sees reflexes, oscillators, and servomechanisms as the fundamental units of behavior. Sensitive to afferent neural and hormonal influences, the diencephalon serves to potentiate and depotentiate the response mechanism in highly specific ways. As we have pointed out already, the prepotent response of the non-predatory cat when its lip is touched is to withdraw or else actually rub its face against the stimulus. When the lateral perifornical area on the opposite side is stimulated, these non-predatory responses are depotentiated, and head-orienting and biting responses are

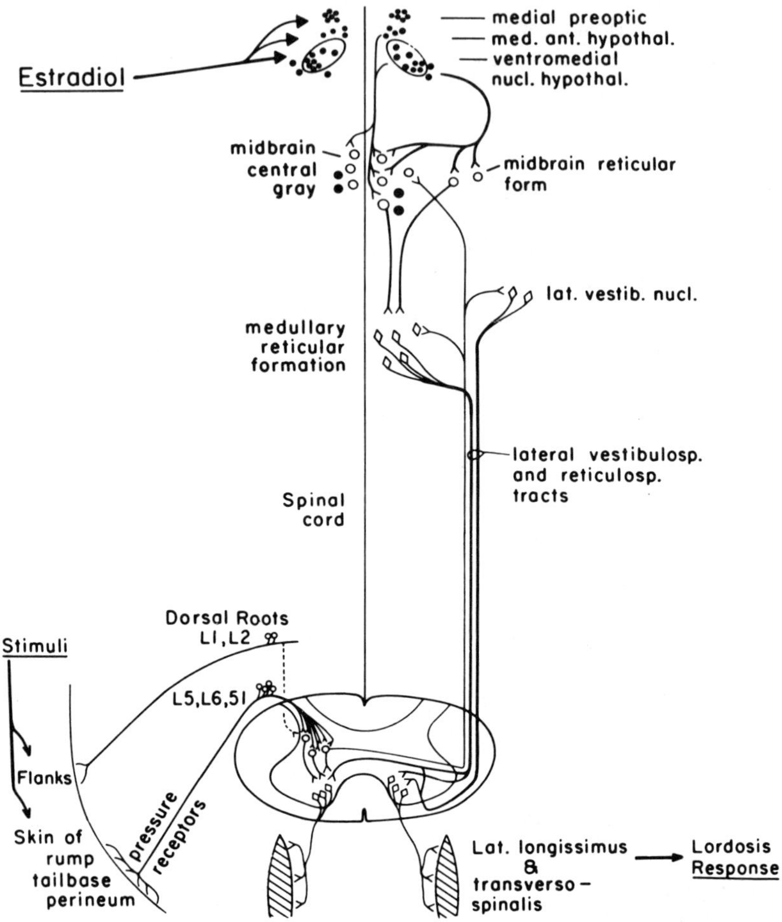

Figure 4.10 Neural circuitry involved in the lordosis response of female rat to flank, rump, and perineal stimulation by male rats after she is made sexually receptive by estrogen (estradiol) in the hypothalamus (Pfaff, 1980.) Reprinted by permission.

potentiated on the contralateral side. On the ipsilateral side, where there is no depotentiation, the withdrawal or face-rubbing remains. So a highly specific unilateral pathway is involved in this instance.

The same is true even when the motivated behavior involves a learned instrumental response (Beagley & Holley, 1977). For example, if rats are taught that they can press a bar for food only when a light shines in one or the other eye, it can be shown that, with unilateral LH stimulation, the satiated rat will press the bar and eat only if the light shines in the contralateral eye. Shining the light in the ipsilateral eye does not elicit bar-pressing or eating to LH stimulation on the same side. Thus, the brain stimulation motivates the trained rat on one side and leaves it satiated on the other.

In Gallistel's concept, the same neural hierarchy involved in such simple acts as walking is involved in motivated behavior. The potentiation or depotentiation of the response mechanisms of the caudal neuraxis by rostral structures is aroused by three main types of events: (a) external arousing or releasing stimuli, (b) an endogenous oscillatory process or biological rhythm, and (c) an error signal in the servomechanism operating in homeostasis. A fourth possibility is "autonomous accumulation" due to deprivation of the opportunity to perform the act, or what Lorenz thought of as the basis for the "vacuum reaction." Gallistel outlined the principles of the response hierarchy in which the hierarchy is a lattice work, so that several rostral mechanisms can potentiate the same caudal response mechanisms. In addition, rostral mechanisms can potentiate and depotentiate each other, giving a relative hierarchy or heterarchy. Both of these principles recognize that motivated behavior is not stereotyped, and both allow for considerable variation in the responses used to achieve the same end-point, or the goal of motivated behavior.

In Teitelbaum's concept, there is also a hierarchy in the neuraxis (Teitelbaum, Schallert, & Whishaw, 1983). His empirical work, however, has uncovered a different classification of response mechanisms. He views lesions that affect motivated behavior (e.g., LH lesions) as transections that cut off rostral from caudal structures. In recovery, some degree of rostral control is restored. As the recovery progresses, more and more of the caudal response mechanisms are brought under rostral control. This is somewhat the same process that occurs in normal development, in which the basic response mechanisms emerge first and are gradually transformed into larger units of response under the organizing or integrating influence of the rostral mechanisms. This is the process that Teitelbaum calls the encephalization of motivated behavior (1971). He illustrates it in the case of hunger when he shows that depressing the cortex with KC1 in the recovered lateral hypothalamic rat reinstates the syndrome of aphagia and adipsia (Teitelbaum & Cytawa, 1965; Cytawa & Teitelbaum, 1967).

With the lateral hypothalamic lesion, the rat is close to the "zero-state" of motivation because the rostral mechanisms are not able to organize the caudal response mechanism (Teitelbaum, 1982). Instead, only the basic response mechanisms or motor subsytems remain as fragmentary elements of motivated behavior. The motor subsystems so far uncovered are: mouthing, orienting, head scanning, postural support, and locomotion. It is because the motivational mechanism at the rostral end of the neural hierarchy cannot organize the caudal response mechanisms, following an LH lesion, that we see aphagia and adipsia and also sensory neglect, akinesia, and catalepsy. Teitelbaum disconnects this hierarchical mechanism with lesions, neurotoxins, and antagonists and agonists of neurotransmitters and then watches it put itself back together again as recovery proceeds. Or he sees the units become synthesized and integrated in the course of normal development, much the way Twitchell (1970) has done in the case of the grasp reflex.

Although the LH lesions affect both motivational and sensori-motor systems together, it seems likely now that even more rostral integrative mechanisms may control them separately. As pointed out earlier, by implantation of fetal substantia nigral tissue into the caudate, it is possible to restore the akinesia and catalepsy deficits without restoring the motivational deficits following 6OHDA lesions in the LH (Dunnett & Björkland, 1983; Dunnett et al., 1983). Thus, although the motor subsystems are basic response mechanisms in motivated behavior that are integrated and controlled by rostral brain mechanisms, we still need to learn more about what those rostral mechanisms for motivation are and how they work to prime specific motivated behaviors.

We need more of the kinds of detailed analysis of the structures and pathways involved of the sort that Pfaff (1982) has provided in the case of sexual behavior and Miselis (1981; Hyde & Miselis, 1983) is developing in his anatomical tracing studies in hunger and thirst. Then we will be able to reap the full benefit of the broader conceptual schemes of Gallistel and Teitelbaum. Only then will we be able to specify how motivation so selectively and flexibly controls the response mechanisms to yield adaptive, motivated behavior.

Reward, Affect, and Hedonic Response

While selective and flexible adaptive motor responses are the hallmark of motivated behavior, other outputs of the central-neural mechanisms are also involved. Some of these outputs are relatively simple and directly observable, such as affect, affective display, and emotional expression. Others, like reward and reinforcement, must be inferred from behavior, and this has been classically done in studies of both animals and humans. Hedonic experience, however, can be directly dealt with only in humans where it can be reported subjectively or registered more objectively as a magnitude estimation or the mark on an analogue scale. One of the great contributions of the study of the neurobiological basis of motivated behavior is that it opens the way for the investigation of the even more difficult question of the physiological and neurological basis of reward, affect, and hedonic experience.

Nowhere is the relationship between the mechanisms of homeostasis, motivation, reward, affect, and hedonic experience clearer than in the case of temperature regulation. As pointed out earlier, there are neural mechanisms controlling physiological responses to temperature challenges at all levels of the neuraxis, but the major integrator is in the preoptic/anterior hypothalamic area. Even when these regions are damaged and physiological responses to temperature challenges are impaired, however, animals are still capable of behavioral temperature regulation and will respond to turn on a heat lamp when challenged with cold (Satinoff & Rutstein, 1970). It is not until the lateral hypothalamus is damaged, and a number of other motivations are impaired, that thermoregulatory behavior fails (Satinoff & Shan, 1971). On the other hand, physiological thermoregulatory responses are only minimally damaged by LH lesions; thus, there is a dissociation of physiological and behavioral mechanisms, although not a complete one.

In the intact animal, the two systems must work closely together. For example, when Corbit (1973) heated or cooled the preoptic/anterior hypothalamic area of the rat by flowing warm and cool water through an implanted thermode, the animal readily learned to press a lever to give its brain a brief (15 s) exposure to the opposite temperature. The warmer the brain temperature, for instance, the more frequently the rat pressed a lever to have a brief shot of cool water through the implanted thermode (Figure 4.11). Quite clearly, the cool water was acting as a reward in the same way that electrical self-stimulation reward does, and the rat was working hard to get it. The same applied to brief heating of the preoptic/anterior hypothalamus when it was kept at a cool temperature. The animals also learned to heat or cool their skins in response to the experimenter's cooling and warming the brain, and *vice versa.* But they could discriminate temperature change in the brain from temperature change in the skin. For example, trained to make one response to cool their brain after it was warmed and a different response to cool their skin, when given a choice, they prefered to cool their brains when their brains

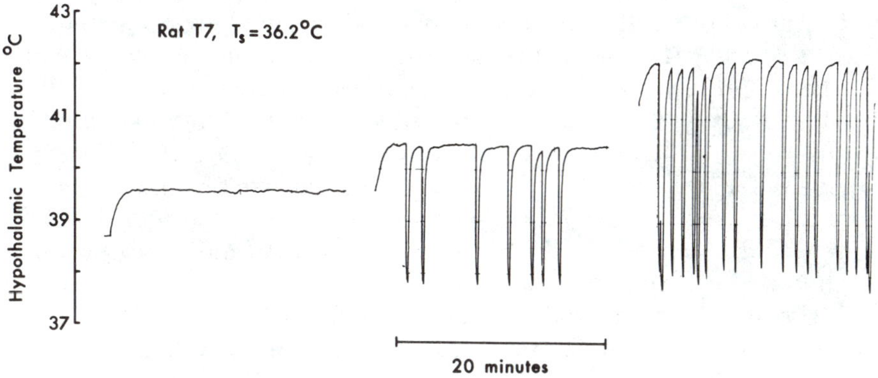

Figure 4.11 Increased rate of responding for a momentary 15°C lowering of brain temperature as a function of increasing basal brain temperature by means of a thermode implanted in the preoptic/anterior-hypothalamic area of the rat (Corbit, 1973.) Reprinted by permission.

were warmed and their skin when only the skin was warmed (Corbit & Ernits, 1974).

Cabanac et al. (1972) and Hawkins (1975) experimented with raising and lowering of core temperature of human subjects immersed in warm and cold baths. By these procedures, they were heating and cooling their subjects' brains as well as the rest of their bodies and studying their hedonic responses, for if they only warmed or cooled the skin and did not change core temperature, they got only minimal hedonic effects (Fig. 3.12). As pointed out earlier, the raising and lowering of core temperature was rated as unpleasant by human subjects. This led them to judge hand baths as most unpleasant when they were the same temperature as the tub and most pleasant when they were at the opposite extreme. Even more striking was the fact, in Hawkins' experiment, that subjects took long showers at these opposite extreme temperatures and judged as most pleasant water temperatures that were judged unpleasant at neutral body temperatures.

Thus, core temperature (brain temperature) is defended physiologically and behaviorally. The motivation to make behavioral adjustments is strong, the reward or reinforcement of thermoregulatory behavior is positive, the somatic and autonomic affective responses are clearly evident in vascular and other changes, and in humans, the reported hedonic experience is intense. All of these responses occur together. Furthermore, animal studies with brain lesions and stimulations, make it clear that the same or closely related neural mechanisms are at work to produce these different responses, even though components can be dissociated by appropriate lesions.

Hoebel (1984) has made the same argument about the relation of the neural mechanisms involved in the regulation of food intake and reward. The same sites in the LH yield both self-stimulation and feeding behavior, and variables that influence feeding behavior influence self-stimulation in the same way (Hoebel & Teitelbaum, 1962; Margules & Olds, 1962). Furthermore, in his recording studies in the lateral hypothalamus of the monkey, Rolls (1982) found that neurons that were responsive to taste stimuli when the monkey was hungry were also activated by sites that yielded self-stimulation. In some cases, the effective self-stimulation sites were the same as the recording sites, thus indicating that there is convergence of the mechanisms of hunger and self-stimulation reward, right down to the level of single LH neurons.

Hoebel has diagramatically portrayed (Figure 4.12) some of the complex relations of feeding and reward. He sees a dual mechanism.

(a) *Activation of the LH leading to feeding and reward,* such as occurs with taste stimulation of the hungry animal or direct electrical LH stimulation. The reward effect may be mediated through the LH con-

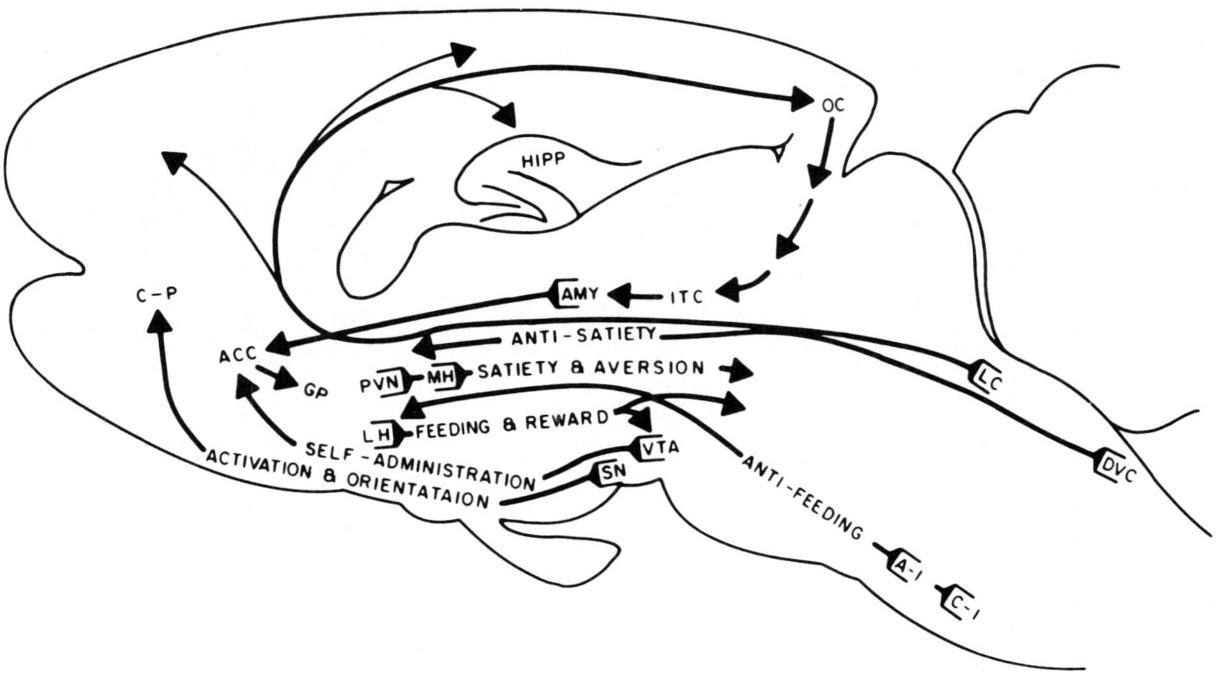

Figure 4.12 Lateral view of the rat's brain, schematically showing the areas and pathways involved in the control of feeding behavior and reward, based on the effects of lesions, electrical stimulation, and self-injection of neurotransmitters, their agonists, antagonists, and peptide modulators. (See text for explanation.)

Abbreviations: ACC, nucleus accumbens; AMY, amygdala; A-1, norepinephrine cell group; C-1, epinephrine cell group; C-P, caudate-putamen; DVC, dorsal vagal complex; FC, frontal cortex; GP, globus pallidus; HIPP, hippocampus; ITC, infratemporal cortex; LC, locus coeruleus; LH, lateral hypothalamus; MH, medial hypothalamus; OC, optic cortex; PVN, paraventricular nucleus; SN, substantia migra; VTA, ventral tegmental area (Hoebel, 1984.) Reprinted by permission.

nections to the ventral tegmental area (VTA), where rats self-stimulate and work to self-inject opiates and neurotensin or show place preferences when these peptides are injected there. Projection of VTA dopamine cells to the nucleus accumbens is also thought to be part of the reward system. Rats will self-inject amphetamine in the nucleus accumbens, presumably because it releases dopamine there. Epinephrine and norepinephrine from C-1 and A-1 cells of the brainstem are inhibitory in this scheme, and their activity in the LH leads to reduced feeding and reward.

(b) *Activation of the PVN-MH leads to satiety and aversion,* according to Hoebel's concept. These mechanisms are inhibited by input from the dorsal vagal complex (DVC) through taste or as a consequence of depletions in the gut or liver. They are also inhibited by norepinephrine, resulting in increased feeding and reward.

In addition, noradrenergic pathways from the locus coeruleus (LC) arouse the hypothalamus and forebrain, and dopaminergic pathways from the substantia nigra (SN) facilitate the motor mechanisms in the caudate, putamen, and globus pallidus for the execution of behavior appropriate to feeding and reward. The diagram and the concepts are speculative, but they summarize a large number of experimental facts and they portray some of the complexities we must deal with in trying to see how excitatory and inhibitory mechanisms lead to the control of feeding behavior and to reward and reinforcement.

It is too early to develop a concrete conception of the neural basis of reward and hedonic experience. All we have are models like those suggested in temperature regulation and general schema such as Cabanac (1979) has provided, or putative pathways and mechanisms such as Hoebel has attempted.

These models are useful guides, but they need to be tested empirically so that detailed anatomical pathways and physiological mechanisms underlying behavior can be worked out. At the same time, they need to be extended to a wider range of motivated behaviors, including non-homeostatic and acquired motivation. Then what we learn about the basis of one kind of motivation can lead to a testable hypothesis about the basis of another kind of motivation. In addition, as we learn more about motivated behavior, we should be able to uncover the neurological and physiological basis of reward and reinforcement, the expression of affect, and hedonic experience.

As we shall see in the next chapters, the self-stimulation model offers us one of the best approaches to uncovering the details of the neural basis of reward and reinforcement. It has become behaviorally sophisticated and quantitative, and at the same time, has reached the point where the detailed tracing of the specific neural pathways and neurotransmitters involved is developing rapidly.

Summary

We have described the properties of a central neural mechanism for the arousal and satiation of motivated behavior that is controlled by peripheral afferent neural and metabolic input. This is the same mechanism that, on the one hand, operates in physiological regulation, and on the other hand, that we believe makes up the neurological and physiological basis of affect, reward and reinforcement, and hedonic experience.

The core of this mechanism is a brain state produced by a combination of changes in the internal environment and afferent neural input. Flynn's perifornical stimulation of the hypothalamus is an example of the experimental induction of the brain state that primes the cat to attack a suitable prey object like a rat. Pfaff's description of the effect of estrogen on the ventromedial and anterior hypothalamus in priming or potentiating the lordosis and sexual receptivity of the female is an example of a natural biological rhythm that produces the brain state. A similar example is Epstein's finding of the dipsogenic effect of angiotensin II on the subfornical organ in the anterior wall of the third ventricle. Candidate neurons that make up the central brain state in hunger have been identified in the lateral hypothalamus and related areas by Rolls, in his finding that individual neural units respond to the taste and sight of food only when the animal is hungry.

The central-neural mechanism is a hierarchy of integrators at various levels of the neuraxis. Decerebration studies in temperature regulation, sexual behavior, and feeding behavior reveal integrating mechanisms in the spinal cord, brainstem, and diencephalon. Without the diencephalon, however, responses tend to be fragmentary and incomplete. In the case of feeding behavior, however, as Grill has shown, the decerebrate rat can accept or reject foods, depending on their taste and its state of deprivation. The decerebrate is also capable of cephalic insulin responses and is sensitive to insulin, but it cannot learn taste aversions or seek food. Neural pathways from the taste system and to and from the abdominal viscera are being traced into the caudal medulla, and from there to the hypothalamus and amygdala, and then back down to the caudal medulla. How such a hierarchy might work is diagrammed by Flynn for the case of elicitation of aggression by perifornical stimulation, where concomitant stimulation of both rostral and caudal structures can result in either the facilitation or the suppression of evoked attack.

The complexities of peripheral and central-neural interactions are explored in the example of feeding behavior. Information about the status of new energy supplies entering the alimentary tract and being absorbed from the gut, and the depletion of energy stores in the liver and fat depots reaches the brain over afferent neural pathways and perhaps also directly reaches areas of the brain sensitive to the level of available energy, as Nicolaidis suggests in his ischymetric hypothesis. The central-neural mechanisms involved, in turn, control both metabolism and visceral activity, which also have their consequences for the control of feeding behavior and satiation. Thus, there are reiterated peripheral–central–peripheral loops that participate in the control system. These feedback loops must, in the end, influence the major central brain mechanisms for feeding and satiety, systems most likely involving excitatory and inhibitory mechanisms in both the lateral hypothalamus and medial hypothalamus in their functions as the major short-term and long-term integrators of energy metabolism and feeding behavior.

The details of how such rostral integrators control the caudal response mechanisms have not been worked out, although remarkable headway has been made in elucidating the pathways in the case of lordosis in the female rat. Both Gallistel and Teitelbaum have addressed this issue, and their concepts are briefly presented.

Finally, the question of how the neurological and physiological mechanism for motivated behavior yields reward and reinforcement, affect, and hedonic experience is discussed. Although we know only fragmentary details and rely heavily on the model of thermoregulatory behavior, we try to frame the questions in terms of the conceptualizations of Hoebel and look ahead to the next chapters, which will explore the challenging opportunities opened up by recent progress in the study of rewarding electrical self-stimulation of the brain.

5

The Measurement of Brain Stimulation Reward

Background

Ever since its discovery in 1954 by Olds and Milner, the phenomenon of self-stimulation behavior has attracted the attention of neuroscientists interested in the brain and motivated behaviors. Like the early work with electrolytic lesions, electrical stimulation of the brain (ESB) held out the hope of revealing a part of the neural mechanisms of motivated, ethologically significant behaviors. In this regard, Neal Miller wrote about a 1961 article by Olds:

> In the Olds' chapter, we have seen, as might be expected from the drive-reduction hypothesis, that the rate of bar-pressing reinforced by central stimulation in at least some locations can be manipulated by changing the intensity of certain drives. The fact that the effect of certain drives is at least partially specific to the reward effect of stimulation opens up the possibility for further research. (Miller, 1961, p.576)

The following years saw numerous studies on the relationship between rewarding brain stimulation and natural reinforcers. Some differences between natural and brain stimulation reward were delineated—for example, the apparent lack of satiation seen with ESB self-stimulation (Olds, 1958b; Valenstein & Beer, 1964) or its surprising lack of resistence to extinction (Howarth & Deutsch, 1962; Culberton, Kling, & Berkeley,

1966). Some differences, such as the extreme sensitivity to extinction, were partially attributed to superficial aspects of the brain reward, such as its immediate delivery without the need for the subject to go over to a food or water dispenser (Panksepp & Trowill, 1967a, 1967b). Other differences seemed more constitutional, like the lack of any relationship of ESB self-stimulation to satiation owing to the absence of any nutritive consequenses of ESB. Mogenson and Cioe (1977) provide a good review of these studies.

Looking back from the present perspective, we can see that one problem for early workers in this field was the lack of any way of relating the effects of ESB at one site to its effects at another site. Although many workers behaved as though they assumed that nearby lateral hypothalmic sites activated pretty much the same neural substrate, it was unclear how ESB at this site related to septal or even to lateral preoptic sites of self-stimulation. Every major region had to be treated and analyzed as yielding a functionally separate phenomenon. Early attempts to solve this problem involved study of the neuroanatomical connections of the ESB self-stimulation sites. The locations of many of the electrode sites themselves gave the first clue as they revealed the importance of a major fiber system in the ventral brain, the medial forebrain bundle (Olds, 1956; Olds & Olds, 1963). Subsequent lesion studies attempted to trace out the interconnections within the medial forebrain bundle self-stimulation sites or between the medial forebrain bundle and other sites by interrupting the pathway carrying the reward signal away from the electrode. For reviews of this early literature, see Valenstein (1966), Lorens (1976), Routtenberg (1976), or parts of chapter 6 of this book.

A successful lesion or transection that cut a reward-relevant pathway was judged by its ability to block ESB self-stimulating behavior. However, complications of behavioral measurement arose. For example, consider the placement of a lesion in the posterior medial forebrain bundle (Olds & Olds, 1969). Some animals exhibited decreases in the rate of responding for the ESB, but these decreases were difficult to separate from overall decreases in behavioral competence. This problem with using rate-of-response measures persisted in the field despite early warnings of the inadequacy of rate measures (Valenstein, 1964). The result of this measurement problem is that self-stimulation behavior had to be discussed as a whole and not with regard to the ESB reinforcing effect alone. This is difficult because, unlike feeding behavior, ESB self-stimulation behavior is an artificial laboratory phenomenon, and much of the excitement in it comes from what studying this odd behavior might tell us about the neural processes underlying reinforcement in general. Therefore, the subfield of ESB self-stimulation research must focus on better measures of reward if it hopes to teach the general field of psychobiology anything of interest.

Another method for getting at the question of the reward substrate is to look carefully at the anatomical projections from one self-stimulation site to another. For example, Routtenberg (1970) identified axons from the frontal cortex that descend in the medial forebrain bundle and into the brain stem. He suggested the attractive hypothesis that these axons might subserve at least a part of the reward of self-stimulation at the two regions. His anatomical evidence came from a study that used a stain for degenerating nerve fibers. The degeneration was produced by making a lesion through a frontal cortex self-stimulation electrode, thereby ensuring that the degenerating fibers were the same ones that were activated during stimulation. Of course, since the lesion destroys reward-relevant and irrelevant fibers with equal facility, it could well have been some other pathway, perhaps a cortical–cortical connection that was crucial to self-stimulation. In fact, more recent evidence (Corbett, Laferriere, & Milner, 1982a, 1982b; Stellar, Illes, & Mills, 1982) suggests just such a possibility—namely, that frontal cortex–sulcal cortex connections and not frontal cortex–hypothalamic connections are crucial to ESB self-stimulation of the frontal cortex. This example illustrates the difficulty of associating any one of the complex connections of the nervous system with the particular function of the reward of ESB. Unfortunately, these and other problems prevented the establishment of a good anatomical framework for organizing observations from different electrode sites in earlier research.

A major advance was made with the histochemical maps of Ungerstedt and others (Ungerstedt, 1971a; Lindvall & Björklund, 1974). The concordance between these monoamine maps and effective sites of ESB self-stimulation gave the field its first substantive anatomical basis. To compound the excitement, neurochemical ideas implicating monoamines in self-stimulation were generated at about the same time. Unfortunately for the field, the first specific hypothesis, stating that the activation of norepinephrine cells was the major neurochemical/anatomical basis for self-stimulation (Stein & Wise, 1967, 1969; also see Stein, 1975 for a review), was incorrect. Contemporary thinking, with improved psychopharmacological agents and anatomical techniques, now focuses heavily on dopamine-containing cells (Wise, 1982).

It is illustrative of the problems faced in the study of self-stimulation and motivation in general that some of the early studies (e.g., Stein & Wise, 1967) supportive of the norepinephrine hypothesis were later criticized (e.g., Roll, 1970; Rolls, Kelly & Shaw, 1974) for the same reasons of inadequate behavioral measures that plagued the early lesion work. Although discussion on this point continues (Stein, 1980, p. 113), it is worth more than a moment's pause to reflect upon this shortcoming. Although it is reasonable to expect that technical advances in the diversity and precision of pharmacological agents would alter thinking about the neurochemical basis of self-stimulation, it is disappointing to see in the literature the consistent oversimplification by many researchers of the problem of measuring ESB reward. In the opinion of the authors, the resulting contradictions and reversals of opinions have damaged the prestige of self-stimulation research, in particular, and the field of neurobiology of motivation in general.

Along these philosophical lines, it may be useful to compare the history and current status of research on motivation, and specifically self-stimulation, to the long and distinguished history of research on the neurobiology of vision. It seems to us that the early visual sciences had at least two major advantages over self-stimulation research. First, it was obvious in vision what were the inital anatomical components of the system (e.g., retina, optic nerve and tract, lateral geniculate nucleus, etc.). Although the later elaboration of the role of the visual cortical areas in acuity and/or form vision was somewhat controversial, the good agreement on the initial anatomy offered striking opportunities to trace out subsequent anatomical and functional projections. The recent Nobel prize-winning work of David Hubel and Torsten Weisel on the primary visual cortical areas testifies to the success of this area of research.

The second advantage for visual science came from work in perception where psychophysical methods of stimulus analysis were established early. Used in both humans and animals, these techniques set important constraints on our understanding of the quantitative operating characteristics of the visual system. In many places, these perceptual characteristics match beautifully with the biological substrate. For example, the psychophysically determined relationship between the frequency (color) and the intensity of light required to reach the threshold of seeing in dark-adapted subjects matches quite closely the absorption spectrum of rhodopsin when corrected for the absorptive characteristics of the media of the eye. This gives rise to the belief that rhodopsin is the photopigment of scotopic vision. Another example of this match is the parallel between decreases in the visual acuity with lateral distance away from the fixation point, and the decreases in density of photoreceptors, accompanied by increases in size of ganglionic receptive field with distance from the fovea (Kling & Riggs, 1971). The match between structure and function in these two examples from vision research illustrates a precision that gives a satisfying "engineering" quality to this field; that quality has often been missing in self-stimulation research.

If the current neurochemical hypothesis about the role of dopamine-containing neural systems in ESB reward (Wise, 1980, 1982) is basically correct, or if the current neuroanatomical attempt to identify the neurons directly excited by the electrode succeeds (Gallistel, 1983), then we would have some anatomical underpinning for a new, more precise era in self-stimulation research. Accompanying this neuroanatomical development, and completing the parallel with vision research, as discussed above, is the development of quantitative or psychophysical studies of reward based on the controllability of electrical stimulation from the perspective of stimulus generation. This offers the opportunity to solve many of the reward measurement problems that plagued earlier research and offers the tremendous advantage of being capable of generating a list of quantitative characteristics that specify, to some extent, the nature of the neural substrate that mediates reward (Gallistel et al., 1981). For example, the measurement of the conduction velocity and direction of conduction of some of the reward-relevant neurons (Shizgal, Bielajew, Corbett, Skelton, & Yeomans, 1980) suggests that the directly activated lateral hypothalamic neurons are myelinated and descend (Bielajew, 1983a) in the medial forebrain bundle into the ventral tegmental area. Recently, this research effort has shown signs of generating a set of complementary results from different laboratories (Hoebel & Novin, 1982, pp. 405–443). These findings hold promise of revealing the nature of some of the neurons directly excited by an electrode in the medial forebrain bundle. These findings are discussed in detail in chapter 6.

This and the next two chapters constitute the primary discussion of ESB reward. This discussion is organized somewhat differently from other considerations of self-stimulation. We begin and end this chapter with a discussion of problems of ESB reward measurement. In the first part, we review examples of self-stimulation methodologies to illustrate the critical problem of reward measurement and its separation from performance factors such as motor deficits. Then we illustrate briefly the tradeoff methods in psychophysical techniques, how they work, and what they accomplish. In the next chapter (6), we examine the anatomical substrate of brain stimulation reward by focusing on the problem of identifying the axons that are directly excited by lateral hypothalamic ESB and carry away the reward signal. Finally, we focus on the dopamine hypothesis (chapter 7), its supporting evidence from drug self-administration as well as ESB studies, and the current research efforts. Functional considerations such as the relationship to hunger and feeding are considered briefly in the light of current measurement and anatomical understanding, but this discussion does not take place until the last chapter of the book (chapter 8).

The Problem of ESB Reward Measurement

Measurement of the reward of brain stimulation is not a simple matter. What are the reasons for this? At first, ESB reward measurement seems easy enough. A rat or other animal can be trained to perform some arbitrary operant task, such as pressing a lever, that results in brain stimulation. As Teitelbaum has noted (1977), performance of the operant guarantees that a motivational state is present and that the stimulus is reinforcing. Skinner (1938) and others have shown in fundamental and classical work that response rate will, over some range, depend positively on amount of reinforcement obtained by the subject. Furthermore, this basic observation has been confirmed in every laboratory that has studied brain stimulation reward, given an appropriate appreciation for a variety of threshold (cellar) and ceiling effects.

The problem enters, in a major way, when one manipulates the brain in some manner, for if the brain itself is different, the rules that translate a fixed level of reinforcement into operant behavior may well be different. Thus, the first criterion for any prospective measurement of reward is that it be able to separate reward from motor or performance effects or, at least, to be relatively unaffected by changes in motor competence caused by brain lesions, drug treatment, or other experimental manipulation. The second criterion should be that the above property be verified in an actual experiment in which motor competence and ESB reward are independently manipulated and the effect on the reward measure is noted. "Reward" can be altered by reducing the pulse frequency or pulse number (if square wave) or reducing the intensity of the brain stimulation burst given as a consequence of performing the operant. Such a manipulation should not greatly alter the basic motor capabilities of the animal, but will clearly reduce behavioral responding unless some other aspect of the stimulation is increased (e.g., the duration).

To a first approximation, "motor competence" can be altered by increasing task difficulty. Two ways to do this might be either by putting extra weight on the response lever, making it harder for the subject to press, or by giving the animal a subparalytic dose of a peripheral cholinergic blocker, like curare, that interferes with the action of the neuromuscular junction. These motor manipulations should not alter the impact of brain stimulation on the neural tissue beneath the electrode tip. However, they should alter the complex function that translates a given amount of ESB reward into a given amount of behavior. It must also be noted that motor debilitation may well induce a new cost to responding that subtracts from the positive or reward aspects of the operant situation. This is a complication in the separation of motor and reward effects; it is discussed in chapter 7. In conclusion, both the reward and motor manipulations must be tried on any new measure of self-stimulation behavior before it can be claimed to be a measure valid for either reward or motor assessment.

The above arguments should not be taken to preclude the use of lever-pressing as a measure of reward. A number of laboratories have quite successfully used a simple continuous reinforcement lever-pressing paradigm as a reward measure. One example is the double pulse studies of Shizgal, Bielajew, Corbett, Skelton, & Yeomans (1980) and Yeomans (1975, 1979) who inferred a number of characteristics of the neural substrate mediating reward from psychophysical manipulations of the parameters of brain stimulation. However, it must be understood that in none of these studies did they make a lesion or other physiological manipulation of the brain beyond changing the brain stimulation. Thus, we can be fairly sure that no motor competence problems arose to confound their interpretation.

What follows is an assessment of several paradigms for investigating self-stimulation, weighing the advantages and disadvantages of each. These are intended to serve as a representative, and not as an inclusive, survey and provide a framework for discussing the principle of performance–reward separation. It will also be clear from the survey that the search for a rate-free paradigm is an old one, resulting in a number of techniques that have had mixed success. It is also a new one and goes to the heart of important issues in the generation of self-stimulation behavior.

Continuous Reinforcement Lever-Pressing

We begin with this paradigm because it is the oldest, the most heavily used, and superficially, the simplest of all paradigms. Olds and Milner's original paper in 1954 used lever-pressing as the behavioral response by which they initially confirmed the stimulation's rewarding properties. At first, they employed an informal place preference in an open field, rewarding the animal for entering or remaining at a particular location. This place preference, it was thought, could be too easily confused with reflex freezing reaction to brain stimulation; subsequently lever-pressing on a continuous reinforcement schedule was instituted as a superior response (Olds & Milner, 1954; Mogenson & Phillips, 1978). It is superior not only because it is an operant response with a long history in psychology, but because it is extremely easy to implement and automate. Experimenters need only to attach the response lever to a stimulator that generates fixed-duration bursts and to record in a given period of time the number of lever presses. Alternatively, one can record each response on a cumulative recorder. In this record (Figure 5.1), the slope of the line then indicates rate, with steeper slopes showing higher rates.

This procedure then generates a single numerical measure known as *rate of response*. Many things were shown to affect rate of response, including stimulating current (Olds, 1958c), gonadal hormones or food deprivation (Olds, 1958a; Hoebel, 1975), immediate prior exposure to brain stimulation (Olds & Milner, 1954; Howarth & Deutsch, 1962; Gallistel, 1969a, 1969b), occurrence of seizures (Reid et al., 1964), and motoric effects of the ESB (Edmonds & Gallistel, 1974). Today few people would accept all of these factors as altering reward. Clearly, motoric side-effects can limit rate of response. In a somewhat more subtle way, the effects of immediate prior stimulation are thought to alter (increase) response rate, in part, due to changes in arousal and motivation (Gallistel

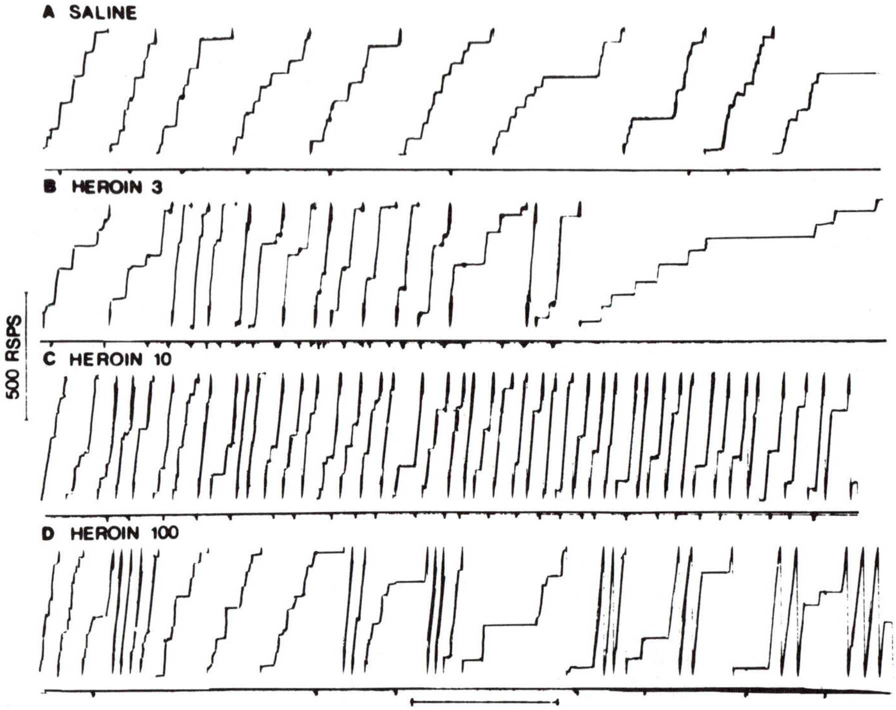

Figure 5.1 Cumulative record of lever-press responding (y-axis) for ESB plotted aginst time (x-axis), with animal responding on a continuous reinforcement schedule. *Note.* In this typical graph, the slope of the line gives a measure of response rate. In this study, heroin was shown to increase response rate (dose is in ug/kg, i.v. infusion, over 28 seconds). The heroin infusions were triggered by the animal responding on a different lever and are indicated as the vertical pips on the horizontal line beneath each graph. These authors also employed other measures, such as autotitration, in this study. (Bozarth & Wise 1981).

1973, 1983). Some of these performance/motor-related factors may account for the observation that, with two levels of stimulation, the level for which rats will respond at higher rates is not always the most preferred, and in fact, may be clearly less preferred in a choice test (Hodos and Valenstein, 1962; Gallistel, 1969b). Simply put, too many factors affect rate of response to make it very useful as a measure of brain-stimulation reward (Mogenson & Cioe, 1977; Valenstein, 1964).

Even if these problems of interpretation are set aside, operant research has long since gone beyond measuring performance on the simple continuous reinforcement schedule as a reliable quantitative measure of natural reward. Difficulties occur in instability of the behavior (Reynolds, 1968) because the rate of reinforcement is dependent almost completely on the rate of response in this schedule. For example, as the animal responds more rapidly, it gets more reinforcement. This encourages more rapid responding, which then leads to still more reinforcement. The sequence described here is a positive feedback loop, the consequences of which are that the behavior, once started, tends to go to a maximum limit or behavioral ceiling set by either the motoric capacity or some other variable perhaps linked to the ESB itself (e.g., aversiveness). Ironically, in an effort to produce good, stable, vigorous self-stimulators, researchers may be setting stimulation parameters to produce this ceiling.

One alternative to the continuous reinforcement schedule is to restrict the maximum number of reinforcements received to some number that is clearly less than the behavioral capacity. This is called an intermittent schedule and has the advantage of preventing the ceiling phenomena described above. One of the most favored intermittent schedules is the variable interval schedule in which, every so often, independent of the rate of responding, a reinforcement is set up so that the next response delivers it. A given mean setup time (e.g., 5 seconds) with a known variance about that mean can be programmed so that the probability of a reinforced lever press is known. This schedule produces steady rates of responding in which motoric rate-limiting side-effects of the stimulation are reduced because most of the responding occurs in the absence of a brain stimulation reinforcer. Furthermore, a time-out period can be given during the actual ESB burst to prevent any distraction or disturbance in behavior at the time of receipt of ESB from artificially reducing response rate. Another good method is to use discrete trials in which responding delivers ESB, terminates the trial, and begins an intertrial interval. Again, responding occurs in the absence of (i.e., before) ESB, and so cannot be impaired by elicited motor or other performance-impairing side-effects of the ESB.

To end this section, we would like to mention the obvious fact that the rate of responding will depend on the demand characteristics of the task. For example, it is clear that rats that are lever-pressing for brain stimulation reward require more time for a response than rats that are nose-poking for the same reward. In the nose-poking situation, a rat simply inserts its nose in a hole to interrupt a photocell beam, usually on the other side of a hole in a cage wall. The task requires little major skeletal muscle activity other than maintenance of posture. Slight movements of the head or even the nose are usually sufficient to alter the shadow cast on the photocell device to generate a response count, and rates can be very high. The behavior typically has a high spontaneous activity level, and the amount of reinforcement required to maintain some low level of responding is quite a bit less than for lever-pressing. However, this subtlety is not always appreciated. In the summary statistics of a fairly recent ESB study (Ettenberg, Koob, & Bloom, 1981), a level of drug was observed to abolish the "harder" lever-press responding in the presence of the "easier," maintained nose-poke responding. This was taken as evidence of the drug's action on motor function, an idea of some merit. However, the drug may also have acted selectively on reward but not reduced the level of reinforcement enought to knock out the easier task. The point is that one cannot tell which of these ideas is true. This example points out the dangers of taking the simple approach to reward measurement.

The Input–Output Curve, Rate-Intensity, and Threshold

Reacting to the problems of the simple rate procedure discussed above, many researchers studying self-stimulation turned to a method in which a number of measurements of rate of response are made at different levels of brain stimulation. The most common example of this method is the rate–intensity procedure, which involves measuring the rate of response on a continuous reinforcement schedule at different stimulation intensities or currents. The result is a curve that typically plots increasing behavior on the ordinate vs. increasing current on the abscissa. An example is shown in Figure 5.2. It is referred to here as an *input–output curve.*

This input–output curve has the important advantage that behavior is sampled at a number of levels, thereby giving an opportunity to make observations over the entire range of behavioral capacity. Thus, the method permits one to avoid the problem of accidentally testing at currents well into the behavioral ceiling, in which minor changes in a single high current level (e.g., from 300–350 μAmps stimulation) produce little behavioral change. With this curve, it is always possible to focus attention on the sensitive range in which behavior is able to change in response to manipulations that alter stimulation effectiveness.

The real power in this input–output curve lies in the ability it gives the researcher to observe systematic changes in the shape or placement

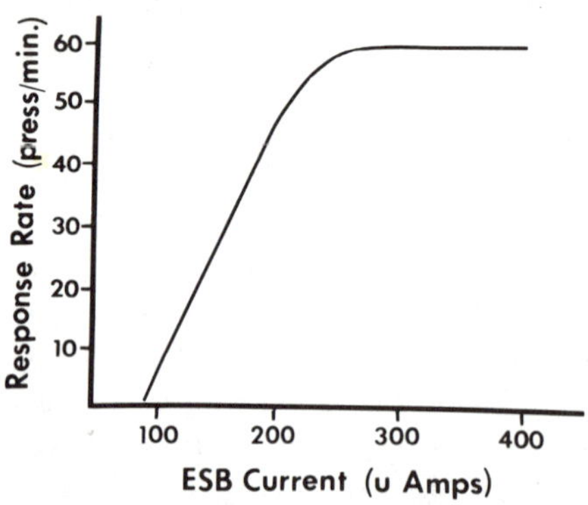

Figure 5.2 Rate–intensity curve with a maximal response rate of 60 presses/min. Note that, in the current range of 300–400 μAmps, changes in ESB will not affect responding, whereas, changes in the range of 100–250 μAmps will alter responding.

of the curve. For example, suppose that one gives a drug to a self-stimulating animal and compares the rate–intensity curve under drug conditions to the curve obtained in the control, drug-free condition. The rate–intensity function might reveal a change in the point of origin (threshold), or in the slope, or in the asymptote. One might observe multiple changes. Perhaps one or more of these changes would be seen better if the data were plotted on a logarithmic scale or on an inverse scale. These are all possibilities that are open to the experimenter gathering measurements at a number of stimulation levels. These possibilities are not available to those measuring rate at only one point on this curve. Consequently, input–output function analysis is vastly superior to the simple rate measure discussed previously.

The Variable Parameter in an Input–Output Curve

Rate–intensity functions are the oldest widely used measures after the simple rate measure. This is true partly because early stimulation employed *A.C.* stimulators in which intensity and duration were the only parameters available to be varied. Intensity, at first, seems appealing and simpler. It allows all timing factors of reward delivery to be kept constant. In actual fact, this procedure is far from simple. Increasing intensity of current expands the effective field of stimulation within the brain, bringing into play "new," previously unstimulated neural elements. With a lateral hypothalamic electrode placement, current spread to the medial hypothalamus may, for instance, generate *aversive* side effects (Shizgal & Matthews, 1977). In this case, further increases in current will bring the growth of rate–intensity curve to a stop, imposing an asymptote uncharacteristic of the reward system itself. This is especially likely if the electrode is medially placed within the lateral hypothalamus. If the electrode is placed too far laterally, current increases may bring with them growing motor effects due to direct activation of the internal capsule, which lies lateral to the lateral hypothalamus. These motor effects or disturbances will limit the ability of the subject to respond with high rates by producing forced movements of the head and upper body during ESB.

If a square wave stimulator is used, then five parameters can be independently varied: stimulation current, pulse duration, pulse frequency, number of pulses, and duration of the stimulation burst. Of these, pulse frequency, pulse number, and burst duration are related such that specifying any two also determines the third. As discussed previously, increasing the current, especially in the hypothalamus, brings with it the danger of directly activating motor or aversive side-effects. Increasing stimulation pulse duration is similar to the current variation in that longer durations allow for a greater time for the pulse current to flow, which will add previously unexcited neurons and thereby expand the stimulation field. The two remaining parameters, pulse frequency and number, can be classified as parameters that affect only timing properties. That is, they determine the number of action potentials and the temporal density of those action potentials set up by a given burst, but do not add new neural elements to the stimulation field. Although it is certain that any parameter variation has complex effects remote from the stimulation site, number and frequency of pulse parameters are thought to be the most straightforward, at least at the electrode tip. Indeed, many of the advances in understanding the psychophysics of the ESB reward substrate have come from manipulations that vary the temporal arrangement of stimulation pulses.

Threshold and Half-Maximal Criterion

The simplest use of an input–output function such as a rate–frequency curve (Figure 5.3), may be the calculation of *threshold*. Here, the experimenter simply examines the point where the input–output function begins to rise from a behavioral zero. Alternatively, one may first determine the operant or baseline rate of responding when no stimulation has ever been given, and then establish some criterion (e.g., 10 presses/min) for when this rate has been exceeded and "real" responding is occurring. The amount of ESB needed to sustain this value of rate is then found on the input–output curve, and the associated ESB parameter level is called threshold. For a threshold level of 10 presses/min on Figure 5.3, the associated pulse frequency is 24 Hz. Notice that it is not necessary to generate the whole curve to find this threshold. Starting at a low level of frequency and increasing on each trial, only a few steps may be necessary before criterion is exceeded. However, the problem of keeping the subject continuously near extinction presents a practical difficulty. Therefore, many people prefer to either gather the whole curve (i.e., from zero responding to behavioral asymptote) or use a descending approach starting at some parameter value that is known to generate vigorous responding. Alternative forms of threshold-finding also exist (e.g., the Békésy tracking method), but will not be discussed here. They all have the same goal of finding threshold.

Other points besides threshold could be employed as the behavioral criterion. For example, one could select an arbitrary criterion of 35 lever presses/min as criterion. A less arbitrary behavioral criterion might be *half-maximal performance* (Figure 5.3). This gives a measure that is always at the center of the variable range of behavior and so avoids ceiling and cellar effects. It also is a point of vigorous responding that gives the opportunity to ensure that behavioral activation is adequate. However, the half-maximal criterion depends upon calculations based on maximal level. As previously discussed, maximal responding may be influenced

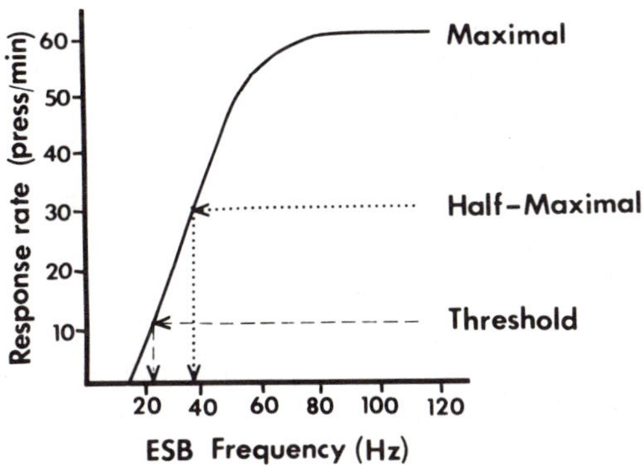

Figure 5.3 Rate intensity curve wih half-maximal and threshold behavioral criteria depicted as dashed horizontal lines. *Note.* Behavioral criterion for threshold is somewhat arbitrary, but is usually chosen to be just above spontaneous response level. Alternatively, one could consider the place where a straight-line fit to the rising portion of the curve would intersect the x-axis, as suggested by Miliaressis, et al. (1982). The vertical dashed line shows the calculated locus of rise statistic (37 Hz) that is based on the half-maximal measure.

by a variety of non-reward factors. Certainly, any report of stimulation levels required to sustain half-maximal behavior must be presented along with the maximal behavior upon which those calculations were made, so that changes in this factor can be seen as well.

A Discrete Trial Procedure

The input–output function is the dose–response curve of ESB research. Like a dose–response curve in pharmacology, it provides rich information. However, to this point in our discussion, the data in the input–output curve have come from the simple rate of response measures in a continuous reinforcement paradigm. This is important to remember because it is easy to think of the statistic derived from half-maximal responding as being rate-free since its units are in terms of ESB parameters and not behavior. However, this statistic is still based on simple rate of response, and if that measure is flawed (particularly at maximum) some of this error could creep into it. A better behavioral measure for the basic data of the curve is obtained when control of the density of reinforcement is substantially taken away from the subject. One of many ways to do this is to impose a discrete trial situation in which, on each trial, the subject works for a single burst of rewarding stimulation. Following this reward, the subject then enters an intertrial interval before a new trial can begin. Any direct rate-limiting consequences of ESB are eliminated because the motor or distraction effect occurs after responding for ESB has been measured. This is an important advance in reward measurement technology and can be used to generate input–output curves.

As an example of discrete trial procedures, we here consider a *runway paradigm*, which has been used by a number of laboratories (Edmonds & Gallistel, 1974, 1977; Franklin, 1978; Stellar, Kelley, & Corbett, 1983). Here, the rat waits in a start box to be released by the opening of a door into a straight alley. At the other end of the alley is a lever which, if pressed, yields brain stimulation. Following each run, the rat is returned to the waiting box and then begins another trial by being placed in the start box (Figure 5.4). Time taken by the rat to go from the start box to reach and press the lever is taken and converted to a running speed score. It is important to note here that the rat is responding (running) before stimulation is given. As previously discussed, the animal's behavior is largely governed by its prior history of experience at the reward lever. It is *not* governed by direct motor stimulation consequences or other rate–limiting side–effects of the stimulation!

Discrete trial paradigms like the runway are also useful in controlling one other factor often overlooked in brain stimulation reward measurement: the *priming* effect. Gallistel and others have shown clearly that brain stimulation in the medial forebrain bundle not only reinforces behavior, but that the same stimulation also energizes those previously reinforced behaviors—that is, rewarding brain stimulation generates an after-effect that arouses the subjects and makes responding for ESB more likely and more vigorous (Gallistel 1973). This was called the priming effect and was demonstrated convincingly in the runway paradigm with hypothalamic ESB. Here, the addition of pretrial ESB just before the

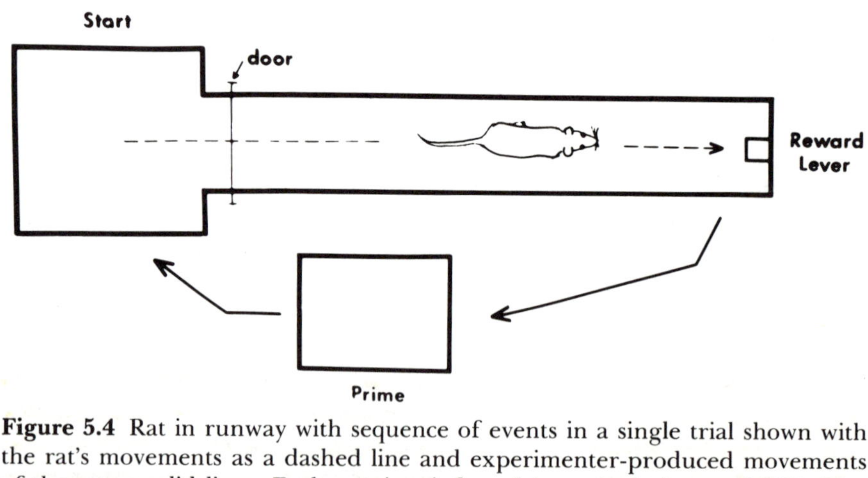

Figure 5.4 Rat in runway with sequence of events in a single trial shown with the rat's movements as a dashed line and experimenter-produced movements of the rat as solid lines. Each run is reinforced by a single burst of ESB. The prime box is the site of pretrial ESB, which is administered non-contingently on the rat's behavior. It is designed to generate a fixed high level of arousal. (Stellar, & Neeley, 1982.) Reprinted by permission.

subject is placed in the runway start box was shown to produce a large increase in running speed for a *fixed* reward (Gallistel, Stellar, & Bubis, 1974). This priming effect decays slowly over a period of several minutes with large bursts of priming ESB. The priming effect is discussed in more detail in chapter 8, and concerns us here simply as an obstacle to measuring reward.

Since priming after-effects are common with ESB of the medial forebrain bundle (Reid, Hunsicker, Kent, Lindsay, & Gallistel, 1973), one can easily see how a paradigm, such as continuous reinforcement, that does not control the density of ESB is exposed to the problem of an uncontrolled energizing or priming effect on behavior that could confound reward measurement. This is also true in an input–output curve. Here, the priming effects of ESB reward at the high end of the curve are likely to be much greater than at the low end of the curve. This exaggerates the behavior at the high end relative to the low end and introduces a small error in the calculation of the ESB level required to sustain half-maximal responding, for example. One possible exception to this problem is situations in which the animals are well-primed with warm-up ESB trials at the start of each period of data collection, and are typically tested at levels well above threshold. Under these circumstances, it may be safe to assume the animals are well-primed at all times.

The Reward Summation Function

One of the better techniques of reward measurement lies in the combination of the discrete trial procedure of the runway paradigm with the method of generating input–output function by varying the frequency or number of pulses. In essence, rats are trained to run down a runway for a single burst of ESB pulses. After being extensively familiarized with ESB reward bursts of different sizes, an input–output curve is then collected, with number of pulses per reward burst as the variable parameter and running speed as the behavioral measure. The curve has the form of previously discussed input–output functions; it has a starting point or threshold, an area of rise, and a maximum or asymptote. Because it is imagined that the underlying neural substrate is adding up or summating the number of pulses over the duration of the reward burst, the input–output curve is typically called a *reward summation function*.

The runway-based reward summation function has been shown empirically to have some very interesting and useful properties. As originally described by Edmonds and Gallistel (1974), the reward summation function can shift in two characteristic ways under altered testing conditions. First, in response to a decrease in the effectiveness of the stimulating pulse (e.g., produced by lowering the current), the reward summation function can shift to the right (i.e., toward higher values of pulse number).

Such a shift means that more of the less effective (low current) pulses were required to produce the original behavioral effect. This is true at every point on the dotted curve shown in Figure 5.5A. An important fact is that the same asymptote was reached in the shifted curve. This means that the subject can respond as fast as before, providing it is given a great enough number of stimulation pulses. The additional fact that the entire curve maintained the same shape is a good indication that the complex process that translates stimulation-generated reward into motor performance was unchanged. As an analogy to this proces, consider an employee working for a monetary payoff when the purchasing power of the currency is suddenly devalued by 50%. The employee's work may well fall off, but a greater number of now-devalued units of currency will restore performance. In this analogy, pulses equal currency. The decrease in the effectiveness of pulses (or currency) is what is meant by a reward effect.

The second type of shift occurs in response to a manipulation that alters the process of behavior generation or, in other words, creates a motor or performance effect. For example, Edmonds and Gallistel (1974) gave a sub-paralytic dose of methocarbonal, a curare-like compound, or they introduced an obstacle such as making the runway slant steeply uphill. These manipulations caused the curves to shift down (Figure 5.5A) on the axis. The original behavioral maximum was not achieved following the "motoric" manipulation. However, the place on the graph where the curve rose from threshold to maximum was unchanged, as shown by the fact that the calculated number of pulses required to sustain half-maximal remained the same. Edmonds and Gallistel (1974) termed this the "locus of rise" of the reward summation function and proposed it as a selective and empirically verified measure of stimulation pulse effectiveness in generating ESB reward.

In summary, then, manipulations that logically should have no effect on the summation processes of adding up stimulation pulses, such as physical obstacles, do not significantly alter the locus of rise. However, manipulations that do degrade pulse effectiveness, such as reduced stimulating current, shift the locus of rise. Exactly the opposite is found if one looks at the simple speed value reached at the maximum. Motoric manipulations do change behavioral maximum; pulse reward effectiveness manipulations do not (Figure 5.5B).

One very interesting observation made by Edmonds and Gallistel (1974) is that reducing the pretrial priming stimulation appears as a performance effect in this analysis. That is, it decreases asymptote and does not shift locus of rise. *This means that the arousal or motivational effects on behavior may be separated from reward effects and classed with the other performance factors.* This is exactly the way priming is treated in Gallistel's writings (for example see Gallistel, 1973).

The runway-based reward summation function has been used in a number of drug and lesion experiments (Edmonds & Gallistel, 1977; Franklin, 1978; Stellar & Neeley, 1982; Stellar et al., 1983). Here the nature of the physiological manipulation is unknown and may well produce both reward and motor effects that, without a good measurement technique, would be hopelessly confounded. As previously stated, the failure to separate motor and reward effects has caused much trouble in self-stimulation psychopharmacology, and the motor–reward distinction remains a practically and theoretically potent issue today. Another advantage of this reward summation function technique is that quantitative estimates can be made of pulse effectiveness changes. For example, if a drug injection induces a shift in the locus of rise toward higher pulses (Figure 5.6), and if that shift is a doubling of the required number of pulses, then one can say that the effectiveness of the pulses was reduced by half. One can then calculate how much pulse effectiveness degradation could be seen before motor effects (behavioral maximum shifts) appeared, compare results to other studies, and generally move toward an escape from the qualitative method of reasoning in favor of a quantitative one.

In this move toward quantitative thinking, an important and interesting complication of the technique is that one must pay attention to the shape of the curve. For example, in Figure 5.6 the high drug dose produces a shift that differs from the others in slope. This is not true of the intermediate dose. Different slopes of the curve make more complex the interpretation of the locus of rise measure by removing the assurance that the function translating ESB reward levels into performance is unchanged. Some insight into this problem may come from looking at the work of Milliaressis and associates, who have examined similar reward summation functions generated in a simple lever-pressing paradigm in which the animals received ESB on a fixed interval 1-second schedule of reinforcement (Miliaressis, Rompré, & Durivage, 1982). They found that, as they moved their electrode from one site to another within the brainstem, reward summation curves were generated, at times, with varying slopes. To handle this, they proposed that all of the curves including ones of shallower slope (as in Figure 5.6, 0.5 mg/kg) could be analyzed by fitting a regression line to the preasymptotic portion and calculating the point where this regression line intersected with zero level of behavioral performance (the x intercept). They also looked at y intercepts, as well. In their reasoning, the shallower slope could be caused by a stimulation -related motor impairment from direct activation of motor systems in the brain stem. It should be noted that a major difference between the Miliaressis, et al. analysis and Figures 5.5 and 5.6 is that these figures are plotted on a log scale; where as Miliaressis, et al. use a natural scale. This does not change the important concept of focusing on the slope of the reward summation function.

In a subsequent report, (Rompré, Phillipe, & Miliaressis, 1983) this

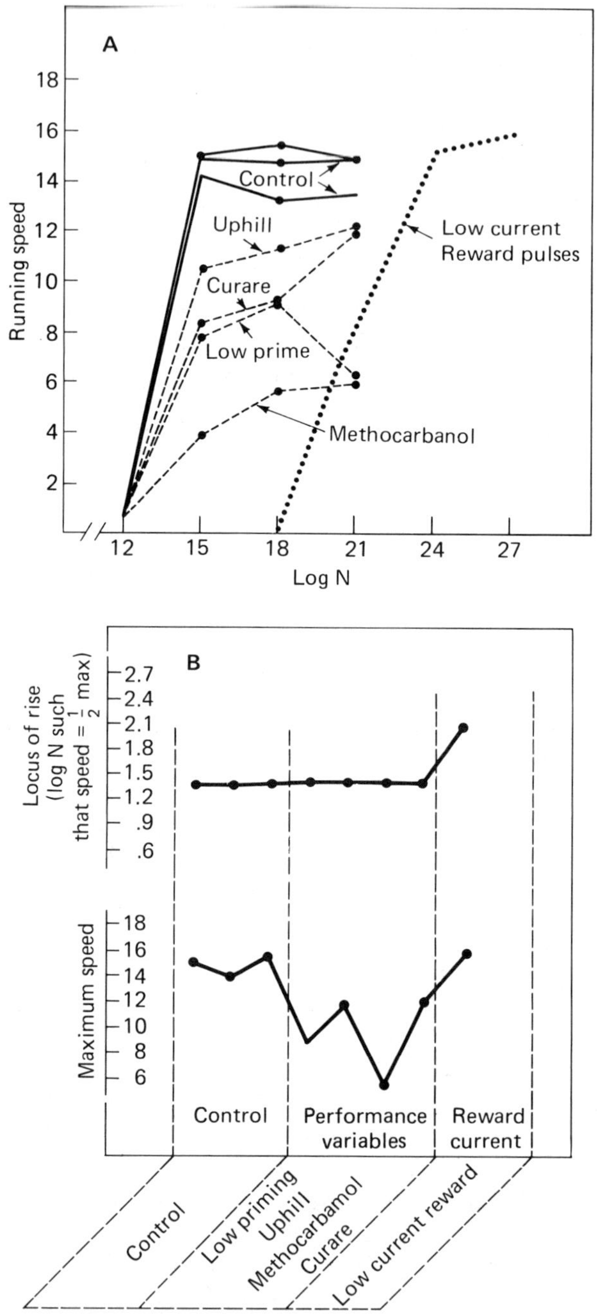

Figure 5.5 A. Reward summation function. Running speed is given in arbitrary units, and number of pulses in an ESB reward burst is given as its logarithm. Various baseline (control) and physiological manipulations are shown. Only the

group showed that in their paradigm a slope change could be produced at one brain site by adding simultaneous, identical stimulation (same frequency of pulses) on a second electrode placed directly within a brainstem motor structure. Thus as the "reward" from the first electrode grew and behavioral output went up, the "motor" impairment also grew, flattening the slope of the curve but not changing the point of intersection with zero level of behavior. This is important because the locus of rise analysis shows the high-dose curve of Figure 5.6 (0.5 mg/kg) as having a further shift in locus of rise over the medium-dose curve. Following the Miliaressis et al. (1982) method of analysis, the high dose would produce no further increase in the behavioral zero point, and therefore, no further degradation of reward pulse effectiveness. However, one must remember that in the runway paradigm, motor after-effects following the delivery of ESB have no direct effect on response strength (running speed); this is due to the long post-reinforcement intertrial interval. Clearly, these subtle refinements deserve attention and research as we move from a qualitative to a quantitative mode of analysis.

A second observation, minor by comparison, can be made from Figure 5.6. This concerns the low reward or low ESB current curve (dotted) of the figure. This curve has the same slope as the control baseline curves, but at a shifted position. It reveals a potential lower safe limit on the operating range of the technique. Below this point, pulse effectiveness could be so degraded that one may not be able to give a great enough number of pulses to compensate for decreased pulse effectiveness without encountering other physical limits of the neural substrate mediating the reward effect. For example, if burst duration is held constant at some value (a typical method), then the frequency of pulses increases with number, and it is clear that no physical system has a limitless frequency carrying capacity. Instead of trying to produce a big curve shift, experimenters may want to focus on producing smaller shifts that are within the limits of the technique to handle. If the drug effect degrades pulse effectiveness too much, one cannot compensate with increased pulse frequency and conduct the analysis.

Finally, let us consider one more refinement of a different kind dealing with the separation of mixed reward and aversive ESB sites. In a recent

---

low current reward condition should and does alter the pulse effectiveness in generating ESB reward. B. Curves (shown in A) analyzed into the locus of rise (top) and maximal performance (bottom) statistics. Note that performance-impairing manipulations do not alter locus of rise, but the reward current manipulation does. Also note that the performance-impairing manipulations do alter the maximum running speed, but the reward current manipulation does not. (Edmonds & Gallistel, 1974.) Reprinted by permission.

paper, Neeley and Stellar (1983) showed that some reward summation functions from lateral hypothalamic sites reach a maximal level and then turn down so that at still higher frequencies of pulses, lower levels of behavioral performance are seen. Neeley and Stellar were able to show that this turndown is produced by an increasing hesitation or latency to press the lever after having run the runway. They employed a photocell placed just before the reward lever so that they could measure both time to reach the lever after door opening and latency to press it once having arrived in the area of the lever. With higher pulse frequencies, they never saw decreases in time to reach the lever, even in the face of increased latencies to press. Furthermore, they demonstrated that the size of the latency to press at any pulse frequency was correlated with the same animal's tendency to escape from the same stimulation in another apparatus. This suggests that the increased latency or hesitation to press may be caused by the anticipation of aversive consequences of the ESB burst. Measuring just the running speed to reach the lever (break the photocell beam) provides a less contaminated measure than the conventional total running speed. Once again, this demonstrates the need always to search for refinements in behavioral measures.

The runway also has major limitations when compared to more traditional testing in a Skinner box apparatus. Aside from the increased

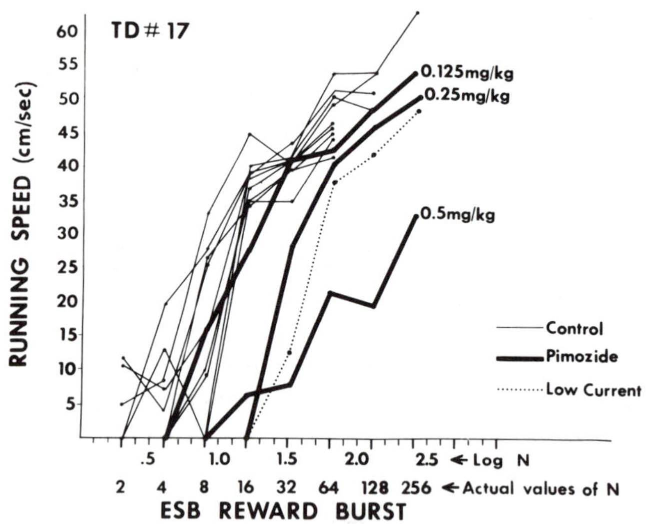

Figure 5.6 Reward summation functions collected from a single animal under control and drug conditions. Note that at the intermediate dose of pimozide (0.25 mg/kg), the curve appears to be shifted to the right. This is also seen with the low current reward curve. As in Figure 5.5 and in the text, this implies a pure shift in ESB reward pulse effectiveness without a performance impairment. The same cannot be said for the high drug dose of 0.5 mg/kg. (Adapted from Stellar et al., 1983.) Reprinted by permission.

mechanical complexity (e.g., a door with a release mechanism), one major practical limitation is the time required to collect a curve. A typical trial (Figure 5.4) requires 2–20 seconds for a run down the runway and lever press by the rat, 20 seconds for the intertrial interval, 10 seconds for priming stimulation, and 5 seconds before the door opens again at the start of the next trial. The total time for one trial then equals 37–55 seconds, depending on the rat's speed of running. Typically, 11 trials are run for each condition of number of pulses, with the first four being discarded as a period of adjustment of behavior. Given a warm-up and extinction condition and a minimum of five points to determine the input–output curve (77 total trials), each curve takes over an hour to generate. Automation of this technique through computers to permit a number of runways operating in parallel is the only practical way to gather large quantities of data.

We now turn our attention to other techniques of measurement. These first three methods have told a story of the development of input–output curves and the need to control ESB density. In our opinion, the runway-based reward summation function is one of the best methods available, although not the easiest to implement. In this chapter, it serves now as a basis for comparison to other useful methods.

The Extinction Paradigm

The extinction paradigm is based on a simple rule about conditioned behavior. The rule is that, when reinforcement is terminated, animals will persist in responding for a brief period of time and then gradually reduce responding until they quit. Although the precise shape and time course of this extinction pattern of responding may vary a bit from subject to subject, its overall form is a property of conditioned behavior that has been documented since the time of Pavlov (Kling & Riggs, 1971, p. 569). Since the basic form of the curve has a factor (the initial responding level) that depends upon motor capacity and a second factor (rate and pattern of quitting) that depends upon learning that reward is absent, many experimenters have applied the extinction paradigm to drug studies in the hope of distinguishing reward and performance factors affecting operant responding (Fouriezos & Wise, 1976; Fibiger, Carter, & Phillips, 1976; Fouriezos, Hanson, & Wise, 1978; Gallistel, Boytim, Gomita & Klebanoff, 1982; Beninger & Freedman, 1982; Wasserman, Gomita, & Gallistel, 1982).

In the context of ESB reward measurement, consider the extinction method as applied by Fouriezos and Wise (1976). They conditioned their subjects to lever-press for ESB on a continuous reinforcement schedule, and then suddenly reduced the current from the stimulator to below threshold for self-stimulation, while measuring rate of response. The pattern of responding for a typical animal is shown in Figure 5.7A. The animal begins responding in extinction at the same basic rate as when stimulation was administered after each response, then quits. This result was then compared to drug conditions in which the stimulation was not altered, but the drug was presumed to block its rewarding effects. If the same basic curve is seen, then one argues for a minimal effect on motoric factors. In Figure 5.7B data from groups of subjects (hence less variability) are shown. One group experienced reductions in stimulating current, and the other received the drug, pimozide, with no change in ESB parameters. Clearly, the pimozide extinction curves all begin at control levels of responding, allowing motor effects to be ruled out. Also, note that the highest does of pimozide ultimately reduces responding to a level equal to the lowest current reduction. Whether or not the pimozide curves exactly resemble the true extinction curves was not analyzed in Fouriezos' and Wise's (1976) paper; however, an inviting comparison can be made between the 0.5 mg/kg pimozide dose and the −4 μa stimulation condition in the graph of current reductions.

One problem with this response pattern analysis is that drugs that build

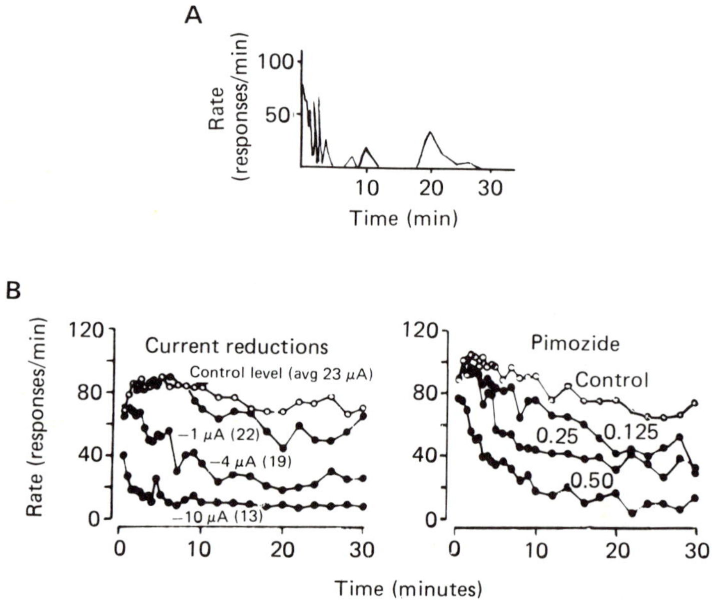

Figure 5.7 All graphs show rate of responding plotted against time. A. The graph shows the response of one animal when the ESB reward current was decreased below behavioral threshold. This is extinction testing. B. The left graph shows a group of rats tested in a similar manner with reductions in ESB current (*AC* waveform), as indicated. The right graph shows the pattern of response seen when the ESB reward was not altered, but the drug pimozide was given at various doses, as indicated. *Note.* The upper figure is adapted from Fouriezos and Wise (1976). The bottom two figures are from Fouriezos et al. (1978). Reprinted by permission.

up a response-debilitating effect over time may produce a response pattern that is similar to extinction. A subtler version of this problem is seen if one considers that the drugs may make the animal very easily fatigable or produce some other situations in which the more the animal works, the less capable of responding it becomes. For example, Gallistel, Boytim, Gomita, & Klebanoff (1982) have shown that sytemically-administered picrotoxin can induce a progressivley increasing pattern of seizures over the course of an ESB session. The result is what they call pseudoextinction. Fortunately, a simple remedy exists to this situation: *task-specific extinction* (Gallistel, Boytim, Gomita, & Klebanoff, 1982; Beninger & Freedman, 1982). In task-specific extinction, a subject is trained to perform for ESB in two dissimilar apparatuses, for example, a Skinner box and a runway. Following extinction in one apparatus, the animal is immediately placed in the other. In typical extinction, the result should be a reinstatement of behavioral responding appropriate to the "new" task. In other words, the animal behaves as though it expects reward in the second apparatus and begins responding and must re-extinguish. With picrotoxin-induced pseudoextinction, the rat does not reinstate responding, but maintains a low level of behavior after the apparatus switch (Gallistel, Boytim, Gomita, & Klebanoff, 1982). This is taken as indicating motor performance debilitation.

An elegant alternative to this method of double extinction is to stop giving the ESB reinforcement, allow the animal to extinguish in a single apparatus, and then reinstate responding in that same apparatus by turning on a stimulus that has been previously associated with ESB reward. This is called stimulus control and accomplishes the same basic goal as switching apparatuses without the need to expose the subject to any arousal or other effects induced by handling. Franklin and McCoy (1979) demonstrated that, in the case of pimozide-induced extinction, a light stimulus could temporarily reinstate responding if that light had previously been paired with ESB reward. Reinstatement of responding argues against motor debilitation effects of the drug administration.

It is encouraging to note that, in all of the experiments cited above, reduced stimulation conditions were tried in order to mimic the decrease in reinforcement expected as a drug effect. This verification strengthens the interpretations one can make from the data, but leaves some questions in the area of motor debilitation. Here, only one group (Gallistel, Boytim, Gomita, & Klebanoff, 1982) explored drug manipulations designed to create performance or motor deficits. They found that, with the double extinction method, low doses of barbiturate anesthetic and picrotoxin injections, discussed previously, both produced patterns of responding that were easily distinguishable from non-reinforcement.

One type of verification that has not been reported is to introduce a simple physical obstacle such as a weighted lever or to selectively block motor function with curare-like compounds. Such experiments proved useful in the runway-reward summation function paradigm and would be important here to refine the motoric interpretations of the extinction response pattern. Such manipulations and procedure verifications are very important where the primary use of the methods has been with dopamine antagonist drugs like pimozide or other neuroleptics that can induce Parkinsonian-like motor debilitation (Marshall & Teitelbaum, 1974). This is especially true since not all researchers agree that there is always a functional equivalence between extinction under dopamine blockade (e.g., with pimozide) and extinction due to low reward. For example, using food reward, *not ESB* Tombaugh, Anisman, and Tombaugh (1982) have shown pimozide to be markedly more effective than non-reinforcement when compared in its ability to produce the response decrement pattern of extinction. On this basis, they argue for an important role for performance impairments from dopamine blockade.

The performance impairments discussed above could be due to quite subtle motor effects. In the light of the Parkinsonism model (Pletscher, 1976) and the well-known motoric mobilizing effects of strong stimuli (Marshall, Levitan, & Stricker, 1976), it is not surprising that rats with dopamine receptor blockade might begin an extinction experiment behaviorally aroused but lose that arousal as extinction proceeds, only to be re-aroused at the start of the second task. Alternatively, an animal with dopamine blockade may find responding possible, but more difficult. This added cost of responding could act as a punisher to discourage future responding somewhat. Again, in the second task, the animal may have to relearn, however briefly, that responding here will also carry this additional cost. Thus, the initial high rates might be preserved in the extinction paradigm, even though a motor effect is continuously present, in addition to the claimed reward effect. The subtlety of the above potential motor effects and the undoubted complexity of the brain systems we are manipulating, demand caution and our best skills at interpretation. Certainly, continued attempts at verification and cross-validation with other methods of reward/performance measurement lie at the base of any such effort. The issue of dopamine's involvement in motor, motivational, or reward function is discussed in chapter 7.

Autotitration or Set–Reset Method

The autotitration technique was first employed by Stein and Ray (1959) and later by Schaefer and Holtzman (1979) to generate threshold data in an automated paradigm. It has been more recently employed by Neill and associates as a "rate-free" measure of self-stimulation in a brain-injection experiment (Neill, Gaar, Clark, & Britt, 1982). The paradigm operates with two levers. Pressing one lever produces a burst of ESB on a continuous reinforcement schedule. However, after a determined number of bursts of ESB, the stimulating current decreases in a measured step. Pressing the other lever will not give any stimulation, but will reset the current delivered by pressing the first lever to the starting level. In the Neill et al. (1982) paradigm, the levers were separated by a partition, forcing the rat to walk about 10 cm from one lever to the other. This imposes a slight obstacle to resetting. The data one collects in the autotitration method are not the rate of responding on the first lever, but rather the stimulation current level at which the second lever was pressed. This is called the *reset current* and is presumed to be a threshold measure.

This paradigm has been employed recently with dopamine manipulations. For example, amphetamine administered systemically lowers the average intensity at which a reset occurs (Neill et al., 1982; Schaefer & Holtsman, 1979). This indicates that the ESB reward effect must be made stronger by amphetamine. Neuroleptics, on the other hand, increase the mean current reset threshold (Schaefer & Michael, 1980). In the Neill et al. (1982) study, a paradox arose when they found that central injections of amphetamine directly into the nucleus accumbens had an unpredicted effect of increasing the mean reset intensity; this was opposite to the effects of peripheral administration. Neuroleptic administration into the nucleus accumbens also produced results opposite to those of peripheral injection. That is, where peripheral injection increased the reset threshold, accumbens injections decreased it.

Neill et al. (1982) advanced an interesting hypothesis to explain the above paradox. In their thinking, the effort that the animal is willing to expend in the task is modulated by dopamine activity in the nucleus accumbens. With the subject more willing to expend effort, the 10-cm walk around the partition becomes less of an obstacle, and one sees more resets (higher mean reset current). This dopamine/effort theory is discussed more fully in chapter 7, but before we go on, there is a basic problem with the behavioral technique.

Fouriezos and Nawiesniak (1982) compared the results of two versions of the autotitration paradigm using frequency of pulses within an ESB burst as the variable parameter. They employed the two-lever paradigm, described above, and a single-lever paradigm. In the single-lever paradigm, the pulse frequency decreased upon lever-pressing (as with the first lever in the two-lever paradigm), but was reset automatically after some fixed interval. This reset was signalled to the subject, but not controlled by the subject. Care was taken to choose an interval so that the rat had always quit responding on the single lever before an automatic reset occurred. Fouriezos and Nawiesniak (1982) then varied the starting frequency in each paradigm and looked at the point at which the subjects quit responding on the stimulation lever and either reset themselves or waited for a reset from the equipment. They showed that starting frequency had a profound effect on the quitting point, as judged by a press on the reset lever in the two-lever paradigm. If the starting frequency was raised, the reset frequency went higher. If the starting frequency was lowered, the reset frequency went down. It was as though the rat was constantly comparing the reward from working on the first lever at the moment with the reward that could be had after a reset. Hence, if the point of comparison changed (the starting value), it is logical that the other point would change as well. What this finding really shows is that the two-lever autotitration paradigm does not give an *absolute* threshold, but a relative threshold—one that is relative to the chosen starting point. On the other hand, the single-lever paradigm did not show such variation. The point at which the subjects ceased responding was the same regardless of the starting frequency.

To go back briefly to the Neill et al. (1982) finding that amphetamine placed in the nucleus accumbens increases the reset threshold, it is possible that this treatment increases the perceived starting point of the variable stimulation parameter (in this case, current.) This would increase, instead of decrease, the mean reset threshold according to the prior discussion. Following this logic, the task then becomes one of explaining why systemic administration, which includes the nucleus accumbens as well as the caudate and other structures, has opposite effects to the treatment of the accumbens alone. This paradox gets into the possible roles of dopamine in the caudate versus the accumbens and, as stated previously, is better left for discussion in chapter 7. The major conclusion, at this point, is methodological. That is, there remain in this simple technique, issues that will take considerably more research to resolve. Once again, this problem reveals the subtleties of reward/motoric assessment in ESB and the need for experimental verification. A measure that is "rate-free" is not automatically one that provides a straightforward base for solid interpretation.

Post-Reinforcement Pause

The paradigm of post-reinforcement pause is yet another method designed to avoid the rate of response measure. It was invented by Huston and Mills (1971) to find threshold for ESB reward by taking advantage of the following long-known facts: First, rats lever-pressing on a fixed interval schedule of reinforcement will exhibit a pause in responding following reinforcement. This produces the common scalloping seen on a fixed interval schedule when behavior is recorded on a cumulative recorder (Skinner, 1938). The second fact is that, if the reinforcement is delivered on a continuous reinforcement schedule, the post-reinforcement pause is not seen and the subject works more steadily (Skinner, 1938).

What Huston and Mills (1971) did was to combine these two schedules. ESB of fixed high current was always adminstered as the reinforcer for lever-pressing on a fixed interval schedule, thus generating responding and post-reinforcement pauses. Then, on all other lever presses, a continuous reinforcement schedule was set in operation. The same response lever was used, but the ESB was first set at a very low current. At this point, the continuous reinforcement schedule was not effective in altering the behavior on the fixed interval schedule. Then, the current of the ESB delivered on the continuous reinforcement schedule was gradually raised until it came to control responding and abolished the post-reinforcement pause characteristic of the fixed interval schedule. Using a criterion of the disappearance (e.g., of 50%) of the post-reinforcement pauses normally seen on a fixed interval schedule, Huston and Mills (1971) found the required ESB current on the continuous reinforcement schedule to produce criterion and called it threshold.

This measure of threshold has been employed by other researchers to look at drug effects on ESB reward (Cassens & Mills, 1973; Cassens, Actor, Kling, & Schildkraut, 1981). The method has potential as an easily automated procedure. Minimum length of the inter-response interval employed as a recognized post-reinforcement pause can be selected from the frequency of occurrence of pauses of various lengths. This interval should almost always occur after a fixed interval schedule reinforcement, but should almost never occur in a continuous reinforcement schedule. If there are any drug-induced changes in motoric effectiveness, these should show up as a basic alteration of responding on the fixed interval schedule. However, this method has not been verified in any previous study. That is, no one has given a simple physical (e.g., weighted lever) or pharmacological (e.g., a sub-paralytic dose of curare) obstacle to responding and examined the effect on threshold. Additionally, no one has altered the stimulation pulse frequency to see if this degradation of the ESB reward produces the appropriate shifts in current threshold. This is especially important since ESB is used as both the "standard" in the fixed interval schedule and the "threshold" measure in the continuous schedule. The absence of these data is a flaw in an otherwise interesting paradigm.

Response Strength Method

In the years since Skinner and his associates first defined and refined the basic rules that govern operant behavior, operant research has taken a more mathematical turn. One of the major molar rules of behavior that has surfaced is the *matching law* (Herrnstein, 1974; deVilliers, 1977). Simply put, this rule states that, given a choice between two concurrent schedules of reinforcement with differing reinforcement rates, subjects will allocate their time in proportion to the reinforcement obtained on each schedule. For example, if one schedule is a variable interval 10-second schedule (VI 10) and the other schedule is a VI 20, the subject will get twice as much reinforcement from the first and spend twice the time responding on the first VI schedule. The equation manifests itself as

$$\frac{R_1}{R_1 + R_2} = \frac{B_1}{B_1 + B_2} \tag{5.1}$$

Where R_1 and B_1 are the reinforcement rate obtained and the rate of behavior observed on one schedule (VI 10), and R_2 and B_2 are observed on the other schedule (VI 20). Note that this work has been done primarily with food or water reinforcement, not ESB.

Heyman (1983), Bradshaw, Ruddle, & Szabadi (1981); Hamilton & Stellar (1983) have used a form of this equation adapted to a situation in which the rats are working on a single lever and on one schedule at a time. In this paradigm, one measures the rate of behavior and of reinforcement on a single lever. All the reinforcement from every other source is seen as competing for the animal's behavioral attention. These researchers adminster a range of VI schedules and obtain various behavioral and reinforcement rates. A theoretical baseline curve is shown in Figure 5.8A. It resembles the input–output curve seen with the reward summation function in that behavior rises over some range to an asymptote. This curve was derived from the equation

$$B_1 = \frac{(k)\, R_1}{R_1 + R_e} \tag{5.2}$$

Where response rate and obtained reinforcement rate are R_1 and B_1, respectively. k is a constant representing behavioral maximum and R_e represents reinforcement obtained from *every* other source (hence the subscript "e"). When k is decreased (Figure 5.8A), the curve will not rise to as high as an asymptote. This would occur in motor debilitation when behavioral capacity is decreased. When R_e is increased (Figure 5.8A), then the rate of climb of the curve is changed and more reinforcement is required to reach each new behavioral point, but the original or baseline asymptote will eventually be reached. To contrast with the theoretical curves given in Figure 5.8A, experimental data are presented in Figure 5.8B and the curves are fit to the data sets using equation 5.2. These experimental data are from a test with amphetamine, a drug that enhanced responding (Heyman, 1983).

To help in understanding this method, consider the following algebraic manipulations. If the reinforcement rate (R_1) were so great that the reinforcement from the VI schedule completely dwarfed the reinforcement from all other sources, then the denominator of Equation 5.2 would be functionally equal to R_1. The equation would then be

$$B_1 = \frac{(k)\, R_1}{R_1} \quad \text{or} \quad B_1 = k. \tag{5.3}$$

That is, behavior would be at its asymptote. Now, if R_1 and R_e were

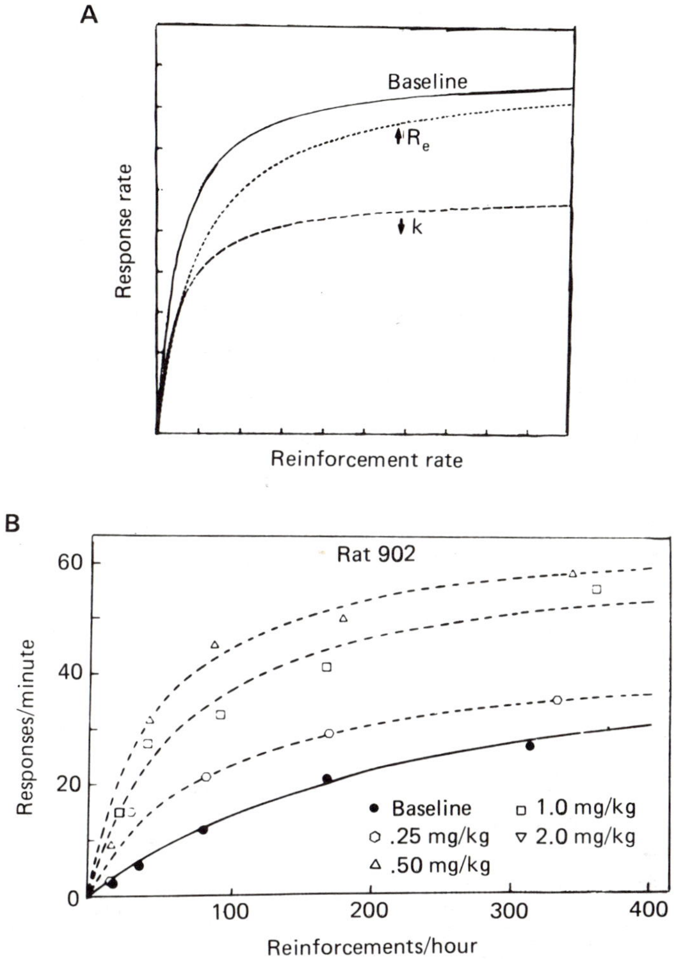

Figure 5.8 A. Theoretically generated curves showing the response strength method (see text) as it is affected by changing the maximum (k) and the reinforcement (R_e) parameters of the equation. B. Actual response strength curves showing lever-press rate plotted against food reinforcement rate. The effect of amphetamine is seen as the dashed line. The fitted curves are computer-generated according to the equation given in the text. Figure B from Heyman (1983). Reprinted by permission.

equal, that would mean that the reinforcement from the VI schedule exactly balanced out the reinforcement from everything else available to the subject (e.g., grooming, sleeping, exploring). Equation 5.2 would then be

$$B_1 = \frac{(k)R_1}{R_1 + R_1} \quad \text{or} \quad B_1 = \frac{k}{2} \tag{5.4}$$

That is, behavior would be at 1/2 asymptote. Thus, R_e is defined algebraically as the reinforcement required to sustain half maximal responding.

This technique is fairly new and promises the powerful advantage of being linked to a vast body of research in operant analysis of behavior, but it has not been tested, much less thoroughly verified in an experiment with ESB. Hamilton and Stellar (1983) conducted a verification experiment with a weighted lever and low stimulation pulse frequency to track changes in the curves after motor and reward debilitation, respectively. To a first approximation, they found that the weighted lever caused shifts primarily in the k parameter (i.e., a lower response asymptote was seen). The low ESB pulse frequency caused a shift primarily in R_e (i.e., a more gradual climb to response asymptote and a greater number of reinforcements to sustain half-maximal responding was seen). These findings are as predicted and raise the hope that this method might fill its promise of reward/motor separation. However, a detailed psychophysical analysis of this paradigm is needed to explore its range and sensitivity with ESB. For another example of the application of the matching law of Herrnstein to research on ESB, see the work of Fray (1981).

The above method is very attractive precisely because it is possible to fit a meaningful theoretical curve to the data. First, the procedure eliminates dependence on a particular point or set of points of raw data between which one must interpolate. For example, in the runway paradigm, discussed earlier, an aberrant point near the half-maximal responding can throw off the calculation of locus of rise, whereas in the response strength method, all the points of data go into the process of determining the curve from which a parameter (e.g., half-maximum or R_e) is calculated. Second, a statistic, percent of variance accounted for, can be calculated that helps one to determine how well the equation fits the data. If the value of this statistic falls below a criterion set by the experimenter, the entire process can be set aside as not working in that case (e.g., in the case of too high a drug dose). In the opinion of the authors, having a theoretical curve promotes the kind of analysis of the method so necessary to permit valid interpretation of the data. Finally, the existence of a large body of literature on the matching law makes it possible to interpret findings in the light of other quantitative operant research. Thus, the method does not operate in isolation.

It is interesting to notice how these two techniques (reward summation function and response strength) cross-fertilize. The response strength points to the value of an analytical equation and suggests that such an equation would be useful with the reward summation function. The reward summation function points toward the kind of empirical verification needed by the response strength method. Indeed, both of the methods could be applied to the same question (e. g., what are a drug's effects on ESB reward vs motor function?) for cross-validation.

Choice and Other Methods

The methods in the preceding sections were chosen as representative. Other methods for studying ESB exist, such as place preference, the two-platform method, or the shuttle box technique. See Liebman (1983) for a detailed and scholarly review of behavioral methods in self-stimulation, and see Valenstein (1964) for an impressive discussion of this problem early in the history of self-stimulation research. Many of these paradigms involve the subjects making some kind of spatial choice between the concurrent alternatives.

Choice in itself, independent of rate, may provide a fundamentally different and selective measure of reward. For example, Findley, Robinson, and Peregrino (1972) offer a rat a choice between self-administering one drug on one VI schedule and another drug on another VI schedule. In their method, pressing a choice lever determines which VI schedule (and therefore which drug) is available. Responding is graded as the proportion of time spent on a particular schedule. Gallistel and Beagely (1971) used a similar choice paradigm in which a rat was offered a choice between obtaining a burst of ESB from one of two levers. Preceding each choice, the rat had to press a lever on the opposite side of the chamber to orient itself and to make the two choice levers active. In this experiment, the goal was to see how preference for stimulation at one brain site over another site changed when the animal was food-or water-deprived. Choice paradigms, especially in the form of the "T" maze have played an important role in the history of animal behavior research (Kling & Riggs, 1971), as well as the history of ESB research (Gallistel, 1969; Valenstein, 1964, Leibman, 1983).

All choice paradigms are based on similar principles and essentially ask the subject where it wishes to place itself or place its effort in the face of alternatives. Since motor impairments are unlikely to affect the absolute choice, though they may affect the rate at which the choice is made, this method appears to naturally get around the problem of motor/reward separation. Indeed, most researchers who employ a choice paradigm do not even collect rate of response data, but rather collect only the data on choices made. However, before celebration of a new selective method can begin, we must await the classical verification experiments. A problem for drug or lesion work is the requirement for two sites of ESB or an ESB-nonESB comparison. To measure reward at one ESB site, a standard is needed for comparison. This limits the use of the paradigm to conditions in which the manipulation (e.g., a drug) does not affect the reward of both levers. Practically, this limitation seems serious.

One way in which the choice paradigm can be employed without the limitations discussed above is as a check on other paradigms. For example, Waraczynski and Stellar (1984) have examined a hidden assumption of the reward summation function paradigm, discussed in detail earlier.

This assumption is that the point on the pulse frequency axis at which the reward summation curve reaches asymptote reflects a *saturation* of the reward process and not a behavioral ceiling effect that would cut off any further upward growth of the curve. In Figure 5.3, the saturation point would be about 70 Hz. If this point does not reflect the saturation of the reward process as pulse frequency is increased, then the locus of rise statistic would be dependent on the motoric ceiling or the performance limitation process that sets asymptote. In this paradigm, the locus of rise is thought to be independent of the motor capacity or other performance process that sets the asymptotic behavior. This is a critical assumption. If the saturation point of the reward summation function is really the point of ESB reward saturation, then the rat should behave in the following manner if tested on the choice paradigm: At ESB pulse frequencies *below* the saturation point, the rat should prefer the higher of the two frequencies when given a choice between them. At ESB pulse frequencies *above* the saturation point, the rat should be indifferent between any two frequencies (i.e., the reward process has saturated). Thus, a systematic comparison of preference between pairs of ESB pulse frequencies should show either of these two patterns of responding. The transition between the two patterns of responding on the choice paradigm should be at or near the saturation point of the reward summation function. This was found to be the case (Waraczynski & Stellar, 1984). For another recent use of the choice paradigm see Mason, Milner, and Giftochristos (1984).

ESB Reward Psychophysics

The goal of ESB reward psychophysics is to quantitatively characterize the neural substrate involved in generating the reward effect of ESB. This sets it apart from all other methods, which seek only to find a level or threshold of ESB reward and to assess a change following drug injection, lesion, or some other physiological manipulation. As might be expected in a method with different goals, reward psychophysics has at its heart a procedure not used previously: the *tradeoff procedure*. Here one parameter of stimulation, for example, the number of pulses in an ESB burst is changed, inducing a behavioral shift. Then, another parameter, stimulation current for instance, is altered until behavior is restored to its original level. These two new values of number and current must then have combined in such a way as to produce the same net effect on behavior as the first two values. Indeed, an entire curve can be constructed of many points where number of pulses and current of pulses have been traded off to achieve behavioral constancy. Because behavioral constancy is always maintained, no consideration need be given to the vastly complicated functions that translate ESB's effects into behavior. For example, using a discrete trial runway paradigm, Gallistel (1978) found that number and current traded off as a reciprocal. That is, doubling the number was compensated for by halving the current (see Figure 5.9). The same relationship was discovered (Shizgal, personal communication) in a lever-pressing situation using a continuous reinforcement schedule. This agreement is due to the fact that the tradeoff function characterizes an aspect of the directly excited neural substrate, not the process that then generates behavior. As an example of this, note the title of the review of this work by Gallistel, Shizgal, and Yeomans (1981), "A Portrait of the *Substrate* of Self-Stimulation."

To make this point more clearly, let us turn to an example from the psychophysics of vision that is often cited by Gallistel (also see Kling & Riggs, 1971). Most students of psychology and physiology take for granted the fact that rhodopsin is the photopigment that serves the process of rod or scotopic vision. Yet the basis for this fact comes from a tradeoff function analysis of the intensity verses the frequency (color) of light energy required to produce threshold of seeing in fully dark-adapted subjects. The resulting curve, plotting light intensity against frequency, shows that the "green" range of the frequency spectrum is the place requiring the least intensity—that is, rhodopsin is most sensitive to green. This and other aspects of the *in vivo* psychophysical curve can then be compared to the same curve gathered on the isolated chemical, rhodopsin, *in vitro*. The *in vitro* curve is called an absorption spectrum and uses as its "threshold" the intensity of light at various frequencies required to isomorize a fixed percent of the molecules. The point is that these two curves are the same when the *in vivo* psychophysical curve is corrected for the absorption of the media of the eye. This means that the same processes are at work in each curve. Thus, the human observer is, in this case, a bioassay for the photochemical properties of rhodopsin in the eye.

How was the psychophysical tradeoff function in the rhodopsin example capable of bypassing the entire complexity of the human observer, including the process that generates the behavior necessary to report perception to the experimenter? The answer lies in how the tradeoff

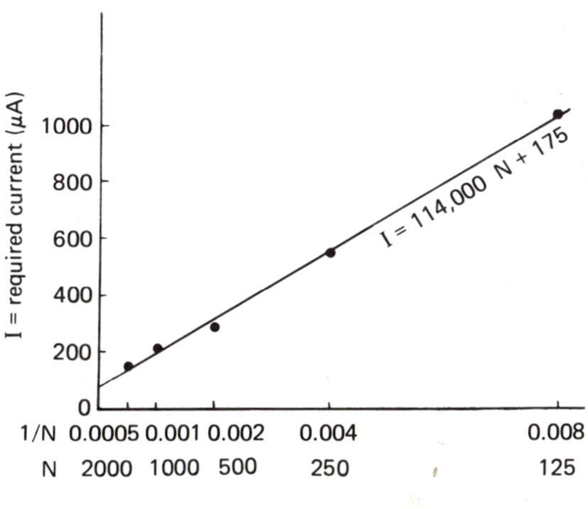

Figure 5.9 A number current trade off function to achieve a constant level of behavioral responding. The number axis is transformed into an inverse scale to show more clearly that the observed relationship between these ESB parameters is reciprocal. (Gallistel et al., 1981). Reprinted by permission.

technique works to hold the output of the first stage (the rods) constant by offsetting a change in one parameter by a change in another parameter of the stimulus. Therefore, all the other later transformations in the subject act on the same first-stage output and act the same. (This assumes that the subject is familiar with and stable in this task.) Therefore, the tradeoff method essentially only "sees" the first stage. So, too, this type of psychophysical manipulation in ESB reward only "sees" the first stage of directly excited tissue.

Much information has come from the tradeoff studies of the ESB reward substrate (Gallistel et al., 1981). Since this information concerns the anatomical substrate, it is reviewed in the next chapter, and some details of the specific methods are discussed there as well. Let us consider here, as a general illustration, only the one example of how refractory periods of the ESB reward-relevant neurons are specified. Refractory periods characterize a neuron along a single dimension: the time required for an axon to recover after firing one action potential before the action potential can be fired again. In self-stimulation, many axons are excited, and so any psychophysical estimate will be a group one. This group statistic is still quite useful even though the characterization can never, in practice, be as clear as for a single axon. For example, on the basis of double-pulse analysis of refractory periods (discussed below), Gallistel et al. (1981) categorically rule out any role for the catecholamine-containing neurons as the *directly* excited substrate, though a role later in the reward process is still possible. They do this based on data showing that catecholamine axons of that small size have such long refractory periods that they could not possibly match the behavioral data (Yeomans, 1975; Gallistel, 1983; cf. Waxman, 1978). This is an important conceptual advance, since many theories (German & Bowden, 1974; Crow, 1972) had posited that direct catecholamine activation was the mechanism of self-stimulation.

The way refractory period data are gathered in ESB is to stimulate with pairs of pulses on the same electrode. If the interval between the pairs is too short, the second member of the pair will fall within the refractory period of the axon and will not be effective in generating a second action potential. Thus, less effective stimulation will be given than if the experimenter allowed slightly more time between the first and second pulse in a pair. With less effective stimulation, less behavior will be apparent. Now, one might think simply to vary the interpair interval and look for sudden changes in behavior as an indication of whether the second pulse in the pair had or had not become effective. Many ESB researchers did experiments based on this assumption (Deutsch, 1964; Rolls, 1971b; Gallistel, 1973). Unfortunately, the quantitative estimates derived were shown very much to depend upon the chosen baseline frequency of pairs (Yeomans, 1975). Baseline frequency should have been irrelevant, but it was not.

The fault in the old simpler method lies in the choice of behavior (e.g., rate of lever-pressing) as the variable to measure or to scale changes in effectiveness of the second member of the pulse pair. Behavior varies with stimulation as an input–output function (discussed earlier). This means that, as more effective stimulation is given (more axons excited, more often), behavior will rise and level off. If the baseline frequency chosen (pulse pairs/second) was at the top of the input–output curve, then little increase in behavior will be obtained by an increase in stimulation effectiveness. On the other hand, if the chosen frequency happens to lie in the rise portion of the input–output curve, then slight changes in pulse effectiveness will produce big changes in behavior. The scale is then unequal in different parts of the frequency range. Worse yet, few researchers took the time to measure the input–output curve to see where they were with their chosen values.

Yeomans (1975) provided a better, more direct scale (i.e., a more nearly linear, interval scale). Suppose the pulse effectiveness of the stimulation increased as a result of an increase in the interval between the members of a pulse pair. (The first pulse of a pair is termed the conditioning or *C* pulse, and the second, the test or *T* pulse; this interval is then called the *C–T* interval.) The increase in pulse effectiveness is due to the fact that more of the second pulses (*T* pulses) in the pairs are getting through and manifesting themselves as an increase in behavior. An appropriate scale for the increase in pulse effectiveness can be found by adjusting the baseline frequency of the pulse pairs (termed the *C–C* interval) to return behavior to its previous level. The size of the *C–C* interval required is then a measure of the increase of *T* pulse effectiveness. Is this a better scale? Before we answer, let us look first at how the data are collected and analyzed.

The heart of the method is a tradeoff, but it is not carried out exactly as described above. In practice, it is easier to simply collect a family of behavior versus *C–C* interval input–output curves, where each curve has a constant *C–T* interval within a curve, but the *C–T* interval varies from curve to curve (see Figure 5.10). One then selects a behavioral criterion (e.g. horizontal line on Figure 5.10), and calculates by interpolation the *C–C* frequency necessary to sustain the required behavioral level for each curve. This procedure of using a family of curves is a common practical method in psychophysical data generation. Here, it generates pairs of values (*C–T* interval vs. *C–C* interval) that will produce equal responding.

Returning to our question about the improvement of this method over the old ones, it is important to notice that this is a "better" scale because an increase in the number of effective *T* pulses is balanced out by a decrease in the number of pairs of pulses (i.e., longer *C–C* interval, since ESB burst duration is constant). Because the tradeoff takes place within a single ESB parameter domain (e.g., intervals between pulses or number of pulses/burst), this gives Yeoman's scale a better chance of escaping the distortations of the other methods.

The derived data from Figure 5.10 can be plotted with the base-

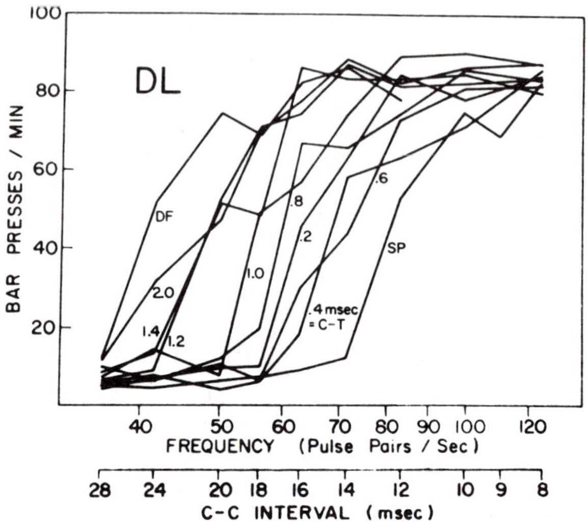

Figure 5.10 Input–output curves for a single subject (DL) in which the interval between the pairs (*C–T*) was held constant while the frequency of the pairs themselves was varied. The range of these curves is bracketed by the condition in which there was no second member of the pair (SP is single pulse condition) and the condition where the second pulse was equally spaced between the first pulses of each pair (DF is double frequency condition). (Yeomans, 1975.) Reprinted by permission.

line frequency (*C–C* interval) against the interval between the pairs of pulses (*C–T* interval). However, to make interpretation easier, Yeomans (1975) transforms the baseline frequency axis into a percent of *T* pulse effectiveness. This is done simply by assuming that 0% effectiveness would occur if all of the *T* pulses were within the refractory period generated by the initial *C* pulses of the pairs, and did not generate action potentials in the axon. This would then be equal to having the same *C–C* pulse frequency condition of single pulses (no *T* pulse delivered). On the other hand, the most effective condition (100%) would be if all the *T* pulses of the pairs were effective. The best way to produce this is to have the *C–T* interval be equal to half the *C–C* interval, so that all the ESB pulses then become equally spaced. The final plot (Figure 5.11) then shows the percent of the *T* pulse effectiveness versus the *C–T* interval.

Although this is the principle of how refractory period analysis proceeds, most researchers do a direct computation of the T pulse effectiveness according to the following formula:

$$E_t = \frac{N_{sp}}{N_{c-t}} - 1. \qquad (5.5)$$

Here, E_t is the *T* pulse effectiveness, N_{sp} is the number of pulses in the

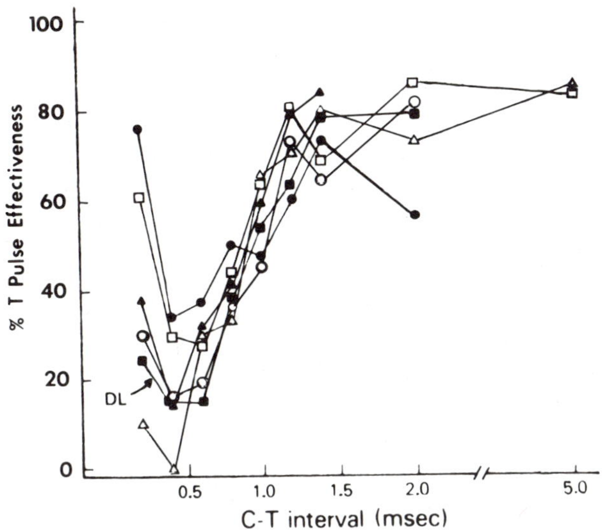

Figure 5.11 The effectiveness of the second pulse (*T*) of a pulse pair is plotted against the interval between the pulses in a pair (*C–T*) for 6 subjects including subject DL from Figure 5.10. Note the rise in T pulse effectivness as the *C–T* interval goes from 0.5 to 1.2 ms. This is taken as the refractory period range for the neurons that are involved with the ESB reward effect. (Gallistel et al., 1981.) Reprinted by permission.

burst of single pulses required to produce a behavioral criterion, and N_{c-t} is the number of pulse pairs in the burst of double pulses required to produce the same behavioral criterion. Number of pulses is simply calculated from knowing the burst duration and pulse frequency. Again, if these two values N_{sp} and N_{c-t} are equal, then no *T* pulse effectiveness is found, and E_t will equal zero. Therefore, 1 must be subtracted from the result of the division in Equation 5.5. Similarly, if all *T* pulses are effective, then half the number of pulse pairs will be required to produce the same effective number of pulses as N_{sp} and the result of the division in Equation 5.5 will be 2. Subtracting 1 leads to an E_t of 1.0, or 100% *T* pulse effectiveness.

Calculation of refractory periods of ESB reward-relevant axons is an illustration of the goals, methods, and successes of the psychophysical method. In any system under study, having quantitative information about some aspect of the substrate offers profound and sometimes unexpected advantages in understanding—for example, the elimination of catecholamine-containing axons as the *directly* activated tissue. However, the psychophysical methods also can be applied to questions addressed by previous methods. For example, the psychophysical relationship between number of pulses and frequency of pulses (Figure 5.9) required to keep behavior constant gives information about the spatial distribution and density of ESB reward-relevant axons under the electrode tip. This relationship has been measured with hypothalamic ESB in animals with large frontal cortex and forebrain ablations and found to be fundamentally unchanged (Stellar et al. 1982). As discussed in the beginning of this chapter, this result suggests that the frontal cortex does not give rise to reward-relevant fibers that pass through the hypothalamus. Thus, the psychophysical method can provide valuable information about the neural mechanisms of ESB self-stimulation. The quantitative precision of this approach to the study of ESB self-stimulation substrate holds perhaps the greatest potential for advancing our understanding of any of the methods for studying ESB.

Summary

The methods reviewed here give a feeling for the types of approaches that have been tried in order to produce reasonable measures of ESB reward. Where possible, any fact about ESB reward should be confirmed with several techniques. There is no substitute for convergent scientific methods. Also, some rules of basic measurement emerge for non-psychophysical paradigms of ESB. First, do not use rate of response as a measure of reward. It is a measure of self-stimulation behavior in its entirety and is not selective enough to distinguish reward from performance effects. Second, use caution with continuous reinforcement schedule methods. It is better to measure the avidity an animal has for ESB when it is *not* receiving ESB—that is, with some method where the animal gets reinforced at the end of an effort (e.g., runway paradigm, VI schedule with time out). Third, and most important, always seek to validate the method against manipulations known to produce relatively selective motor impairments (e.g., physical obstacles, sub-paralytic doses of curare) and ESB reward impairments (e.g., low ESB current or frequency).

As a final thought, we would like to add that no behavioral method is entirely valid or appropriate in all situations. Few methods, even if unvalidated, are entirely without some interesting information, if only for an idea for further work. However, in every field of science, it is the primary responsibility of researchers to understand the tools they use to explore their phenomenon. Judging from its history, the fascinating subfield of ESB self-stimulation could have benefited from more attention to this responsibility. It appears to be doing so now.

6

The Neuroanatomy of Brain-Stimulation Reward

The title to this chapter may be short, but it implies the longest of all creditable bridges in psychobiology: understanding the structure/function relationship well enough to be able not only to point out the neural elements, but also to show how those elements acting together give rise to function. The first part of the process of constructing that long bridge between structure and function involves *analysis* in which the components of a system are isolated and defined. The second part of the process, and much more difficult, involves *synthesis* or the building back to function from the structure (cf. Teitelbaum, 1967). Synthesis in psychobiology is often attempted by making a model and, here, the model is sometimes spoken of as a "wiring diagram." The analogy to electronic circuits is intended where function can be clearly specified in terms of structure. In some cases, such as the process of sensitization and habituation in the gill retraction reflex of *Aplysia* (Kandel, 1979), behavioral neuroscience seems well on its way to such a wiring diagram. Also, as discussed previously in the introduction to chapter 5, vision neuroscience seems to be making some progress toward a circuit–like understanding of aspects of visual function.

By contrast with the above examples, the circuit-like understanding of the ESB reward effect appears far off. A comparable understanding of the reward or reinforcement process in general seems over the horizon and presently out of sight. Additionally, one must face the distinct possibility that such a circuit-like understanding may not, in reality, exist in any manageable form. To make this point, an analogy to the mechanistic understanding of the behavior of an automobile is useful. The property of acceleration is a well-defined, even quantified aspect of the behavior of a car. Yet acceleration depends upon many diverse mechanisms, such as the rate of gasoline entry into the cylinders, the size of cylinders, the timing of firing of the spark plugs, the gear ratio in the transmission to the wheels. Thus, to give a mechanistic account of acceleration requires involving most of the significant components of the car. The neural representation of the process of reinforcement in mammals may well be the same.

With this sobering background, we now turn our attention first to ESB reward and consider the systems that might be directly activated by lateral hypothalamic/medial forebrain bundle stimulation. This directly excited population of cells has come to be called the first stage of ESB reward activation (Gallistel et al., 1981). The second stage occurs after the synapse of the first stage and *may* involve dopamine neurons; however, the discussion of dopamine is largely left for the next chapter, since the evidence is primarily neurochemical. Following the discussion of the lateral hypothalamus, we give some attention to the cortical sites of ESB reward, which are likely to involve very different mechanisms (Corbett et al. 1982a). At the end of this chapter, we review the electrophysiological correlates of natural and ESB reward presentation.

The Lateral Hypothalamus and Medial Forebrain Bundle: Many Possible Substrates

To begin to characterize the neural substrates involved in ESB reward, one has to know first what the possibilities are. Anatomical studies of the hypothalamus and its attendant medial forebrain bundle have been conducted for some time (cf., Krieg, 1932; Nauta & Haymaker, 1969), extending back as far as the nineteenth century. For a brief historical review, see Nieuwenhuys, Geeraedts, and Veening (1982). However, advances in neuroanatomical tracing techniques have made possible a much more detailed and accurate understanding of the fiber contributions of the medial forebrain bundle. This is discussed in two recent papers (Nieuwenhuys et al., 1982; Veening, Swanson, Cowan, Nieuwenhuys, Geeraedts, 1982) that characterize the inputs to and outputs from the medial forebrain bundle. The schematic diagrams from this first paper are reproduced in adapted form in Figure 6.1, A and B.

As can be seen from this figure, the substrate is complex. Yet even a figure as impressive as this cannot represent the finer structure of the depicted pathways. For example, consider the in-dwelling cells of the lateral hypothalamic region, which give rise to many fibers of the medial forebrain bundle. These cells are called path neurons (Millhouse, 1969, 1979; Olds, 1977) because they lie in the path of the medial forebrain bundle. The cells are captured in the Golgi method, which stains the cell's processes completely but selectively. Figure 6.2 is taken from the work of Millhouse (1979) and shows beautifully the rich complexity of these in-dwelling cells. They are highly interconnected and project in the dorsal–ventral and medial–lateral planes, as well as in the rostral–caudal plane of the hypothalamus.

Figures 6.1 and 6.2 still represent only the tip of the iceberg in considering the kinds of anatomical complexity of the medial forebrain bundle. For example, the ventral tegmental area is a dopamine-containing brain region that figures prominently in ESB reward research. One line in Figure 6.1A indicates the outputs of the dopamine-containing ventral tegmental area, which has been shown to project to many forebrain structures, including the nucleus accumbens. Upon closer examination of this "simple" projection, a rich fine structure is revealed. Swanson (1982) studied this projection by injecting the retrograde dye tracer, True Blue, into the nucleus accumbens and also by reacting the ventral tegmental area tissue with a tyrosine-hydroxylase antibody procedure that visualizes catecholamine-containing cells. These methods revealed: (a) most (92%), but not all, of ventral tegmental area projections to accumbens are *ipsilateral*; (b) the ventral tegmental area projection comprises only about 40% of the total innervation of the accumbens from the ventral midbrain region; and (c) only about 85% of these projections from ventral tegmental area to accumbens are actually *dopaminergic* in nature. These figures are very different for the nearby and related central linear nucleus (it is more bilateral), but similar for the well-known substantia nigra, pars compacta. One wonders how the subtleties of this accumbens projection enter into the problem of identifying the reward substrate—and this is only one line in Figure 6.1A.

The realization of such complexity tempers the strength of commitment that can be given to any theory specifying the circuitry of the reward effect of electrical stimulation of the brain (ESB). It also raises the serious question of how one chooses among the diverse and plentiful anatomical and chemical possibilities. Since the question becomes a functional one, the next sections deal with neural activity and behavior.

What Is Activated by the Electrode?

The first logical pass at identifying the brain structures involved in medial forebrain bundle reward might be to ask what structures are directly *activated* by the electrode. Historically, such a question falls in the province of electrophysiology but was prohibitively difficult to answer. This is because it is possible to record from, at most, several small areas

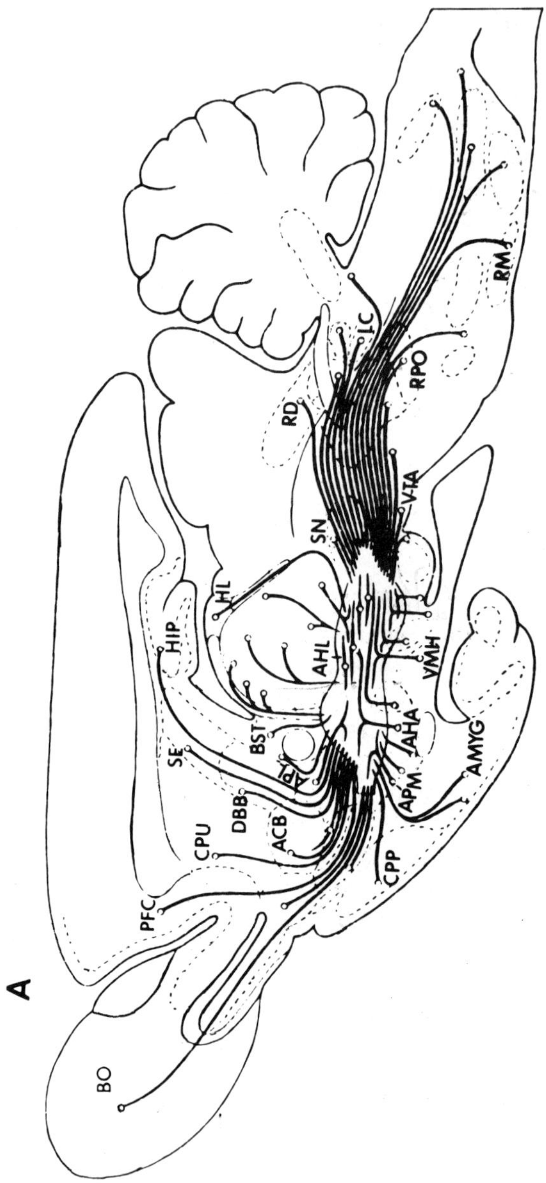
A
BO
PFC
CPU
DBB
ACB
SE
HIP
HL
BST
APL
AHL
SN
RD
LC
RPO
RM
VTA
VMH
AHA
APM
AMYG
CPP

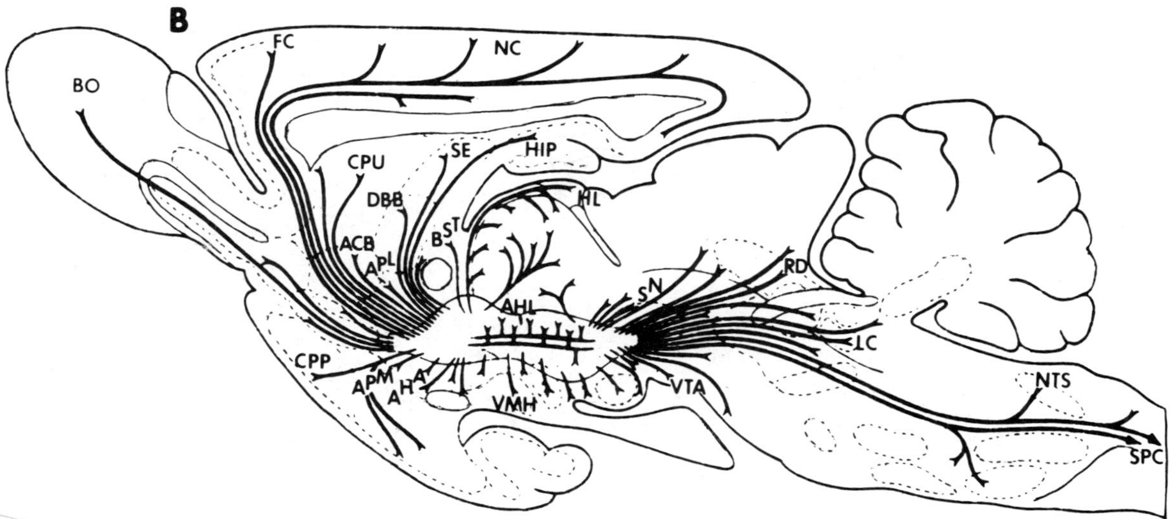

Figure 6.1 Schematic of a saggital section of the rat brain with inputs (A) and outputs (B) of the medial forebrain bundle. Abbreviations: ACB = nucleus accumbens; AHA = anterior hypothalamic area; AHL = lateral hypothalamic area; AMYG = amygdala; APL = lateral preoptic area; APM = medial preoptic area; BO = olfactory bulb; BCA = bed nucleus of the anterior commissure; CPA = periamygdaloid cortex; CPP = prepiriform cortex; CPU = caudatoputamen; DBB = nucleus of the diagonal band (Broca); FC = frontal cortex; HIP = hippocampus; HL = lateral habenula; LC = locus coeruleus; NC = neocortex; PFC = prefrontal cortex; RD = dorsal raphe; RM = raphe magnus; RPO = raphe pontis; SE = septum; SN = substantia nigra; SO = superoptic nucleus; SPC = spinal cord; VMH = ventromedial hypothalamus; VTA = ventral tegmental area; ZI = zone incerta. (Adapted from Nieuwenhuys et al., 1982.) Reprinted by permission.

at once. To build up a complete map of all brain regions activated from a single ESB site would require many subjects and many, many recording sites. Therefore, a whole brain map was not actually constructed until quite recently, when the techniques were developed for measuring regional brain metabolism (Kennedy, DesRosiers, Jehle, Reivich, Sharpe, & Sokoloff, 1975; Sokoloff, Reivich, Kennedy, & DesRosiers, 1977). Essentially this method looks at the glucose requirements of brain tissue, by measuring the local uptake of the radioactivity labelled glucose analog, 2-deoxyglucose (2-DG). Because glucose is the principal energy molecule of the brain and since physiological activation sets up a requirement for energy, the 2-DG technique gives a picture of the regional activations associated with any stimulus, including ESB.

A number of investigators associated with Gallistel's group have done experiments on self-stimulation in rats using this 2-DG technique (Gallistel, Karreman, & Reivich, 1977; Yeomans, Gallistel & Reivich, 1978; Yadin, Guarini, & Gallistel, 1983). Using a computer-assisted analysis program (Gallistel et al, 1982), Gallistel (1983) has reviewed data from previous work (Yadin et al., 1983) and generated a 2-DG map of regional brain activation associated with anterior and posterior medial forebrain

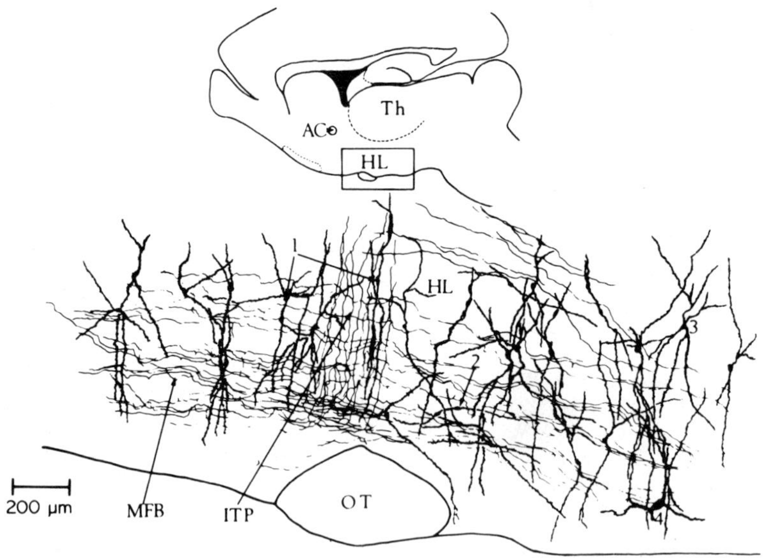

Figure 6.2 A rat brain diagram in saggital view and same orientation as Figure 6.1. The lower portion of the figure is an enlargement of the boxed in portion above showing a camera lucida drawing of Golgi stained neurons in the lateral hypothalamus. One can follow both the dendritic (thicker) and axonal (thinner) processes of these cells. Abbreviations are: AC = anterior commissure; HL = lateral hypothalamus; OT = optic tract; Th = thalamus. (Millhouse, 1979.) Reprinted by permission.

bundle self-stimulation, and with medial prefrontal cortex self-stimulation. This map is shown in Figure 6.3.

The 2-DG map (Figure 6.3) reveals some interesting facts. For example, anterior and posterior medial forebrain bundle self-stimulation have basically the same pattern of activation. In both cases, the diagonal band

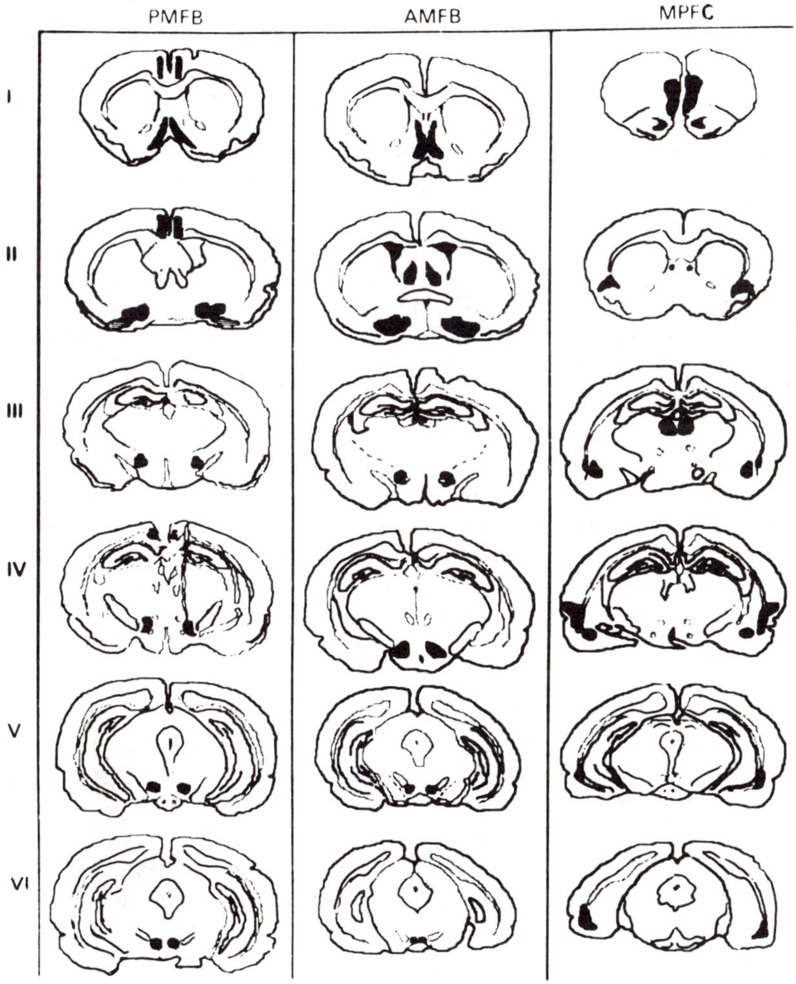

Figure 6.3 Computer reconstructions of labeled 2-deoxyglucose (2-DG) measurements of regional brain metabolism. Self-stimulation electrode sites were: posterior medial forebrain bundle (PMFB), anterior medial forebrain bundle (AMFB), and medial prefrontal cortex (MPFC). Blackened regions indicate places where 2-DG accumulated due to high regional activity. Striped regions indicate somewhat less activity. Note the similarity between AMFB and PMFB but the striking difference between these and MPFC. (Gallistel, 1983.) Reprinted by permission.

area shows strongly at the anterior end of the activation pattern. Moving toward the posterior, the activated regions follow the medial forebrain bundle and finally terminate in the ventral tegmental area. Slight differences do exist between the anterior and posterior placements (e.g., in septum, habenula), but the striking difference is between the self-stimulation sites of the medial prefrontal cortex versus those in the medial forebrain bundle. The lack of overlap between these two self-stimulation sites, suggests that the reward effects from these sites work by quite different mechanisms.

Before going too far, one must realize some limitations of the 2-DG map. The computer diagrams of autoradiographs (Figure 6.3) do not show areas that are inhibited or quite weakly (but perhaps importantly) activated. They rely on the contralateral side as a control and so do not detect bilateral activation, particularly if it is not striking upon casual visual inspection. Autoradiographs also do not detect fast phasic activation, especially followed by inhibition, or cases where inhibition and excitation are simultaneous or spatially mixed on different cells. Finally, and most important, the fact that a structure is activated does not mean it is involved with ESB reward. The structure may be involved with some wholly separate function (e.g., sniffing) that happens to share overlapping or nearby brain regions.

Despite these criticisms, the 2-DG maps suggest a number of important observations to us: (a) the mechanisms activated with medial forebrain bundle stimulation are probably very different from those activated by medial prefrontal cortex stimulation (Yadin et al. 1983) even though these regions share some fibers in common (Routtenberg, 1970, 1976); (b) the medial forebrain bundle may act as a unit regardless of its precise activation site (Yeomans, 1982); (c) the region of the diagonal band and the ventral tegmental area also may figure prominently in the behaviors seen in self-stimulation and perhaps in the reward effect. Thus, the 2-DG map offers a good start, suggesting a focus for other experiments aimed at a finer type of characterization. Electrophysiology is a logical follow-up, but in actual practice was started well before the 2-DG methods (e.g., Rolls, 1974); consequently much data has already been gathered. Before going into this area to search for the individual axons activated by ESB reward, we had better face the question, raised above, of separating relevant from non-relevant activated neurons that might be activated by the electrode. This is accomplished with psychophysical methods.

Psychophysics of ESB Reward: Refractory Periods

The goal of psychophysical experiments, as discussed in chapter 5, is to set constraints on the neural substrate for ESB reward by quantitatively characterizing the functional properties of this substrate. For example, the previous chapter ended with a discussion of neuronal refractory periods. Refractory periods are determined in single axons by applying a pair of pulses, manipulating the interval between the first and second pulse, and observing the effectiveness of the second pulse in eliciting action potential firing. The duration of refractory periods of axons is determined by the physical characteristics of axons such as size and myelination (Waxman, 1978). Therefore, knowing the refractory period enables one to make predictions about the biological nature of the excited cell. The refractory period of the neurons directly excited by the electrode and involved in self-stimulation lies in a range of 0.4–1.3 milliseconds (Yeomans, 1975). This makes it likely that those cells will be small, myelinated fibers (Waxman, 1978). This is an interesting fact in light of the knowledge that catecholamine fibers that had been proposed as the *directly* excited substrate (Crow, 1972: German & Bowden, 1974) are unmyelinated, having refractory periods in the range of 1.8–2.0 milliseconds (Guyenet and Aghajanian, 1978; German, Dalsass, & Kiser, 1980; Maeda & Mogenson, 1981).

Another use of refractory period data is to look for differences between various sites of self-stimulation (e.g., frontal cortex vs. medial forebrain bundle) in a functional–anatomical approach. Here refractory period data are joined by other aspects of the post-stimulation excitability cycle of axons, such as local potential summation, relative (vs. absolute) refractory period, and supernormal and subnormal periods (Yeomans, 1975, 1979; Bielajew and Shizgal, 1982) that enhance the quantitative characterization made by refractory periods alone. For a good review of this material, presented in much greater detail than this discussion, see Gallistel et al. (1981) and Gallistel (1983).

Within this functional anatomy approach, only a handful of ESB sites have yet been tested. Medial frontal cortex sites of self-stimulation have longer refractory periods than do medial forebrain bundle sites (approximate ranges are 0.9–3.5 ms vs. 0.4–1.3 ms, respectively), suggesting that fundamentally different directly activated substrates are involved in the two areas (Schenk & Shizgal, 1982; Silva, Vogel & Corbett, 1982). However, at sites within the medial forebrain bundle—for example, lateral hypothalamic and posterior hypothalamic or ventral tegmental area, the same refractory periods were found (Shizgal, Bielajew, Corbett, Skelton, & Yeomans, 1980; Bielajew, & Shizgal, 1982). Refractory period estimates from the periaqueductal gray also differed from lateral hypothalamus but by a smaller amount than those from the frontal cortex (Bielajew, Jordan, Ferme-Enright & Shizgal, 1981). Nucleus accumbens showed refractory periods that were also quite different from the lateral hypothalamus and more similar to the frontal cortex (Bielajew, Walker, & Fouriezos, 1983). This fact about the accumbens offers some small support for the notion that the catecholamine fibers that run between the ventral tegmental area and the accumbens are not the critical *directly excited* substrate of the self-stimulation electrode. If they were, then one might expect, but not necessarily demand, similar refractory periods from the accumbens and the hypothalamus, which both lie on the dopamine fibers' trajectory (Lindvall & Björkland, 1974).

Finally, the refractory period data are useful when doing electrophysiological studies of the substrate for ESB reward. Here, it serves to link the behavior with the specific cells. Because these refractory period data are determined from behavior, they are selective for the system(s) mediating ESB reward, among many systems excited by the electrode. For example, electrophysiological recordings of a compound action potential were made from the ventral tegmental area with stimulation electrodes in the lateral hypothalamus (Shizgal, Kiss, & Bielajew, 1982). The recorded refractory period range was determined, and this measurement agreed with the measurement of refractory period obtained in the behavioral studies of self-stimulation. This fact bolsters confidence in the behaviorally derived measures by showing that a substrate with the "correct" refractory period exists, but it alone does not prove that this region has reward-relevant fibers, since many systems might have neurons that pass under the electrode and have the same refractory periods. At this point, the real question one wants to ask about the psychophysical method is: Can it provide *direct* evidence of anatomical linkage between two brain regions? The answer to this question is yes; it is discussed below.

Psychophysics: Linkage, Conduction Velocity, and Direction

The problem of anatomical linkage between different sites of self-stimulation can be approached in various ways. The most direct is to have two electrodes situated in different places in the brain. Now, if we restrict our broad interest about anatomical linkage to the specific question of whether the two chosen sites lie on the same axonal pathway, then we can take advantage of the properties of axons and the psychophysical method. In axons that have an orthodromically traveling (i.e., normal direction) action potential, that action potential will be canceled if it should meet an antidromically traveling (i.e., opposite direction) action potential. It is a neurobiological property of axons that colliding action potentials cancel. If canceling occurs, then the output of the axon at its synaptic end will be one firing from the more distal electrode. However, if enough time elapses between the firing of the two action potentials, then two impulses will arrive at the synapse, one from each electrode, and two synaptic firings will occur. What we need now is a psychophysical method that will be able to detect when axons in an ESB reward pathway have fired once or twice. Then we can look for this canceling effect as a diagnostic indicator that the two stimulating electrodes sit (or do not

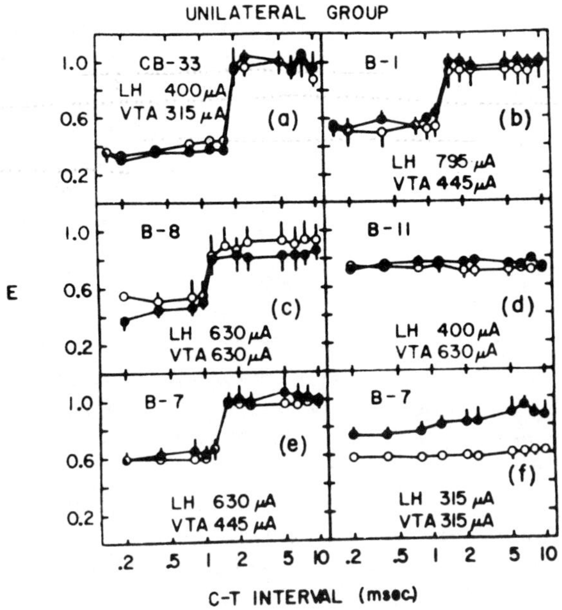

Figure 6.4 Collision effect between ESB pulses from a lateral hypothalamic (LH) and a ventral tegmental area (VTA) electrode. Effectivness (E) of the second pulse (*T*) of a pulse pair (*C–T*) is plotted against the intrapair interval. Closed symbols represent the case where the lateral hypothalamic electrode generated the first pulse of the pair, and open symbols represent the reversed order condition. The point of steep rise of the curves is the transition from collision with its loss of pulse effectiveness to no collision. (Shizgal et al. 1980.) Reprinted by permission.

sit) on the same axonal pathway and stimulate the same axons at different points. The method can be adapted from the psychophysical refractory period measurement, as discussed in chapter 5 and more briefly in the previous section of this chapter. This is discussed below.

The above logic is taken from the work on anatomical linkage of self-stimulation sites done by Shizgal and his associates (cf. Shizgal, Kiss, & Bielajew, 1982). In an impressive series of experiments, this group has developed the logic we have just discussed and has done the initial experiments. Let us begin with an obvious question from the 2-DG map presented earlier. Do axons stimulated by lateral hypothalamic electrodes also get stimulated by the ventral tegmental electrodes? The answer to this question seems to be *yes* (Shizgal, Bielajew, Corbett, Skelton, & Yeomans, 1980; Bielajew & Shizgal, 1982). In these experiments, rats were implanted with electrodes in both regions of the brain and trained to self-stimulate on each electrode. Refractory period estimates were then made for both sites, as discussed above and in the previous chapter. To determine the existence of a canceling effect due to action potential collision, pairs of pulses were applied to the electrodes as in the refractory period studies, except that the first member of each pair was applied to one electrode and the second member of the pair was applied to the other electrode. By varying the time between the pulses, one can look for the collision or canceling effect. However, these data are not merely input–output functions but are tradeoff functions obtained by measuring the required changes in pulse frequency to offset a decrease in the effectiveness of the second pulse in the pair, due to collision. See chapter 5 and Gallistel (1983) for further discussion of the issue of tradeoff functions and scaling. The collision data are then able to be expressed directly as the effectiveness of the second pulse, going from completely effective (score of 1) to not effective (score of 0) as a function of time between the pulses in a pair. Such data are presented in Figure 6.4.

As can be seen from this figure, a sharp rise in the effectiveness of the second pulse occurs at about 1.0 to 2.0 milliseconds. This finding was replicated and the sample size doubled in a second experiment (Bielajew & Shizgal, 1982). Two of the six graphs in Figure 6.4 do not show the collision effect. In one graph (subject B-7), the data showing no collision are a duplication of an earlier successful attempt at finding collision, but at a lower stimulating current. The reason collision was not found under the lower current conditions has to do with the question of alignment of the electrodes within the bundle of axons that passes under the two electrodes. If its electrodes are not aligned, as is shown in Figure 6.5, then no collision will occur at low currents. Raising the current will expand the stimulation field and may compensate for the misalignment to produce some collision. This appears to be the case in subject B-7 in Figure 6.4. In subject B-11, a different explanation must be offered because no collision was found despite fairly high stimulating currents. It should be noted that the absence of a collision effect may simply mean that the increases in current necessary to produce alignment could not

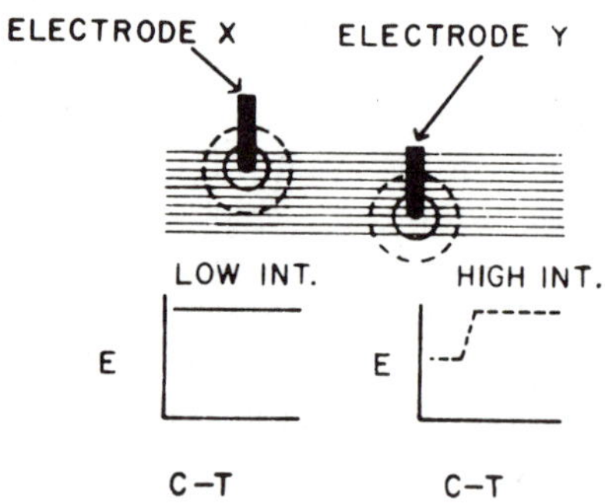

Figure 6.5 Medial forebrain bundle (horizontal lines) with two electrodes misaligned in the path. At low ESB current, no axons in common are excited and no collision is seen in the graph just below and to the left. This case is in contrast with the higher ESB current condition in which the collision effect is seen (lower right). Abbreviations are as in Figure 6.4 (Shizgal et al., 1980.) Reprinted by permission.

be made because of some other consequence of this increase (e.g., aversiveness, motor effect) that disrupted responding. Complete failure to find collision, may indicate an absence of connection between the two stimulating sites. However, as always in science, proof of the negative is difficult. Thus, we rest more firmly on the finding of demonstrated connection between the hypothalamic and the ventral tegmental area than on the absence of such a finding.

Another benefit of the collision effect described above is that it permits one to calculate the conduction velocity to a rough approximation. This is done by dividing the distance between the electrodes as measured histologically by the time required to first see the steep rise in second pulse effectiveness that signals the abatement of collision. One obvious caution is that the distance between the electrodes represents the *minimum* distance over which the axons could course. A glance at the path neurons shown in Figure 6.2 reveals that these axons have a somewhat wavy path through the medial forebrain bundle. In addition, the stimulated axons could travel toward some other location and then swing back when going from one site to another. Therefore, when the conduction velocity estimate is off, it is likely to be too slow. Another important factor contributing to possible error is that the average refractory period of the sites must be subtracted from the collision time. This is necessary because, to be effective, the second pulse must wait not only for the first action potential to pass under its electrode, but also for that region of those axons that carried the action potential to recover from refractoriness before they can be stimulated to carry an impulse again. Thus, any error in refractory period estimate carries over to the conduction velocity estimate.

Shizgal, Bielajew, Corbett, Skelton, & Yeomans (1980) and Bielajew and Shizgal (1982) were completely aware of these sources of error and attempted to set their estimates at the slower end of the probable range by making conservative assumptions about error. Their findings place the conduction velocity in the range of 1.0 to 4.5 meters/second (Bielajew & Shizgal, 1982). This estimate is well out of the range of the catecholamine-containing neurons, which are small, unmyelinated, and have slower conduction velocities in the range of 0.3 to 0.9 meters/second (German et al., 1980; Guyenet & Aghajanian, 1978; Maeda & Mogenson, 1981). This finding is important since, along with refractory periods, it is one of the strongest indications that catecholamine fibers are not *directly* excited by the self-stimulation electrode, although they may well be excited trans-synaptically.

The current stage of this impressive line of work is to address the question of the *direction* of conduction (Shizgal, Bielajew, & Kiss, 1980; Bielajew, 1983a). Here, the same basic logic is applied: two electrodes are implanted, one in the lateral hypothalamus, and one in the ventral tegmental area; the rat is trained to self-stimulate on each electrode, and, as before, a kind of "interference" between the electrodes is examined through psychophysical methods. The difference here is that the "interference" does not come from collision but from hyperpolarization blockade of one electrode or the other. It is known that axons that are conducting action potentials can have those impulses blocked if the action potential is made to conduct through an area of hyperpolarization provided via an extracellular electrode (Ruffler & Vaugh-Williams, 1953; Accornero, Bini, Lenzi, & Manfred, 1977).

In these reports (Shizgal, Bielajew, & Kiss, 1980; Bielajew, 1983a), stimulation pulse effectiveness was examined as a function of the width of the pulse. Normally, the stimulation current return (the anode) is the skull screws. In this work, the normal arrangement was compared to one in which the lateral hypothalamus electrode served as the anode to the ventral tegmental area electrode, and the ventral tegmental area electrode served as anode to the lateral hypothalamic electrode. Because the anode generates a hyperpolarizing field, the following very specific hypothesis was offered if the direction of conduction was *descending*: As pulse width is extended, there will be at some point a decrease in the effectiveness of the stimulating pulses on the lateral hypothalamic electrode when the ventral tegmental area serves as the anode. In no other arrangement will this be found. To restate, the predicted decrease in pulse effectiveness would occur as the hyperpolarizing field in the ventral tegmental area begins to interfere with the descending action potentials generated by the lateral hypothalamic pulses. The interference should not occur at very brief pulse widths because the hyperpolarizing field would have come and gone before the action potentials triggered in the lateral hypothalamus arrived in the ventral tegmental area. But the interference would occur as pulse width was lengthened so that the hyperpolarizing field was present when the lateral hypothalamic-triggered action potentials arrived in the ventral tegmental area.

As can be expected from the space devoted to the previous discussion, the specific predictions were borne out by the data, and the direction of conduction was concluded to be descending (Bielajew, 1983a; Shizgal, Bielajew, & Kiss, 1980). This provides still more evidence against the ascending catecholamine neurons as *directly* excited by the stimulating electrode. Caution should be exercised in concluding that no portion of the directly excited axons mediating the rewarding effect generated by the electrode travel in an ascending or rostral direction. All that we can say is that the major portion seems to travel from the lateral hypothalamus to the ventral tegmental area, in a descending direction.

The application of the method of collision to investigate the anatomical linkage of self-stimulation sites has not been restricted to the lateral hypothalamic and ventral tegmental area sites. Medial prefrontal cortex and lateral hypothalamic sites (Schenk & Shizgal, 1982), periaqueductal gray and lateral hypothalamic sites (Bielajew et al., 1981), and medial prefrontal cortex and posterior-medial frontal cortex sites (Silva, Vogel, & Corbett, 1982) have been tested. None of these studies found evidence for direct axonal connection, although the periaqueductal gray and lateral hypothalamic site study did find appreciable summation between the reward effects at these sites, suggesting, perhaps, a trans-synaptic link. Such summation was not found between medial prefrontal cortex and lateral hypothalamic sites, again suggesting that the mechanisms of ESB reward in these two sites are different.

The collision effect was also not seen between lateral hypothalamic and ventral tegmental area sites of stimulation when the behavior tested was stimulation-elicited escape behavior, not ESB reward-seeking behavior (Bielajew & Shizgal, 1980). This was true even though the collision effect had been demonstrated for the ESB reward-seeking behavior in the same animals with the same electrodes. The Bielajew & Shizgal (1980) paper reinforces the belief that the collision effect is a real *functional* anatomical technique and suggests a different anatomy for ESB-induced reward and aversive effects.

Psychophysics: Other Structural and Anatomical Properties

Many other characteristics of neurons and the neural system(s) mediating ESB reward could be described. Gallistel et al. (1981) list 14 quantitative and physical properties in their review paper. We have discussed fewer than half of these from their list. Examples of undiscussed properties are: the properties of the directly excited axons, such as their ability to integrate the current delivered in ESB pulses (Matthews 1977; Yeomans, Matthews, Hawkins, Bellman, & Doppelt, 1979) or the length and magnitude of the supernormal period following action potentials triggered by ESB (Yeomans, 1979). These and other properties will help in the electrophysiological identification of the ESB reward-relevant neurons (Shizgal, Kiss, & Bielajew, 1982). Still other psychophysical characteristics, which depend upon the summation or integration of many ESB pulses, will perhaps aid in the identification of the second stage or the indirectly excited neurons involved in ESB reward.

Finally, the acquisition of important information continues. We are now able to determine the approximate distance that current spreads from a lateral hypothalamic electrode (Fouriezos, 1980), and perhaps even determine something of the postion of the electrode with regard to the edge of the ESB reward axon bundle (Yeomans, Prior, & Bateman, 1982).

In summary, what do we know from the psychophysical study of self-stimulation? The answer is that we know characteristics of the neural substrate like the refractory period (0.4–1.3 meters/second), the existence of axonal linkage between two areas (lateral hypothalamus and ventral tegmental area), the conduction velocity along this path (at least 1.0–4.5 meters/second), a major direction of conduction (descending), and more. Every bit of new information helps to define the systems' operating characteristics. Additionally, these quantitative traits, like descriptions of a criminal by a witness, aid the electrophysiologist in the identification and apprehension of the specific individual axons involved in ESB reward. Once identified electrophysiologically, the cells can be examined for their anatomical connections, neurochemical characteristics, and so forth, thus opening new research opportunities. Although these psychophysical traits set very powerful constraints on the system(s) involved in ESB reward and, in combination with electrophysiology, hold great promise, other approaches also yield important information that can reinforce these conclusions.

Lesion Studies of ESB Reward

A number of investigators have used the technique of electrolytic or other lesions of the brain to get at the question of the anatomical substrate of ESB reward. The basic argument is that if the lesions disrupt the self-stimulation behavior, then one has damaged a part of the relevant system. A serious limitation of this argument is that the damage could be on a system that converges to the relevant system but is not itself directly stimulated. This point is often raised when a lesion *enhances* self-stimulation behavior (Asdourian, Stutz, & Rocklin, 1966; Lorens, 1966), but may be missed when the lesion decreases behavior. In light of the healthy scientific preoccupation with positive results, it is interesting that much of the interpretational clarity and value of lesion studies, as discussed below, comes from examples in which large lesions gave the seemingly negative result of failing to alter or abolish self-stimulation behavior. Such lesions are useful in eliminating possibilities of specific connections or pathways that are thought to be critical to ESB reward, especially if they are shown in combination with effective lesions.

Another relevant point formed the theme of chapter 5; namely, that rate measures of self-stimulation behavior are of questionable value in investigating ESB reward (Hodos and Valenstein, 1962). Since ESB self-stimulation is a laboratory phenomenon, although dependent on naturally existing brain systems, most researchers today are not really interested in the neural substrate of self-stimulation behavior as an end in itself. Rather, they are interested in the substrate of ESB *reward* as studied through self-stimulation behavior. Unfortunately, most of the lesion studies on self-stimulation have used rate of response measures and thus can only comment on self-stimulation behavior as a whole. To repeat, a brain lesion-induced decrease in rate of response could be due to a loss of reward effectiveness of ESB, or it could be due to a decreased ability of the subject to perform the task required as a result of a motoric or other nonreward deficit. Worse yet, if high stimulating currents are used to get a "good" starting behavior, then a lesion that does not affect self-stimulation may have actually somewhat reduced the effectiveness of the ESB in generating reward, but not reduced it enough to go below that required to sustain asymptotic responding (see Figure 5.2 for an illustration of asymptotes). In other words, ceiling effects could play a role here if many levels of stimulation are not tested.

In a review of the literature to 1976, Lorens (1976) lists some 26 lesion studies. Except for a few studies in the 1960s most of the papers cited reported self-stimulation electrodes in the lateral hypothalamus. In most of these studies, lesions of the medial forebrain bundle *anterior* to the self-stimulation site had a small effect on self-stimulation behavior (Morgane, 1962; Lorens, 1966; Olds & Olds, 1969; Unemoto, 1968; Keesey and Powley, 1973). One study (Boyd & Gardner, 1967) did find a larger effect of anterior lesions. The lesions in their study were in the lateral preoptic area. Six rats were tested, four of which showed a decrease in responding and then exhibited only partial recovery.

In contrast to the anterior lesion effects, electrolytic lesions placed posterior to the medial forebrain bundle site of self-stimulation were generally much more effective in disrupting self-stimulation behavior. By itself, this observation might not mean much, since the medial forebrain bundle is known to be more compact in its posterior portion (Nauta & Domiseck, 1983) and so might be more susceptible to damage. However, in combination with the psychophysical data, a consistent picture begins to emerge. A more recent study (Stellar & Neeley, 1982) employed a reward summation function paradigm and so could separate ESB reward from motoric impairments. This study agrees with earlier findings on the relative importance of anterior and posterior lesions. One should note that the reward summation function approach may be especially useful here because lesions of the lateral hypothalamus are known to produce sensory-motor integration deficits even when the lesions are unilateral (Marshall & Teitelbaum, 1974).

In a recent study (Janas & Stellar, 1984), two groups of anterior lesions were tested using the knife-cut technique to make the lesion. This technique enables one to transect more completely the medial forebrain bundle while doing far less damage in the orthogonal direction (rostral–caudal) and so is an improvement over the electrolytic lesion method. Also, the reward summation function was employed in this study. Janas and Stellar found that large, unilateral knife cuts going from the anterior commissure to the base of the brain failed to disrupt self-stimulation behavior (Figure 6.6). What may be even more interesting is that, if the knife cut was placed a bit more posterior, so as to cut through the lateral preoptic region, then a significant change in ESB reward pulse effectiveness and in asymptotic response vigor was noted. This result focuses

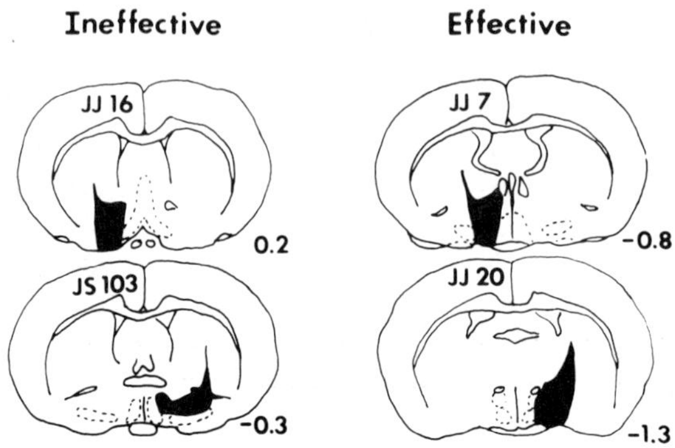

Figure 6.6 Histological analysis of two groups of anterior medial forebrain bundle knife-cuts in the frontal and saggital planes of section. One group was ineffective in altering the reward pulse effectiveness on the reward summation function measure, and the other group was effective in degrading reward pulse effectiveness and in producing decreases in performance maximum. Distance from Bregma is indicated in millimeters and negative means posterior. The effective knife-cuts passed through the lateral preoptic area, but cut many others fiber systems as well. (Janus & Stellar, 1984.)

our attention on the lateral preoptic area, but it should be noted that some fiber systems originating outside the lateral preoptic area course between these two knife cuts. Also, it is not possible, from this study alone, to say if the relevant fibers that were cut were ascending or descending. Making this conclusion depends upon including data from other methods. Finally, it is curious that Stellar and Neeley (1982) did not find much effect of anterior lateral hypothalamic electrolytic lesions. One explanation for this difference may be that the electrolytic lesions were not big enough. The knife cuts were approximately three times the cross-sectional area of the lesions. Another explanation may concern exact lesion placement since one recent sudy also found lateral preoptic area lesions significantly depressed self-stimulation responding (Munoz, Sprick, & Huston, 1983). Unfortunately, this study used rate of response as the behavioral measure.

The lack of dependence of hypothalamic ESB reward on connections with neural tissue much farther anterior than the anterior commissure is also illustrated in a more radical set of studies by Huston and his associates (Huston & Borbely, 1973, 1974; Huston, Pritzel, & Buscher, 1981; Huston, 1982) in which the entire forebrain anterior to the hypothalamus was surgically removed. Huston and Borbely (1974) ablated all of the neocortex and most of the forebrain rostral, lateral, and superior to the thalamus. Indeed, these rats were termed "thalamic rats" because the thalamus was the highest remaining structure not directly damaged. What was remarkable about these rats was that, despite enormous behavioral impairments, they could be trained to rear or to elevate their tails to turn on ESB. The operants had to be on-body responses, but the animals could learn the task. This demonstrated that some degree of operant behavior remained and that ESB on the lateral hypothalamic electrode retained some ability to generate a reward signal to the animal (Huston and Borbely, 1973, 1974).

In the above studies, one might well ask to what extent the brain structures underlying ESB reward were impaired but not totally ablated by the extensive forebrain damage. That is, was the lesioned animal operating on some brainstem system that originally generated only a portion of the reward effect? This question cannot be answered by the Huston studies because simple rate of response was used as the behavioral measure. For that matter, the reward summation function, also would be inadequate to answer this question unless before and after measurements could be obtained in the same animals. The reason for this is that the reward summation function is a signature in a particular animal of the self-stimulation system and it is dependent on the particular ESB site, the chosen stimulating current, and so on (see chapter 5).

To investigate the question of how much of the original ESB reward system survived the lesion, Stellar et al., (1982) prepared rats with unilateral forebrain ablations equivalent to those done by Huston and Borbely (1974). The unilateral ablation permitted the use of runway running, a more sophisticated operant, and much more sophisticated ESB reward measures—the trade off function, which is not troubled by the problem of electrode site specificity, as discussed above. However, the unilateral nature of the lesion does not control for contralateral projections; this is discussed later. Stellar et al. (1982) measured the ESB pulse number versus pulse current tradeoff and the ESB total burst charge versus burst duration tradeoff.

While a complete discussion of these tradeoff functions is beyond the scope of this book, several aspects of those functions can be described briefly. The number–current tradeoff function measures the way increasing ESB current expands the stimulating field and thereby fires *more* relevant axons. It does this by looking at how the ESB pulse number can be decreased as current is increased to keep behavioral responding at the same level. In another realm, the charge–duration tradeoff function measures the decrease in efficiency of *integration* of ESB pulses as duration of the burst of pulses is lengthened and the pulses are correspondingly spread out. It does this by assessing requirements for pulses of higher current as the burst duration is lengthened.

In the Stellar et al. (1982) study, neither the number–current nor the charge–duration tradeoff function was different in a group of unilateral forebrain-ablated rats when compared to a group of unablated intact rats. The findings mean that neither the neurons under the electrode tip nor the neurons integrating the action potentials were appreciably damaged by the unilateral ablation. This reinforces and extends the conclusions offered by Huston (1982). Recently, Cole (1984) presented more evidence to support this position. Working with rats implanted with electrodes prior to any ablation, she showed that subsequent unilateral forebrain ablations that included frontal cortex, rostral caudate, accumbens, and olfactory tubercle had only small degradative effects on the reward pulse frequency threshold for ipsilateral lateral hypothalamic electrodes. It seems that lateral hypothalamic self-stimulation can survive well without the major forebrain terminations of the medial forebrain bundle, and this once again focuses our attention on the neural structures below the rostral forebrain.

In summary, the results from the lesion studies and the psychophysical studies interlock and provide support for the hypothesis advanced in the next section of this chapter. The interlocking is important because each set of studies has questions of interpretation arising from our limited knowledge of the subtleties of brain function. Consider the fact that, in lesion studies, some recovery of self-stimulation is often seen following medial forebrain bundle damage that disrupts self-stimulation. This could reflect a recovery of ESB reward substrate that was temporarily disrupted by a local dysfunction (e.g., edema, altered blood brain barrier), or it could reflect a regeneration process. For example, we now know that medial forebrain bundle neurons show some regeneration following transection (Foerster, 1982). However, the agreement betwen lesion and psychophysical studies gives us some grounds for setting aside these recovery or regeneration processes when drawing our main conclusions.

The Descending Path Hypothesis

The most parsimonious explanation of the above literature on lesions and two-electrode psychophysics is that the primary ESB reward pathway descends in the medial forebrain bundle, that it courses into and/or through the ventral tegmental area, and that the axons belong to a small myelinated class of neurons. This last point is necessary to explain the observed refractory periods and conduction velocities (Gallistel et al., 1981). Collectively, these conclusions have been known somewhat informally as the *descending path hypothesis* (Gallistel, 1983; Shizgal et al. 1982; Yeomans, 1982; Wise, 1980) and have inspired further research and thinking. For example, going back to the papers from which Figure 6.1 was drawn, the atlas of the medial forebrain bundle generated by Nieuwenhuys, Geeraldts, and Veening (1982) divides the medial forebrain bundle into compartments based on the diameters of the descending axon. Gallistel (1983, p. 306) has reanalyzed his original 2-DG data on ESB self-stimulation (Yadin et al., 1982) and found agreement between his sites of regional activity and the compartments in which Nieuwenhuys et al. (1982) say contain small descending myelinated fibers.

A second line of evidence corrobarating the descending path hypothesis is the preliminary electrophysiological work of Shizgal et al. (1982). They have measured compound action potentials recorded in the medial forebrain bundle just anterior to the ventral tegmental area that were generated from preoptic medial forebrain bundle electrodes. Although many action potentials are recorded at a time in this experiment, it was possible to achieve a population estimate of both refractory periods and conduction velocity. These electrophysiological findings agreed with the behaviorally determined measures (Shizgal et al., 1982) and so provide evidence that the behavioral estimates are not unreasonable. This reinforces the descending path hypothesis. Finally, other researchers have studied the elctrophysiology of lateral hypothalamic/medial forebrain bundle self-stimulation. For example, Rolls (1974) reports a minimum refractory period estimate of 0.59 milliseconds for a directly excited neuron where the cell was recorded in the amygdala and stimulated from a lateral hypothalamic electrode. This estimate falls well within the 0.4–1.3 millisecond range expected (Gallistel et al., 1981; Schenk & Shizgal, 1982), thus showing that such cells exist, perhaps in many places.

The descending path hypothesis is not meant to be exclusive. It allows that some proportaion of the ESB reward effect from medial forebrain bundle stimulation may ascend or leave the medial forebrain bundle laterally (Kent & Grossman, 1973) for other targets like the amygdala (Rolls, 1974). The hypothesis also does not pertain to other ESB reward sites or to non-ESB rewards such as cocaine self-administration or to the natural rewards of food or water. It does not pertain even to the systems excited synaptically by the stimulated axons. However, the descending path hypothesis represents the first time that evidence has converged from multiple lines (psychophysics, 2-DG, recording, lesions) towards a single unified explanation.

The descending path hypothesis offers a small place to stand when examining other literature and designing experiments. For example, a search is now on for the cell bodies of origin. If they are found, it may then be possible, as mentioned previously, to actually visualize the neurons involved and begin to study their chemistry, physiology, and anatomical connections to other brain regions. In other words, it may be possible to ultimately be in the position to do work like that on invertebrate circuits of behavior as in *Aplysia* (Kandel, 1979). In addition, some (e.g., Gallistel, 1983) hope this approach will ultimately lead to an understanding of the neural basis of other psychological processes such as memory, since it is evident that an animal records the experience of the ESB. If one could begin with a cell that was known to be a part of the circuit carrying the ESB reward signal, then one might be able to follow the circuit and eventually pick up information as to how that signal was preserved in the nervous system. From this point of view, Gallistel (1983) refers to the self-stimulating animal as being a nerve–memory preparation.

Origin of the Descending Path

Before we wander off into speculation about the lofty goals and potential achievments of ESB reward research, we must first come down to earth on one, or perhaps two, specific questions. Where does this descending path originate, and where does it terminate? Let us consider the question of the origin first. This is an issue that is just coming to the fore as researchers now concentrate squarely on the nature of the path. There are two distinct classes of possibilities, which are represented in the first two figures of this chapter. First, the descending path could come from above or rostral to the hypothalamus (the possibilities are listed by Nieuwenhuys et al., 1982, and diagrammed in Figure 6.1). Second, the descending path could come from the indwelling path neurons of the medial forebrain bundle (as described by Millhouse, 1979, and diagrammed in Figure 6.2).

The first possibility has many components, but these are limited by the observation that lesions of the far anterior medial forebrain bundle or many of the forebrain origins of these pathways (see earlier discussions) do not block or substantially reduce the ESB reward effect. Particularly, fibers that pass directly below the anterior commissure do not seem very important. The irrelevant fibers probably include fibers from prefrontal cortex, olfactory bulb, and anterior olfactory nucleus. These fiber systems were never very seriously implicated in hypothalamic ESB reward either because they do not reach back to the ventral tegmental area, (i.e., the olfactory projections, Nieuwenhuys et al., 1982), or because they are eliminated by other experiments, (i.e., the frontal cortex projections, Corbett et al. 1982a; Stellar et al., 1982).

The anterior lesion experiments, discussed previously, have cut some fibers that *have* been implicated in ESB reward. For example, on the basis of 2-DG and psychophysical data, Yeomans (1982) suggests that the diagonal band and the preoptic area are possible origins for this descending path. He diagrammed this hypothesis; his diagram is reproduced in Figure 6.7. The most anterior lesions shown in Figure 6.6 should have partially cut into the projections of diagonal band (horizontal limb), and since there was no effect of these cuts (Janas & Stellar, 1984), this area may not be as important as fibers coming from the vertical limb of the diagonal band, which was spared. The slightly more posterior cuts in Figure 6.6 that went through the lateral preoptic area were found to attenuate the reward pulse effectiveness of ESB, and this makes the preoptic pathway more interesting. However, caution is needed, since many fibers may have been cut by the effective cuts shown in Figure 6.6 and that could involve structures other than the lateral preoptic area. For reference, in going between Figures 6.6 and 6.7, note that the anterior commissure (at −0.3 mm in Figure 6.6) would be located at the anterior border of the third ventricle in Figure 6.7. The above discussion represents the type of convergent analysis between the lesion, psychophysical, and 2-DG data sets that could lead us to the cellular identification of the origin of the descending path. With the addition of electrophysiology (see Shizgal & Rompré, 1984) the convergence becomes stronger.

It should also be noted that many but not all ascending dopamine fibers from the ventral midbrain regions going to caudate and accumbens have moved dorsally and laterally and so might well have escaped the far anterior cut, but perhaps not the more posterior of the anterior cuts (Ungerstedt, 1971a; Lindvall & Björklund, 1974). The exact distribution of these fibers also becomes important. However, we will reserve discussion of the ascending dopamine projections for chapter 7. Other candidate fiber systems selected on the basis of psychophysical data might be subjected to this test of the anterior unilateral lesions. There are descending projections from the medial septum, and the accumbens to be considered (Yeomans, 1982; Shizgal et al., 1982). These and other less prominent projections from the substantia innominata, stria terminalis, central amygdala, and even the paraventricular nucleus, are all candidates because they project to the region of the ventral tegmental area through the medial forebrain bundle (Nieuwenhuys et al., 1982). Most of these candidates are made less likely because they do not show up strongly on the 2-DG analysis (Figure 6.3), but they should be subjected to the criteria

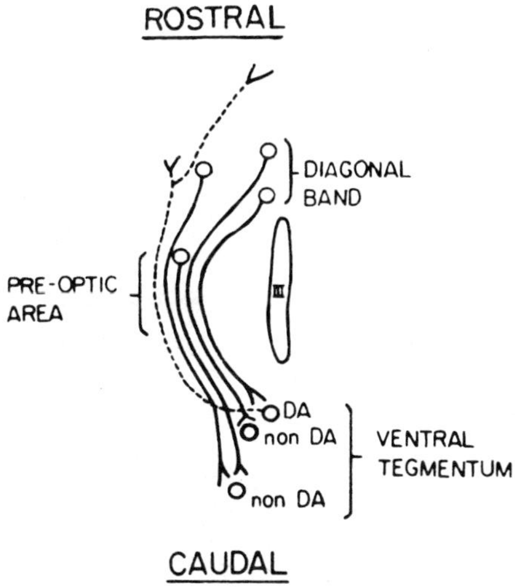

Figure 6.7 Descending path hypothesis in medial forebrain bundle depicted in the horizontal plain. Dashed lines show the ascending dopamine projections to the forebrain. The third ventricle (III) is shown for reference. (Yeoman, 1982.) Reprinted by permission.

set up by the psychophysical, 2-DG, electrophysiological, and lesion data. This work is in progress in a number of laboratories and is a likely subject for writing by researchers in this field.

The second major possibility for the origin of the neurons involved in the descending path hypothesis resides in the so-called "path neurons" themselves (Olds, 1977). As studied by Millhouse (1969, 1979), they originate from the lateral hypothalamic area and throughout the medial forebrain bundle. They appear to send axons in rostral, caudal, and even superior directions. They are heavily interconnected in a reticular fashion and so are quite able to spread excitation rapidly from one cell to another. Olds (1977) thought them to be the neurons of ESB reward and was particularly impressed by the way they collected inputs from a variety of other fibers running in the medial forebrain bundle. Their reticular-like nature may make them capable of the "unity" of anatomy, behavior, 2-DG uptake, and excitability that so impressed Yeomans (1982). It may be only neurons with such a reticulated structure that could survive to generate any reward signal after a bizarre lesion described by Huston (1982). Here, unilateral forebrain ablations and complete posterior ipsilateral transections were made, leaving a "diencephalic peninsula" connected only to the contralateral intact hemisphere. ESB delivered to this "diencephalic peninsula" was able to support self-stimulation behavior (Huston, Ornstein & Lehner, 1978; Huston, 1982). However, as stated earlier, the absence of sophisticated measurement techniques in these experiments makes generalization to intact self-stimulating animals impossible.

Owing to their bipolar nature, these intrinsic neurons of the hypothalamus could support self-stimulation with either anterior or posterior axonal process. Lesions of the posterior portions of the medial forebrain bundle would immediately disconnect anterior ESB sites from their ipsilateral ventral tegmental area, but anterior lesions would leave undamaged the descending limb of neurons serving a posterior ESB site (Figure 6.8). This was precisely the finding of Stellar and Neeley (1982). A com-

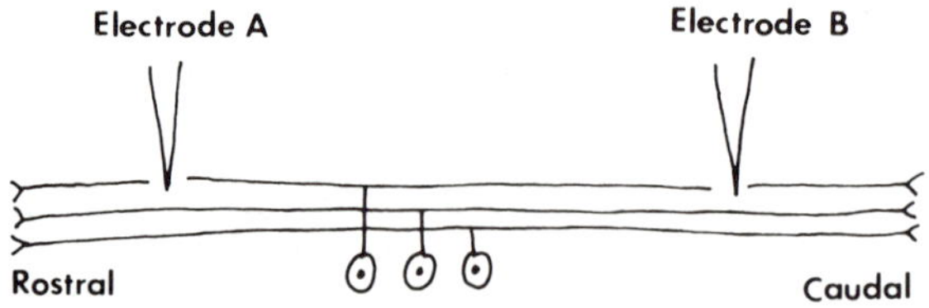

Figure 6.8 Schematic of three bipolar lateral hypothalamic path neurons with electrodes placed at the end of each axonal branch. If the reward path were descending, then rostral lesions (Electrode A) would not effect the ESB reward generated at Electrode B. However, the reverse would not be true.

plication comes from the Janas and Stellar (1984) study in which anterior medial forebrain bundle knife-cuts were found to be effective in attenuating ESB reward. The differences between these studies were discussed previously, including the fact that the knife-cut occupied a bigger cross-sectional area. Perhaps the knife-cut killed enough path neurons to make a difference while the lesion did not. A better alternative hypothesis may be to suggest that the descending path actually originates in two major places: in the previously discussed lateral preoptic/diagonal band areas and in the lateral hypothalamus from the path neurons.

A final bit of evidence supportive of a role for the path neurons comes from recent work in which these intrinsic lateral hypothalamic cells were lesioned but the medial forebrain bundle fibers of passage were spared (Velley, Chaminade, Roy, Kempf, & Cardo, 1983). This selective lesion was done unilaterally with the agent ibotenic acid, and the rats were subsequently implanted bilaterally with lateral hypothalamic electrodes. Self-stimulation rates at various current levels were found to be seriously impaired or even absent completely on the lesioned side but normal on the intact side and on both sides in control subjects. Fortunately Velley et al. tried a number of levels of ESB current so that we know the effect is not one of raising the ESB threshold only slightly; however they did not use any measures that were able to assess the quantitative extent of ESB reward impairment. Still, the finding is supportive of a role in ESB reward for these path neurons, providing this agent is indeed as selective as claimed. Before these path neurons can be taken seriously as candidates for the ESB reward-relevant axons, either alone or in addition to lateral preoptic neurons, they must be shown to meet the existing psychophysical criterion. Thus, they should be small fibers, myelinated, have refractory periods and conduction velocities in the correct range, and so on. This is an interesting subject for further research. However, caution is needed because one recent report did not find this impairment of self-stimulation with a similar technique (Munoz et al., 1983, abstract only).

Some Subtleties and the Termination of the Descending Path

The descending path hypothesis of hypothalamic ESB reward as articulated above and as either implied or discussed by others (Shizgal et al., 1982; Yeomans, 1982; Wise, 1980; Gallistel, 1983; Bielajew, 1983) is not a particularly complex or subtle concept. The fact that it took almost 30 years from the original discovery of ESB reward by Olds and Milner (1954), to formulate it with a reasonable amount of solid supportive evidence reflects the complexity of studying ESB reward phenomenon. Nevertheless, the brain is almost always more intricate than models of its structure and/or function make it out to be, even if those models are hard-won.

To take a glimpse at the type of refinements one might ultimately want to make in this hypothesis, let us consider the question of *bilateral crossed connections* of the descending path. The work reviewed by Huston (1982) on the "diencephalic peninsula" and briefly discussed above, makes an argument for bilaterality in the descending path by simply eliminating most other alternatives and showing that the rats still self-stimulate. Additionally, the striking lack of change in the psychophysical properties tested in *unilaterally* forebrain-ablated animals (Stellar et al., 1982) also suggests involvement of the contralateral hemisphere in the ESB reward effect from a unilateral electrode. Finally, from the lesion work, it appears that even the most effective posterior medial forebrain bundle lesions (Stellar & Neeley, 1982) are not completely effective at abolishing self-stimulation. Crossed connections could explain this observation.

Bilateral stimulation studies also lend general support to the notion of the existence of some crossed connections, although not specifically in the directly excited neurons. For a long time it has been known that the reward effect of two bilateral lateral hypothalamic ESB electrode placements will summate or add together (Ungerleider & Coons, 1970). As part of the control procedure employed by Shizgal, Bielajew, Corbett, Skelton, and Yeomans (1980) in testing for collision, rats were implanted bilaterally in the lateral hypothalamus. Pairs of pulses were given, and the effectiveness of the *second* pulse of the pulse pair was determined when it was delivered on the contralateral electrode. The effectiveness was 25% to 80% of what one would see if maximally effective second pulses had been given on the ipsilateral electrode. (See the earlier discussion of linkage for methodological details.) Thus, a 25% to 80% bilateral summation may exist. This is even more striking when one compares the results to unilateral summation. Consider the two subjects in Figure 6.3 in which rats with electrodes on the same side of the brain did not show collision; their summation was between 60% and 80%. This was within the range for the bilateral summation cases. It should be noted that summation does not always exist between ESB reward sites. For example, Schenck and Shizgal (1982) found poor summation (mean = 18%, SER = 6.5%) between medial prefrontal and lateral hypothalamic self-stimulation sites. Although the significance of the numbers of 25% to 80% bilateral summation is not clear in terms of the relative amount of crossed connections, these data are suggestive, and the matter deserves further investigation.

Little work has been done on the actual anatomy of bilateral crossed connections of the hypothalamus. In one study (Huston et al., 1981), a preparation was made with a unilateral ESB electrode and a posterior transection disconnecting the brain stem. In addition, the other hemisphere was given a forebrain ablation. These rats self-stimulated, and when the retrograde neuronal tracer, horseradish peroxidase (HRP), was delivered at this same site, fibers could be traced leaving the hypothalamus and crossing the midline through the thalamic commissure and the supraoptic decussation. Labeled cell bodies were found in the contralateral lateral hypothalamus (see also Huston, 1982).

In a thorough study on a more standard preparation—an *intact* rat—Gerfen, Staines, Arbuthnott, and Fibiger (1982) injected HRP into the dopamine-containing substantia nigra. They found cell bodies in many places in the brain, but pursuant to our interest here, they found a significant number of cells in the contralateral lateral hypothalamus. This must mean that some neurons within the lateral hypothalamus send descending crossed projections into the area of the substantia nigra. Phillipson (1979) conducted similar studies on the ventral tegmental area and found many afferents coming from the lateral hypothalamus, the preoptic area, and the diagonal band. Apparently, however, few contralateral cells were found, unless the HRP was deposited in the midline caudal structures within the ventral tegmental area. Unfortunately, in Phillipson's paper, the section discussing contralateral connections was very brief. From our perspective, the question of descending and specifically crossed projections to the ventral tegmental area deserves more attention. In one anatomical paper (Simon, LeMoal, & Calas, 1979) only afferents from posterior regions were discussed, and the hypothalamus/basal forebrain was not even studied.

The second property that one might want to consider in relation to the descending path hypothesis involves the point of path termination. Yeomans (1982), Wise (1980), and others have speculated that the dopamine and perhaps non-dopamine cells of the ventral tegmental area are the most prominent targets of the descending path (see Figure 6.7). The 2-DG studies (Gallistel, 1983) tell us that these cells are certainly activated (see Figure 6.3). In addition, low threshold ESB sites nicely track the dopamine cell groups in this area (Corbett and Wise, 1980) as shown in Figure 6.9. Further, pharmacological studies suggest an involvement of dopamine in reward and in motor function (Kelley & Stinus, 1983; Wise, 1980). However, there is some disagreement (see Figure 7.7) in which the ESB reward path is postulated to largely bypass the dopamine neurons (Neill et al., 1982). The issue of dopamine involvement in ESB reward is a long and interesting story that is taken up in chapter 7.

Despite the massive amount of evidence supporting dopamine's role in ESB reward, there are some reasons to pause and think carefully before assigning the dopamine-containing cells the role of the second stage in ESB reward of the hypothalamus. The first reason was articulated by Peter Shizgal in an informal symposium preceeding the 1983 Neurosciences meeting (both authors were attending). This is that the excitability characteristics of dopamine neurons are such that they appear to be low-pass filters when compared to the characteristics of the directly excited, ESB reward-relevant axons (Gallistel et al., 1981). For example,

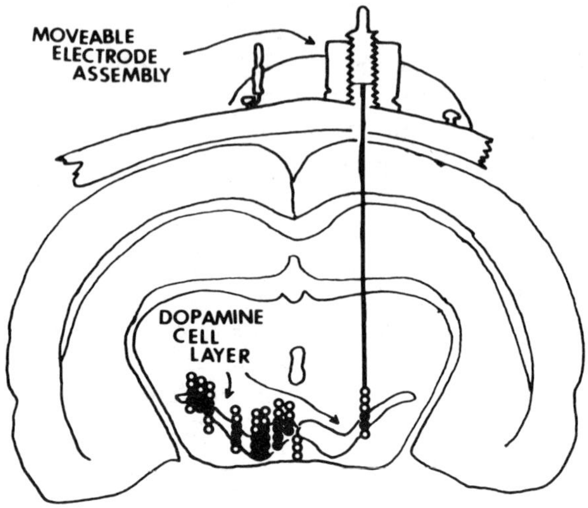

Figure 6.9 Movable electrode study that found a close agreement between sites of low threshold ESB self-stimulation and the anatomical distribution of the midbrain dopamine neurons. Closed symbols indicate low threshold and high rate self-stimulation electrode sites. Open symbols indicate sites of high threshold and low rate, or no ESB self-stimulation. This figure was provided by D.Corbett and is based upon his work with R.Wise (1981).

dopamine neurons have a low maximum following frequency beyond which they fail to follow applied stimulation pulses. As Shizgal pointed out, it seems odd from an engineering perspective to have a neural system with higher frequency capacity (the descending path) feed into one with a lower capacity as a second stage. However, some kind of faithful frequency compression could occur, allowing the firing of dopamine neurons to represent any level of input, but on a different scale. This general principle of transformation and compression is not strange to psychology. It is one of the oldest principles whereby a dimension of a peripheral physical stimulus, such as light intensity, is represented as a perception, such as brightness (e.g., first the Weber-Fechner law and then Steven's power law, Kling & Riggs, 1972). However, the existence of precedent is not, in itself, a strong recommendation for belief in a notion.

Some light can be shed on the issue of the dopamine cell's potential for consideration as the second stage of ESB reward activation by looking at the electrophysiology of the dopamine neurons. First, neurons in the ventral tegmental area were studied electrophysiologically and dopamine neurons were identified by their neurochemical properties. The dopamine neurons were found to have a specific set of electrophysiological characteristics—refractory period, rate of firing, duration of action potential (Guynet & Aghajanian, 1978; Yim & Mogenson, 1980, German et al., 1980). Then, using these indicators, Maeda and Mogenson (1981) showed that ESB pulses, given to the lateral hypothalamus, profoundly influenced the activity of these dopamine neurons exciting some, inhibiting others. All of this work was done in anesthetized animals.

Others (Steinfels, Strecker, Haym, & Jacobs, 1982; Steinfels, Haym, Strecker & Jacobs, 1983) have investigated the activity of dopamine neurons in freely moving animals. Unfortunatly for our purposes, these studies were not performed on the ventral tegmental area, but were performed on the nearby substantia nigra. This is interesting because this structure is a site of ESB reward, but it is not the focus of activity in the 2-DG autoradiographic studies discussed above. Steinfels et al. (1982, 1983) found that the substantia nigra neurons do not change their activity very much with behavior, but rather seem to provide more of a tonic background level upon which behavior is superimposed. They do not, for example, fire off a burst of action potentials just as a hungry animal sees or eats food. Thus, these neurons do not seem to behave like natural food reward or reinforcement detectors. However, caution is required because it is not clear that we know what a "reward detector" behaves like, although Rolls (1977) seems to have no difficulty in finding reward-relevant neurons in the hypothalamus.

It is also not clear that we have yet devised adequate tests of behavioral conditioning and other aspects of the operation of an operant reinforcer. Finally, the area studied was not the ventral tegmental area, which may have different characteristics. Also, Steinfels et al. (1982, 1983) did find impressive changes in substantia nigra unit activity when the animal oriented toward a stimulus (e.g., the experimenter opening the chamber door), but the change was a decrease in firing rate.

The Frontal Cortex: ESB Reward from Another Site

Self-stimulation behavior of the frontal cortex is different in a number of ways from that of the hypothalamus, suggesting differing substrates for the two systems. In comparison with hypothalamic self-stimulators, some of those differences are: Animals implanted with medial frontal cortex electrodes press at lower rates, show less behavioral arousal or excitement, and show slow acquisition of self-stimulation behavior when first tested (Routtenberg & Sloan, 1972; Douglin & Glassman, 1979). To start with the last of these phenomena, medial prefrontal cortex-implanted animals require a number of sessions of "practice" before they will press for ESB. This "practice" may be enforced on them by confining the rats in a chamber and administering non-contingent ESB. Such a procedure will greatly facilitate response acquisition (Corbett et al., 1982b). On the basis of this observation, one could conclude that the ESB does not acquire its rewarding properties until some unspecified process such as kindling has occurred. In support of this notion, diazepam and phenobarbital treatments, which suppress seizure development, will block the above "practice" effect (Robertson, Laferriere, & Milner, 1982b). However, these same treatments do not diminish already established self-stimulation behavior, suggesting that established self-stimulation does not depend upon seizure activity for its reward effect.

The slow acquisition may also be attributable to another process. Frontal cortex lesions are well known for their ability to interfere with the learning of complex operant behaviors (Kolb, Nonneman, & Singh, 1974). ESB may have some similar effects as lesions by enforcing a disorganizing rhythmic pattern on the subtle and complex regional activity of the brain. Cortical ESB has been shown to disorganize language in humans, leading to temporary aphasia for the duration of the stimulus (Penfield & Rasmussen, 1950). In a test of this notion, Corbett, Silva, and Stellar (in press) have shown that previous practice with the lever-pressing operant can greatly facilitate the acquisition of medial frontal cortex self-stimulation. They have also shown that, in a period ranging from day 1 to day 15 following the establishment of self-stimulation, rates of response rise steadily; but the locus of rise measure of reward pulse effectiveness taken from the reward summation function does *not* change. This means the ESB reward is not increasing over the same period while rates are still improving. As a possible corollary to this finding, it has been shown that frontal cortex self-stimulation produces a moderate motoric or behavioral suppression effect on a variety of neurological tests (Wilcott, 1981; Corbett & Stellar, 1983). This motor-suppressive effect does not dissipate with acquisition of and experience with self-stimulation. However, it is possible that the animal may learn strategies to improve responding, and this could account for part of the improvement seen in the 1- to-15-day period discussed above.

The motor-suppressive effect of medial frontal cortex ESB may also help to explain the slow response rates for this ESB site as opposed to the hypothalamus sites. Another subtler consideration is that the temporal characteristics of the frontal cortex ESB reward itself may be longer or more prolonged than those of hypothalamic ESB reward. Although no direct measurements have been made on temporal integration in the frontal cortex, it is known that in comparison to lateral hypothalamus, refractory periods are longer and the summation of reward effects is poor between the hypothalamus and frontal cortex ESB sites (Schenk & Shizgal, 1982; Silva et al., 1982). This points to differences in the substrates between the two systems as discussed previously. If the reward effect generated by a brief ESB burst given to the frontal cortex were to last a long time, then this could explain the slow responding along the line of "one shot and you're good for the whole day," a comment from one researcher in the field (Corbett, personal communciation).

Few studies have been done on the functional anatomy of the efferent path of ESB reward from the medial frontal cortex. One study by Corbett et al. (1982b) shows that ipsilateral accumbens or medial forebrain bundle lesions do not alter frontal cortex self-stimulation, but transection of fiber pathways leading out of the medial frontal cortex in a lateral direction does drastically suppress self-stimulation behavior. These transections leave the animal normal in feeding behavior and in general appearance. They probably cut pathways going to the sulcal cortex (Beckstead, 1979; Nauta, 1964), which is especially interesting since the sulcal cortex is another region of the frontal cortex that supports self-stimulation (Clavier & Gerfen, 1979), and ESB delivered to the sulcal cortex can facilitate the ordinarily slow acquisition of medial frontal cortex self-stimulation (Robertson et al., 1982a). Thus, it appears that the reward effects of ESB in the medial frontal cortex may look more to other cortical regions than to subcortical regions for the relevant circuitry. This thought is confirmed by the work on 2-DG shown in Figure 6.3. Inspection of this figure reveals little or no subcortical activation outside the medial dorsal nucleus of the thalamus that serves this region of the cortex. However, activation is found in rhinal or sulcal cortex, the claustrum, and the amygdala (Gallistel, 1983).

As a final note, we would like to observe that medial frontal cortex is connected to the sulcal cortex (Beckstead, 1979) and the sulcal cortex has projections to the entorhinal cortex, which connects through the perforant path with the hippocampus (Nauta, 1964; Nauta & Domiseck, 1983). These are all ESB reward sites and are all linked anatomically. Work in this area may yield another ESB reward path that could provide an intersting contrast to the medial forebrain bundle. Perhaps we will someday be able to see how the cortical and subcortical mechanisms operate in parallel and/or work together at certain anatomical points (e.g. the amygdala).

Single Unit Recording

A powerful way to study the substrate of ESB reward is to look at the neurons activated by the ESB. This gives anatomical information, since the location of both the stimulating and recording electrode is known. By testing properties of the neuron, such as whether the recorded action potentials are rigidly time-locked to the stimulation, one can get information about whether the connection is direct or transsynaptic. If direct, then refractory and conduction velocity estimates can be obtained as well as other properties such as accommodation, supernormal and/or subnormal periods. If the connection is indirect, then the sign of the stimulation effect can be found, (i.e., excitatory or inhibitory), and temporal integration properties can be explored. Often, periods of excitation are followed by inhibition, or vice versa (Rolls, 1974). In general, then, this is a method by which a great deal of information can be gathered; however, the problem remains of identifying ESB *reward-relevant* neurons from coactivated but reward-irrelevant ones. Here, psychophysical measurments can play a strong role by providing a list of expected characteristics of the neural systems determining ESB reward. For a recent discussion of these issues and recent work, see Shizgal et al. (1982) and Shizgal & Rompre (1984).

As of this time, very little has been done in correlating specific properties of the ESB reward substrate determined by psychophysical methods with single unit recording. One study by Matthews (1978), looked for strength–duration properties of units that were determined behaviorally in a previous study (Matthews, 1977). He found, in the brainstem, a variety of units that together could account for the characteristics observed behaviorally, but he was not able to use this information to pinpoint a specific region as being potentially ESB reward-relevant. Two reasons accounted for this: One was the fact that he did not have a good, specific set of places to search. For example, the 2-DG data of today were not available then. Second, he was not able to employ the conduction velocity or many of the other parametric facts available today (Gallistel et al., 1981) to strengthen the identification. Refractory period information determined by others (e.g., Rolls, 1971) have been used (Gallistel, 1983) to make a few inferences about the substrate for self-stimulation, but this is minor compared to the role to be played by research that purposefully brings together electrophysiology and ESB reward psychophysics.

Another advantage of the unit recording method is that one can test natural stimuli, if the animal is awake and relatively free to behave while the recording is being done. Rolls (1974, 1975, 1976, 1977) and his associates have conducted such experiments in the rhesus monkey. Looking anterior in the medial forebrain bundle, Rolls (1977) has found lateral hypothalamic units that respond to food and water. Some of the hypothalamic units responded best only to the sight of food, and others (fewer) responded best to the taste. Specificity was seen in that units could be found that responded best to water, but little to a 5% sucrose solution. Responses could be excitatory or inhibitory to these natural stimuli. Often these units could become conditioned. For example, glucose was administered orally in a syringe, and after several trials the sight of the syringe itself elicited the unit response. These effects diminished with repeated presentation as the animal satiated, and Rolls (1975) proposed that these units are controlled by deprivation state. Self-stimulation was found, with low thresholds at these sites, indicating a possible tie-in with ESB reward. Other evidence of a tie-in comes from noting that these same units that responded to food would also often respond to stimulation at rewarding ESB sites in the sulcal cortex, accumbens, and dorsomedial nucleus of the thalamus (Rolls, 1976, 1977).

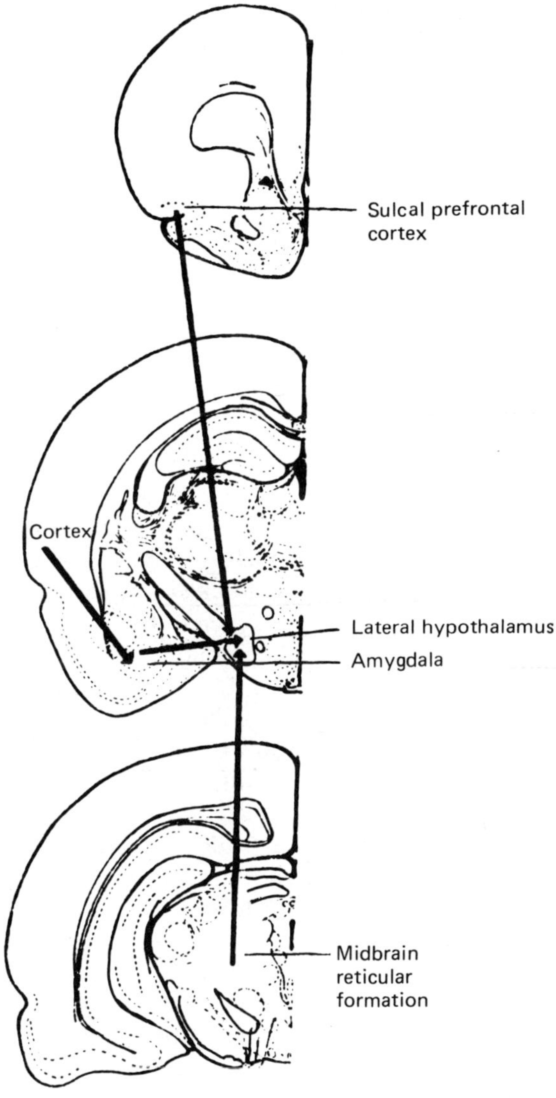

Figure 6.10 A summary of electrophysiological data showing convergence on the lateral hypothalamus from various ESB sites. (Rolls, 1979.) Reprinted by permission.

The anatomical interpretation of this research is represented in Figure 6.10, which shows a schematic of how several sites of ESB might relate to each other. This diagram is based on observations of where rewarding ESB electrodes were located that could drive units in the lateral hypothalamus (Rolls, 1975). It raises the issue of connections that go into the brainstem, where ESB reward effects can also be found (Milliaressis et al. 1982). It also raises the issue of how the sulcal cortex and amygdala might relate to the hypothalamus. Remember that previous ablation work, some of it psychophysical (Huston & Borbely, 1974; Huston, 1982; Stellar et al., 1982), showed the hypothalamus to be capable of sustaining unaltered self-stimulation after the loss of sulcal cortex and amygdala. However, this does not mean that these systems are not tied together in the intact animal, even if lesions can demonstrate a certain independence.

Summary

Discussion of the anatomy of self-stimulation has now led us into several other topics. We have gone beyond the hypothalamus to consider other ESB reward sites, and raised the problem of how various ESB sites relate to each other. We have also raised the larger problem of how ESB reward sites relate to natural rewards of food or water. Let us take the ESB site-to-site relation problem first. The conclusion here is that sites along the medial forebrain bundle look very much like they are activating the same neural systems. This is a necessary conclusion from the descending path hypothesis but would remain a likely possibility based on refractory period, 2-DG, and other data, even if the descending path hypothesis were denied. One complication is that the behavior of animals with various placements along the medial forebrain bundle varies a bit from site to site. The hope of the descending path hypothesis would be that these behavioral variations are explained by *side effects* such as partial activation of the nearby fibers of the internal capsule or aversive effects from current spread to the ventromedial hypothalamus.

To look at sites outside the medial forebrain bundle, the ESB of the medial frontal cortex seems to be activating a very different system with little overlap with the hypothalamic system. This may come as a surprise to some, considering the well-known connections of the frontal cortex and the hypothalamus that, among other things, has led to the identification of regions of the frontal cortex with the limbic system. However, as noted above, this absence of dependence one on the other for an ESB reward effect does not mean that these areas are not tied to each other in some subtle but important way. If we could identify, with certainty, individual neurons in one region, for example, the medial forebrain bundle—which mediated the ESB reward effect, then we could follow them anatomically and begin to get a handle on the area-to-area interaction problem and perhaps address the problem of function.

The problem of relating ESB reward at an any site to natural rewards is even more difficult. We will briefly consider this question in the next chapter from a pharmacological perspective and in the overview chapter of the book on a largely phenomenological level. To try to approach this question on a neural level seems impossible at this time. Yet it is interesting to note that many researchers acknowledge privately that it was just this problem of investigating that neural basis of natural reward or reinforcement that led them to the field of self-stimulation research in the first place. One irony in this is that if the current round of psychophysical and other experiments aimed at identifying the properties of the neural system(s) mediating ESB reward are successful, then the field may go even further away from psychological concerns and into neurophysiology as we try to identify the neurotransmitter(s) of the directly excited neurons or determine other neural properties. We may become bioengineers of the ESB reward-relevant neural systems. Although this seems to be moving away from the question of function, the hope is that once we are in possession of a critical mass of solid neurobiological facts, we will be able to build back to behavior (synthesis). The further hope is that this can be done in a powerful and careful way that will yield a high-quality, circuit-like model of at least part of the ESB reward effect.

7
Dopamine and ESB Reward

In this chapter, we explore the role(s) that dopamine systems might play in ESB and other rewards, principally through the study of pharmacological evidence. Again, our discussion is concerned with the problem of behavior–physiology linkage. Although here the problem seems particularly subtle and complex. There are multiple components to be considered in the structure and function of dopamine systems. Difficult questions arise about the effects of dopamine on behavior, such as the separation of motor arousal and reward, or even the adequacy of these terms to describe dopamine's actions. Additionally, research in this area spans a broad range of techniques and methods. It is problematic to know how to compare studies as different from each other as the attenuation of ESB self-stimulation by dopamine blockade, dopamine agonist self-administration, food reward extinction induced by dopamine blockade, open field locomotion, or akinesia and catalepsy induced by dopamine lesions. These techniques may reveal different facets of dopamine function, each of which may be fundamentally related or independent.

This area of research is fertile, busy, and always somewhat controversial. For example, see Wise's (1982) article on the reward hypothesis of dopamine function. The article and the following open peer commentary are a good illustration of the interest in and diversity of opinions about dopamine's functions. Generally, interest in a research area can be measured roughly by the number of published papers on the subject. According to our informal survey in one journal, *Pharmacology, Biochemistry, & Behavior,* issues from the years of 1982 and 1983 listed 118 publications concerned with dopamine. Of these, 32 were directly concerned with the issue of reward and/or motor-arousal explanations of dopamine function, with 22 focusing on ESB self-stimulation and the remaining 10 concerned with either food or other natural rewards or with an analysis of response pattern. The other publications focused on more anatomical issues (20), dopamine receptors (14), neonatal dopamine manipulations (8), or relations to other drugs and neurochemical systems (44). With this much activity in one journal and many other journals to consider, it is obvious that any single chapter on this subject can give only a small part of the story.

It should also be remembered that the results of reward studies may depend critically on the behavioral methods employed to assess drug effects. As discussed in chapter 5, simple rate of response measures, whether for ESB or natural rewards, are simply inadequate. They do not discriminate between rate reductions due to performance impairments and those due to a degradation of the reward sustaining the response. Even so-called "rate-free" measures may have surprises built into them and must be verified against physical obstacles, known performance-debilitating drugs, and/or other standard procedures before serving as the basis for interpretations. Finally, modern techniques include measures that are able to provide some quantitative information on both the effectiveness of the reinforcer and on the performance capacity of the subject under drugs. In our opinion, we are in a time when research in this field of dopamine function demands increasingly subtle assessments of changes in both motoric and reward effects. Therefore, it is important that these more delicate questions are approached with more refined techniques. Many advances have been made in the number and selectivity of drugs, in the understanding of receptor–ligand interactions, and in our ability to assay the brain for its neurochemical content. This progress is critical to the advancement of the field, but sophistication in behavioral measurement must not take a back seat to sophistication in pharmacological method or neurochemical technique.

Some Basic Facts

Some basic facts that are widely agreed on seem worth delineating at the outset. The first of these is that mammals, including humans, will act in such a way so as to promote dopamine transmitter release thus mimicking the action of the brain's dopamine-containing systems. For example, they will vigorously self-administer dopamine or its agonists to their brains through oral, intravenous, or intraventricular routes (Wise, 1980). Rats will even inject dopamine agonists directly into the nucleus accumbens (Hoebel, et al., 1982) or the frontal cortex (Goeders & Smith, 1983). Additionally, the same behaviors are seen in humans who self-administer the dopamine agonistic drugs, amphetamine and cocaine, and subsequently report the subjective feelings of pleasure. It is difficult to imagine why these organisms would perform these behaviors unless the action of dopamine in the brain were rewarding. Much of the material presented in this chapter is concerned with showing that dopamine release can have reward properties, but let us consider one interesting experiment here.

Perhaps one of the best demonstrations of the propensity of mammals to seek dopamine activation comes from a study on rats by Fray, Dunnett, Iversen, Björklund, and Stenevi (1983). These researchers took advantage of the newly developed ability to transplant fetal dopamine cells into adult rats that were deprived of dopamine via an earlier 6-hydroxy dopamine (6-OHDA) lesion. These tissue grafts grow into and appear to reinnervate the previously denervated dopamine regions of the forebrain. Fray et al. then implanted those grafts with electrodes and were able to demonstrate that the rats would press levers to obtain electrical stimulation of the implant, which presumably triggered release of dopamine by the activated cells. Furthermore, the rats could be induced to press at increasing rates by giving increasing ESB currents. The rate–intensity function itself and the maximum rates achieved are impressive (Figure 7.1).

This preparation solves many of the problems of studying ESB self-stimulation and drug self-administration. Because the dopamine cell bodies are physically isolated from surrounding brain tissue, there is no question which cells are stimulated by the ESB electrode and whether non-dopamine cells residing in the dopamine cell region are really mediating this reward effect. Such an objection might be made in reference to ventral tegmental and substantia nigra ESB self-stimulation maps (Corbett & Wise, 1980; Wise, 1981), showing the concordance between dopamine-containing regions of the rat brain and sites of ESB self-stimulation (see Figure 6.9). It could be argued that drug self-administration studies also very selectively implicate the dopamine systems in reward (Pickens & Thompson, 1968; Yokel & Pickens, 1974; Yokel & Wise, 1976; Ettenberg, Pettit, Bloom, & Koob, 1982). The difference here is that in the Fray et al. (1983) study, a natural compound (dopamine) is self-administered along a natural route (a synapse), achieving a specificity of activation impossible with systemic or intraventricular injection, and avoiding the artificiality of a cannulae implant into a local brain region.

A second much-agreed-about fact comes from a scientific history older than ESB reward and implicates dopamine in motor function. This is the study of Parkinson's disease, a motor dysfunction syndrome of akinesia, muscular rigidity, and resting tremor. A major cause of Parkinson's disease is a severe dopamine loss in the corpus striatum which is in turn triggered by primary degeneration of the substantia nigra in the basal midbrain (Pletscher, 1976). This disorder, its cause, and its treatment with the compound l-dopa or other dopamine agonistic agents is one of the best success stories of clinical neurochemistry. Here, a behavioral

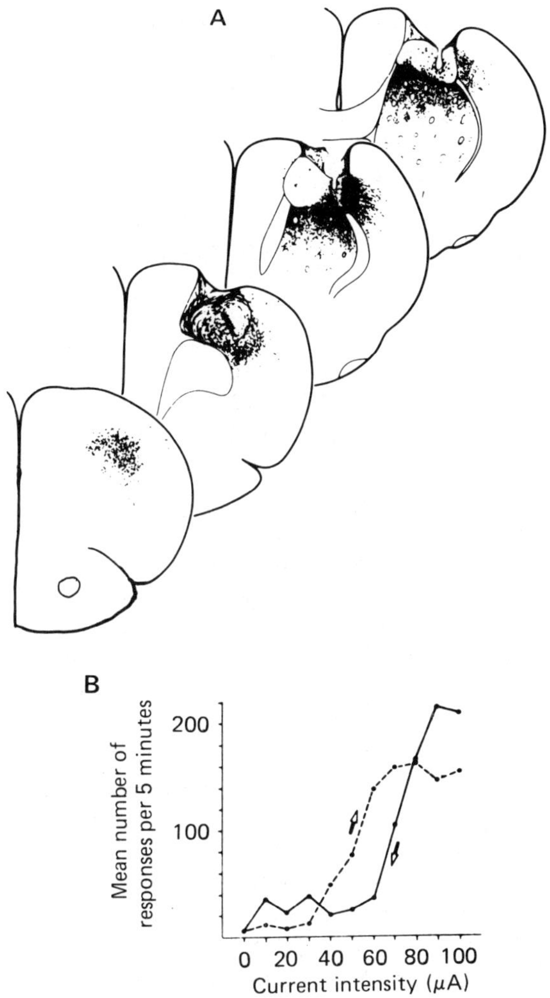

Figure 7.1 Histological and behavioral analysis of an implant of fetal substantia nigra tissue into an adult rat previously depleted of dopamine by 6-OHDA lesion. (A) Histology reveals a novel pattern of dopamine innervation of the caudate and cortex and shows, in the the uppermost brain section, the dopamine cell bodies clumped around a hole in the implanted tissue where the electrode was before it was removed. (B) This graph shows the profile of responding for ESB in a lever press task as the A.C. current was varied in either an increasing or decreasing fashion. (Fray et al., 1983.) Reprinted by permission.

disorder is understood to have at its foundation a particular physiological change. This structure–function linkage was recently and tragically confirmed in some young drug users who injected themselves with a synthetic heroin that was accidentally contaminated with a compound known as MPTP (1-methyl-4-phenyl-1, 2, 5, 6-tetrahydropyridine). They soon presented themselves in a hospital with a severe Parkinsonian syndrome that was shown, in one case examined at autopsy, to have been accompanied by degeneration in the substantia nigra (Langston, Ballard, Tetrud, & Irwin, 1983).

In addition to the major symptoms of Parkinson's disease discussed above, patients with advanced cases also can have wooden or expressionless faces, have great difficulty initiating voluntary movements, and require complete nursing care (Pletscher, 1976). However, they can show expression and vigorous movement in times of crisis or emergency. This observation suggests that the motor circuits are not ablated by the progressive dopamine cell loss, but are only progressively more difficult to arouse. This hypothesis is reinforced by the first treatment of Parkinsonian patients with 1-dopa when that therapy initially became available in medical history. Such patients "awakened" from their motionlessness to a much more normal function when treated (Sacks, 1973).

Animal studies have also revealed motor activation deficits following destruction of the dopamine systems of the nigro-striatal pathway. Here, it is stressed that dopamine deactivation leads to the akinesia seen with Parkinson's disease. For example, Figure 7.2 shows the effects on a rat of profound dopamine-depleting lesions with intraventricular injections of the neuro-toxin 6-OHDA. These rats are akinetic, like Parkinson patients. The rats are also cataleptic, assuming and holding postures for unusually long periods of time, and they possess a lack of sensory–motor integration (Marshall, 1979; Marshall & Teitelbaum, 1974; Teitelbaum et al., 1983). Such akinetic and cataleptic rats can be aroused and show normal behavior following the presentation of strong stimuli (Marshall, Levitan & Stricker, 1976; Stricker & Zigmond, 1976b).

The long-held explanation of the above phenomenon is that the motor system requires dopamine for its activation but does not use dopamine for the actual circuit of behavioral execution. This thinking fits with the well-known replacement therapy of 1-dopa or dopamine agonist administration for the Parkinson patient or the rat made akinetic by 6-OHDA lesions. It also fits with the observation that the dopamine neurons appear not to fire in response to the pattern and timing of movements, but rather maintain a steady level of activity suitable for setting the "tone" or arousal level of the motor system (Steinfels et al., 1982). Finally, the fact that the fetal cell transplant experiments of substantia nigra tissue can ameloriate the akinesia and the sensory–motor deficits of rats (Dunnett et al., 1983) again suggests that tonic dopamine release is more important than behavior-locked phasic release. Certainly, it is hard to

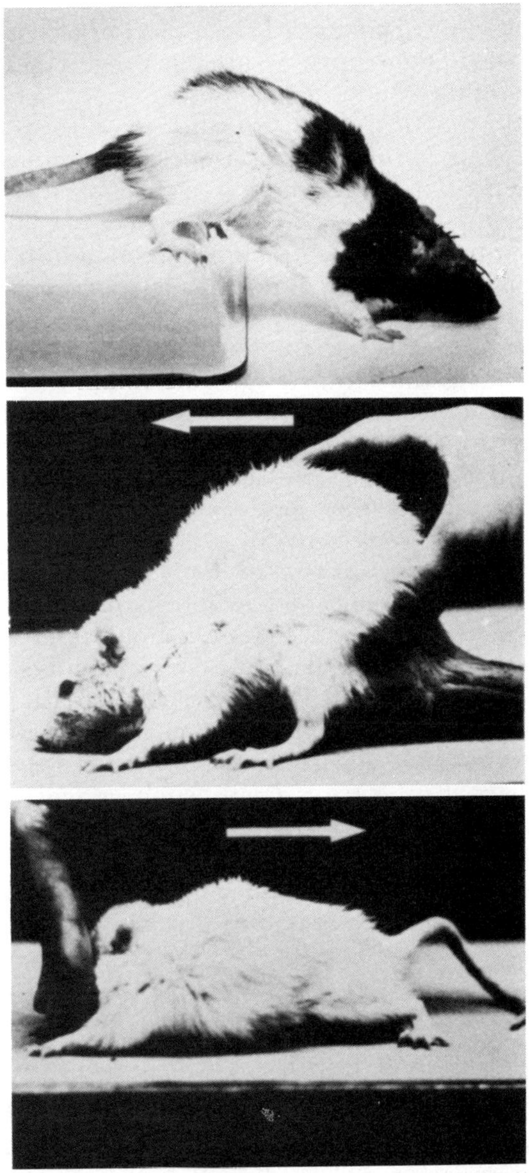

Figure 7.2 Two rats with sustained severe dopamine depletion as a result of intraventricular injection of 6-OHDA. Both rats are akinetic and cataleptic. On the top, one rat is shown in an unusual posture that it maintained for a long time. Below, in two views, an akinetic rat is shown actively resisting displacement. (Schallert et al., 1978, top; 1979, bottom.)

imagine that these transplanted cells fit into a normal circuit since they are placed directly in the corpus striatum and not at the location of the substantia nigra in the ventral tegmentum.

In contrast, dopamine agonists promote motoric activation, and this activation can take many forms. One form is behavioral stereotypy, which consists of repetition of a small portion of the animal's behavioral repertoire in seeming disconnection from environmental control. Stereotypy can be produced by high doses of amphetamine, which has this action because it promotes the release of dopamine from stores in the presynaptic nerve terminals. This stereotypy may be a function of activation of dopamine in the caudate nucleus, since amphetamine does not induce stereotypy in animals with caudate nucleus lesions. Also, following the development of postsynaptic receptor supersensitivity in the caudate after the loss of presynaptic dopamine terminals, stereotypy can be produced by direct dopamine receptor stimulation with apomorphine (Kelley & Stinus, 1984). Because the supersensitivity can be restricted to the caudate by selective depletion, stereotypy can be said to arise from dopamine actions in this structure as opposed to dopamine actions in general.

In lower doses, amphetamine and apomorphine produce locomotion. Often this locomotion contains a preponderance of left or right turns. This has been related to a dominance of dopamine function in the right or left side of the brain, respectively (Glick & Ross, 1981). Although it is now seen as complex, turning or rotation provides a useful model for looking at the dopamine-release or receptor-activating properties of drugs, especially in animals treated with lesions to enhance the natural asymmetry of dopamine. This work has contributed much to the current understanding of the pharmacology and physiology of the dopamine systems and the mechanisms of amphetamine and apomorphine action discussed above. For a fuller review, see Ungerstedt (1971b) and Pycock (1980).

Dopamine Brain Systems

The classic histofluorescence work of Dahlstrom and Fuxe (1964), Ungerstedt (1971a), and Lindvall and Björklund (1974) resulted in the designation of three dopamine cell groups with long fibers and diffuse forebrain projections: A8, A9, A10. Of these, the substantia nigra, pars compacta (A9), and the ventral tegmental area (A10) are the principal structures, with the smaller, more caudal area A8 often considered along with area A9. Amino acid autoradiographic studies of the efferent projections of these regions reveal a topographic projection in which the ventral and medial dopamine cells (ventral tegmental area) project most heavily to the more ventral and medial structures of the forebrain such as medial prefrontal cortex, accumbens, olfactory bulb, septum, and amygdala. The more dorsal and lateral cells (substantia nigra) project to the more dorsal and laterally placed caudate nucleus (Fallon and Moore, 1978). These two types of projections are illustrated in Figure 7.3 A and B and are summarized in Figure 7.3C. The ultra-short (retina and olfactory bulb) or intermediate length (tuberohypophyseal, incertohypothalamic, medullary periventricular) dopamine systems are not considered in this chapter.

In addition to these projections, the dopamine cell groups receive connections from the structures that they innervate. These connections involve other neurotransmitters and serve to regulate the activity of the dopamine cells themselves. This probably accounts for the observation,

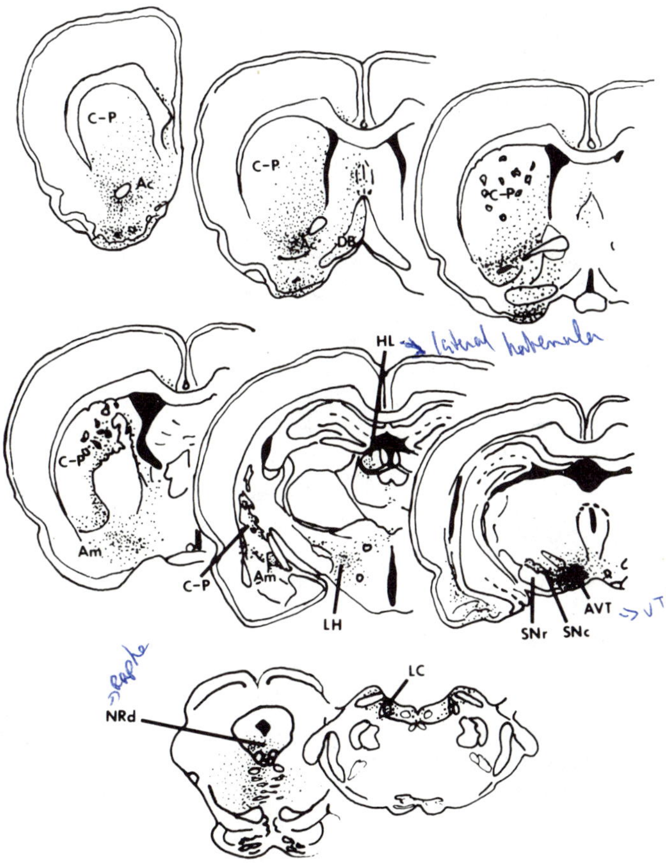

A

Figure 7.3A Anatomical projections (fine dots) of the ventral tegmental area of the rat as they are revealed by the autoradiographic method. Abbreviations as in 7.3C. (Beckstead et al., 1979.) Reprinted by permission.

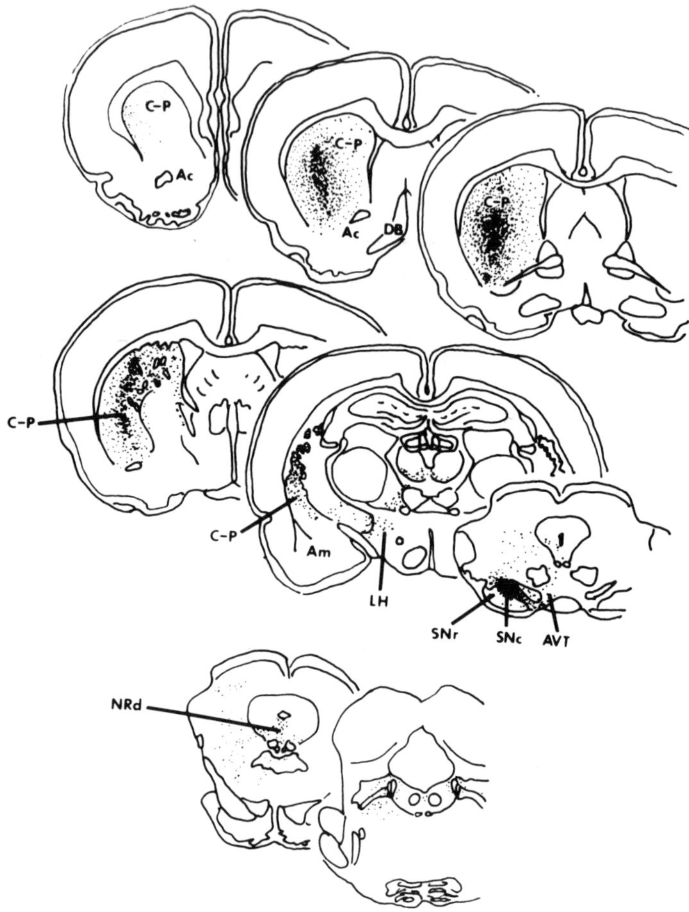

Figure 7.3B Anatomical projections (fine dots) of the substantia nigra as revealed by the autoradiographic method. Abbreviations as in 7.3C. (Beckstead et al., 1979.) Reprinted by permission.

discussed above, that these cells are fairly consistent in their activity pattern. While a consideration of the feedback control of the dopamine neurons is beyond the scope of this chapter, it is important to remind oneself of the existence of the feedback loops, as seen in Figure 7.3D for the substantia nigra. In addition, this figure shows the location of autoreceptors on the dopamine cells that are sensitive to dopamine release. One of these autoreceptors is found on the terminal, another on the cell body, and still another on the dendrites that extend into the reticular zone of the substantia nigra. Autoreceptors contribute to the stability of dopamine release by regulating the synthesis and release as

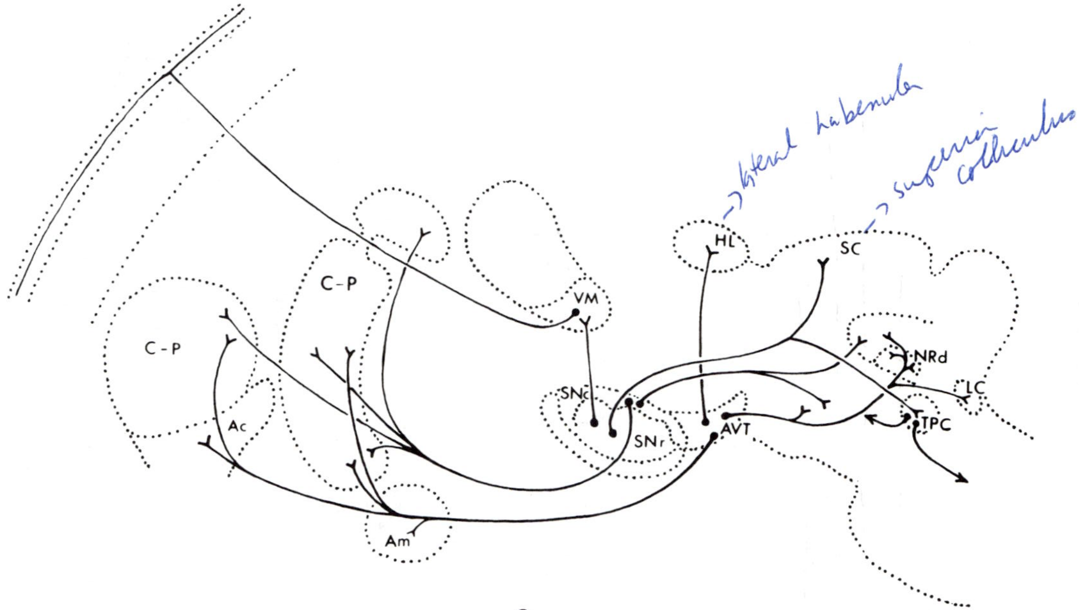

C

Figure 7.3C Summary of the anatomical projections from the ventral tegmental area and the substantia nigra, based on work as shown in Figures 7.3A & B. Abbreviations are: Ac = accumbens; Am = amygdala; AVT = ventral tegmental area; C–P = caudate–putamen; HL = lateral habenula; LC = locus coeruleus; LH = lateral hypothalamus; NRd = dorsal raphe nucleus; SC = superior colliculus; SNr & SNc = substantia nigra (pars reticulata and compacta, respectively); TPC = pedunculopontine nucleus; VM = ventral medial thalamus. (Beckstead et al., 1979.) Reprinted by permission.

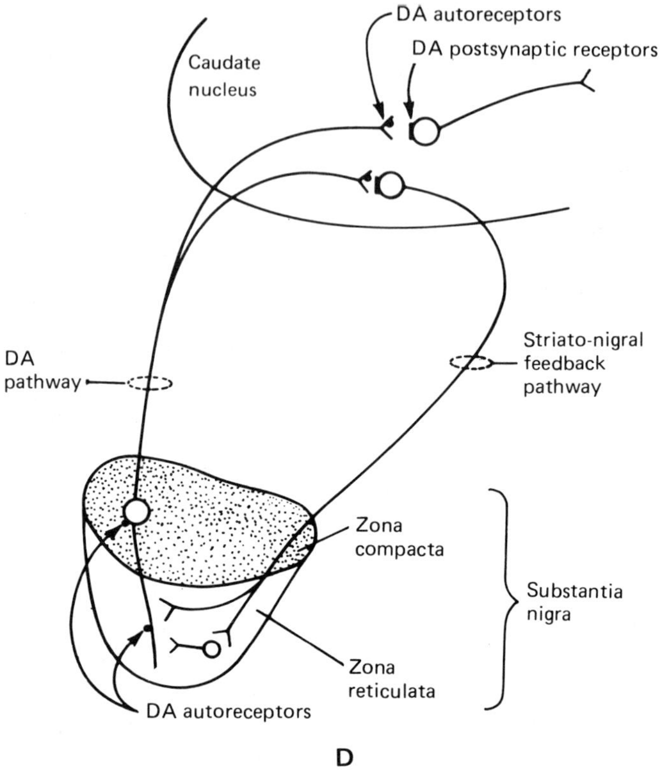

Figure 7.3D Feedback loop controlling activity in the substantia nigra. Also shown are the locations of autoreceptors, which constitute another form of feedback. DA = dopamine (Bunney, 1983.) Reprinted by permission.

well as the rate of firing of the cell. Their activation results in a decrease in dopamine output (Bunney, 1983). The substantia nigra serves as a general model for the ventral tegmental area, although differences exist in the source of the feedback and some cells are thought not to have autoreceptors.

Because the substantia nigra projects to a classically defined motor structure, there is a natural tendency to see the substantia nigra projections as being entirely motor. Correspondingly, ventral tegmental area projections are heavily limbic, and it is tempting to classify them as being motivational. However, this goes against the observation that the substantia nigra and caudate nucleus are ESB sites (Gerfen et al., 1982). Such a dichotomy also over-simplifies the basic anatomy, since the exact boundaries between substantia nigra and ventral tegmental area are poorly defined, and these two regions may really be part of a continuum of cells. Labeled amino acid injection intermediate between these two structures results in an intermediate pattern of terminal distribution (Fallon & Moore, 1978; Beckstead, Domesick, & Nauta, 1979). In addition, interconnections exist between the substantia nigra and ventral tegmental systems, as discussed below. Finally, ESB administered at the ventral tegmental area results in activity in the substantia nigra A9 area (Porrino et al., 1984, Figure 1).

The issue of interconnections between nigral and ventral tegmental dopamine systems is illustrated in Figure 7.4, which is drawn by one of the authors (J.S.) from a recent colloquium given by Nauta on his and other work on limbic–motor anatomy. (See Domesick, 1981; Nauta and Domesick, 1983, for details). The figure shows how activation in the ventral tegmental area may find its way back to the substantia nigra, where motor effects can occur. Nauta refers to this anatomical connection as an example of "handshaking" between the limbic and motor systems. The handshaking concept is important since the tradition in neurology and neurophysiology has been to treat the limbic and motor systems as quite separate entities with essentially non-overlapping structure and

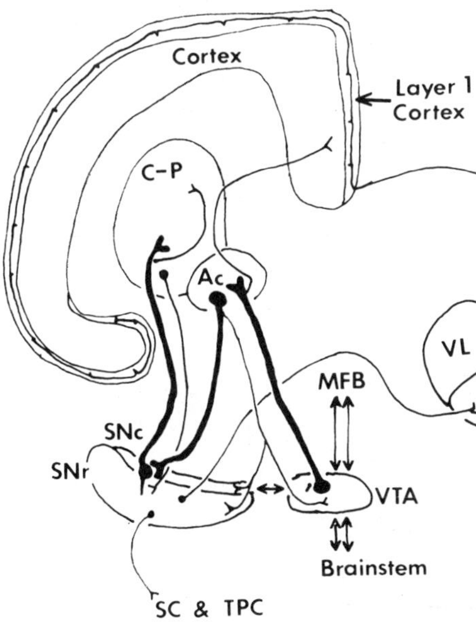

Figure 7.4 Anatomical interconnections of the ventral tegmental area and substantia nigra in the rat, emphasizing with heavy lines the way activation of the ventral tegmental area could lead into substantia nigra activity. MFB = medial forebrain bundle; VL = ventral lateral thalamus; VM = ventromedial thalamus; VTA = ventral tegmental area (see Figure 7.3C for additional abbreviations.)
Note. This figure was drawn from a colloquium of W.J.H. Nauta, Harvard (1982) to emphasize what he described as an example of motor–limbic handshaking. Heavier lines do not indicate a stronger anatomical projection.

function. While the separation between the systems is complete enough to warrant two names, the interaction points may actually be more important to us here, and dopamine is a probable interaction point.

Another of the motor–limbic connections may be seen in a motor structure, the caudate-putamen, where its ventral–medial portion and the accumbens, receive fibers from the limbic structures, the amygdala, and the ventral tegmental area (Kelley, Domesick, & Nauta, 1982). In an interesting subtlety, Yim and Mogenson (1980) have shown that dopamine, at some doses, applied iontophoretically to the accumbens does *not* alter the spontaneous activity of accumbens unless the amygdala is first stimulated and the baseline activity of the accumbens is activated. Then, the typical dopamine-induced inhibition of electrophysiological activity is seen. At the end of this chapter, we return to a consideration of the accumbens. For now, we simply note that the motor–limbic handshaking concept is an improvement in our understanding of the role dopamine might play in behavior generation.

Another improvement in our understanding of the dopamine systems has been the recognition that there appear to exist differing forms of dopamine receptors (Creese, Sibley, Hamblin, & Leff, 1983). The primary evidence for this comes from examining the way various drugs bind to dopamine receptors in radioligand binding studies. Although some disagreement exists as to the exact number, and which ones might be subtypes of others, there is basic agreement on the existence of at least two receptors—D1 and D2 (Kebabian & Calne, 1979; Joyce, 1983). The D1 receptor is the classic receptor (Greengard, 1976) which, upon activation, leads to adenylate cyclase activity and the formation of cyclic adenosine monophosphate (cAMP), a second messenger in neurotransmission. By contrast, the D2 receptor either decreases or does not affect cAMP formation.

Different classes of neuroleptics seem to affect the two dopamine receptors differently. For example, the phenothiazines (chlorpromazine) and thioxanthenes (flupenthixol) block both the D1 and D2 receptors, while butyrophenones (haloperidol, spiroperidol) and substituted benzamides (sulpiride) seem to exert stronger effects at the D2 receptor (Kebabian & Calne, 1979; Creese et al., 1983). The agonist, apomorphine, is also much more effective at the D2 receptor. D2 receptors are found prototypically in the pituitary, which gives rise to the hope that some anatomical and functional separation may occur between these receptor types. However, both types of receptors are found in the striatum. The striatal area is made still more complicated by the appearance of a possible third receptor, the D3 type. A detailed review of this literature is beyond the scope of this book, but see reviews by Creese et al. (1983) or Joyce (1983). Much work is now being done on the potencies of various drugs from the above classes on different behaviors ranging from apomorphine-induced climbing in mice to shock avoidance behavior in the rat

(Roth, 1983; Worms, Broekkamp, & Lloyd, 1983). Although multiple dopamine receptors provide a useful new attack on the problems of structure–function linkage, caution is needed because careful examination has shown it to be unlikely that most drugs act on one neurotransmitter system alone, and other nondopaminergic actions may better explain the differences in behavioral effects of some drugs (Joyce, 1983).

ESB Reward and the Effects of Systemic Dopamine Blockade

Against this background of anatomical and chemical complexity, it almost seems a wonder that we can learn anything specific at all about dopamine's role in behavior from systemic treatment with a pharmacological agent. In addition to any non-specific effects, systemic treatment exposes all of the dopamine receptors on all dopamine systems to pharmacological action. Selectivity is achieved only through differences in biochemical interaction with receptors and possibly with regional metabolism. However, much has been learned by taking this approach and it also shares an important similarity with the clinical practice of psychopharmacology, in which all current treatments are systemic.

A number of studies have focused on the attenuation of responding for ESB that is seen when dopamine receptor blocking drugs, such as neuroleptics, are administered to rats. The question has been: is this attenuation of responding due to a blunting of the reinforcing effect of ESB or to motor incapacitation? Two of the early studies that directly tackled this issue with a rate-free paradigm are the extinction studies of Fouriezos and Wise (1976) and of Fouriezos, Hanson, and Wise (1978). In these studies, it was shown that dopamine receptor blockade (e.g., with pimozide) produced extinction-like behavior. That is, rats treated with dopamine receptor blockers were placed in a self-stimulation situation, and observed to begin responding with normal levels of behavior, but to rapidly cease working for ESB reward. The conclusion of these studies was that blocking the dopamine receptors impaired self-stimulation performance by attenuating the ESB reward effect and not by severely reducing motor capacity.

The above conclusions are reinforced by later studies using the double-extinction method. For example, Gallistel, Boytim, Gomita, and Klebanoff (1982) replicated these earlier findings and showed that after dopamine receptor blockade produced "extinction" in one chamber, placing the rat in a new self-stimulation chamber reinstated responding, only to have it extinguish again. This effect on responding of changing the environment can be restricted to a very specific manipulation of turning on a light that, by prior training, signals the occurrence of a new part of the schedule of ESB availability (Franklin & McCoy, 1979). Here, responding is also reinstated, presumably because the rat expects the signaled second component of the schedule to deliver rewarding ESB even if the first component of the schedule did not. Finally, Beninger and Freedman (1982) have shown, in their version of the double-extinction paradigm, that the pimozide-induced extinction seen in the second lever-press test is accelerated by immediate pretesting (and extinction) with lever-pressing but not with a motorically demanding task of wheel-running. These effects all argue against the notion that dopamine blockade produces a severe motoric handicap, but encourage the notion of a loss of reward strength of ESB. This type of a selective reward role is advocated by Wise (1982) in his *anhedonia hypothesis* of dopamine receptor blockade. Supporting these conclusions and extending them somewhat, Wasserman et al., (1982) have shown that delivery of free non-contingent bursts of ESB has the normally expected arousal function of temporarily increasing response vigor. They propose that this motivational or arousal function, termed *priming,* survives the dopamine blockade.

Other studies also support a role for dopamine in ESB reward. For example, in a twist of the conditioned taste-aversion phenomenon, Ettenberg and White (1981) were able to produce conditioned taste preference using pairings between a novel flavor and rewarding ESB that was self-administered. Then they demonstrated that pimozide, administered during the time of the flavor–ESB pairings, decreased the size of the conditioned taste preference. Presumably this occurred because the pimozide blocked the rewarding properties of the ESB enough so that the conditioned taste preference could not develop. In this experiment, one worries about conditioned taste aversions induced by pimozide, but Ettenberg and White saw no evidence of this in their control groups. Because the taste preference was tested well after the drug wore off, no motor effect of pimozide was or could have been seen. Of course, this is the point of the paradigm; and though it enables one to point to a role for dopamine in ESB reward, it does not permit the measurement of any motoric component of dopamine receptor blockade.

Still another paradigm in which dopamine blockade was found to disrupt ESB reward is the autotitration of threshold or set–reset method (see chapter 5 for details). In this paradigm, the subject presses a lever for ESB reward, but the ESB current or frequency progressively decreases with every fifth or so lever press. This decrease occurs until the animal stops and presses a second lever that does not deliver ESB but resets the ESB current or frequency to the maximum allowed. The current or frequency at which the reset lever-press occurs is noted and is called the reset threshold. Systemic administration of dopamine-blocking drugs elevates the reset threshold, and this is taken as a decrease in ESB reward effectiveness (Stein & Ray, 1959; Zarevics & Setler, 1979; Neill et al., 1982). Although some inconsistent effects have been found (Schafer & Michael, 1980) with this method, the basic picture confirms the developing dopamine story with regard to ESB reward.

It should be noted that this set–reset technique and the previous method control away, rather than measure, any motor effects of dopamine blockade. This is both a strength and a weakness of the procedures. It is a strength because ESB reward effects can be assessed without contamination by performance factors. It is a weakness because one does not see the motor factors, and the temptation is to neglect them in formulating theories of dopamine function. Finally, there is some doubt that this method actually measures threshold uncontaminated from extraneous variables, such as the choice of starting level to which the stimulation is reset (Fouriezos & Nawiesniak, 1982; see also chapter 5).

In some small conflict with the selective view of dopamine function stated above, there stand a few quantitative studies of ESB reward that simultaneously measure reward and performance capacity. For example, in one experiment, Stellar et al. (1983) tested the effects of pimozide on the reward summation function in a runway. They looked simultaneously at the locus of rise measure of ESB reward pulse effectiveness and the asymptotic running speed measure of behavioral capacity (see chapter 5 for details of this method). They found evidence for a loss of ESB reward effectiveness following dopamine receptor blockade, but it was not selective. A clearly significant performance impairment was seen at the higher drug doses (0.5 mg/kg pimozide). This was judged by the failure of running speed in the runway to reach the same asymptote or maximal levels as attained in baseline conditions, despite increases in the amount of ESB offered. It should be noted that this higher dose (0.5 mg/kg) is well within the range of doses tested by the extinction studies and is 10 times lower than a dose reported in one study of extinction (Wasserman et al., 1982).

Another study (Hamilton & Stellar, 1983), attacked the problem of pimozide's selectivity on ESB reward using a very different quantitative method. Here, the rat pressed a lever to receive ESB on a variable interval schedule of reinforcement. The density of the variable interval schedule was changed five times to produce a number of observations relating response rate to obtained reinforcement rate. This method (called response strength, see chapter 5) yields a function similar to the reward summation function method, in which reward and motor effects of drugs can be discriminated. Using this method, Hamilton and Stellar (1983) found that pimozide produced a reward impairment, but a performance impairment was also seen, especially at the high dose (0.5 mg/kg).

One quantitative study (Franklin, 1978) using a reward summation function method did not report a motor impairment with dopamine blockade. However, in this study, the baseline locus of rise was very high. This meant that the effectiveness of ESB pulses was low, and that many pulses were required to get the rat to perform the task (running the runway). When moderate to high doses of neuroleptics, including pimozide, were given, they knocked the reward effectiveness down to the point at which the animals would not run and no reward summation function was gathered. Since no function was gathered, Franklin was prevented from determining the performance-monitoring statistic, maximal running speed. Then Franklin was forced to rely on the extinction-like nature of the responding on the initial ESB condition to conclude that motor impairments were absent at these doses. Stellar et al. (1983) note that the locus of rise statistic for their study was significantly lower than in the Franklin study, indicating more effective stimulation pulses. The reason for differences in reward pulse effectiveness has to do with choice of stimulating current, pulse width, electrode site, and other factors. Had more effective ESB pulses been used in baseline in the Franklin (1978) study, maximal running speed could have been measured and performance impairments might have been seen at the higher doses.

Similar results to the above studies were found in the method termed *self-regulation of duration* (Liebman, 1983), which enables the animal to regulate ESB duration by responding in one way to turn on ESB and responding in another way to turn off the ESB. Responding can take the form of pressing one of two levers (ON or OFF) or entering one of two sides of a shuttlebox. A decreased vigor of ON responding in the absence of decreased OFF responding is seen as reflecting a selective loss of ESB reward effectiveness, while in a novel addition to the response measurement capabilities discussed thus far, an increase in OFF responding is seen as reflecting an increase in *aversiveness* of the ESB (Hoebel, 1975). However, if both ON and OFF responses decrease, then the possibility of a motoric impairment exists. In tests with the dopamine receptor blocker, haloperidol, selective decreased ON responding was seen at low doses, but at higher doses, both ON and OFF responding was decreased (Edwards, Wishick, & Sinnamon, 1979; Liebman, Hall, & Prowse, 1982). In one study (Atrens, Ljungberg, & Ungerstedt, 1976), haloperidol always decreased both types of responding. While it is possible that haloperidol acts to both blunt reinforcing and punishing properties of ESB, a motor debilitation effect cannot be excluded.

A number of ESB studies have focused directly on this motor- or performance-debilitating effect of neuroleptics, aiming to demonstrate its existence rather than to show reward effects. For example, Ettenberg, Cinsavich and White (1979) took three groups of rats and put them on real extinction (no reinforcement). In two of these groups, an intermediate (0.25 mg/kg) and high (0.5 mg/kg) dose of pimozide was given. The pimozide groups extinguished faster than the group without pimozide, indicating that a simple blunting of the reward of ESB is not a complete explanation. Further, they showed that pimozide decreases the spontaneous response level of a behavior (nose-poking) that was *never* reinforced. They reason that, if only reward effects were decreased, then pimozide should leave the response level of unreinforced behavior unaltered; but if performance capability were impaired, one might expect the response rate decreases that they found.

Other studies (Rolls et al., 1974; Fibiger et al., 1976) attempting to show that dopamine blockade produces a motor impairment suffer problems of interpretation because they rely on demonstrating preserved responding on simple tasks of chewing and eating food or licking water while more complex responses of lever pressing for ESB are attenuated. The problem is that tasks of different complexity are difficult to compare because different levels of reinforcement are likely to be required for tasks of different difficulty. This is especially true when one of the tasks involves a behavior such as *feeding* which has reflexive components and may be controlled in a very different way by the food reward. The use of feeding as a control is discussed in more detail in an upcoming section on food reward and dopamine.

Even when both tasks are operants, one may not be safe in comparing them because simpler, easier tasks are likely to require less reinforcement to maintain them than more complex, difficult tasks. Therefore, this type of test does not discriminate between motor or reward decrement explanations of lost performance. A recent example of this is a study (Ettenberg, Koob, & Bloom, 1981) that compared the effects of a neuroleptic on responding for ESB on two different tasks, lever-pressing and nose-poking. Although this paper was criticized on methodological grounds (Corbett et al., 1983; Bielajew, 1983b; Wise, 1983) and Gerhart and Liebman (1981) did not find this result, the above argument is perhaps the most interesting. To replay the point, Ettenberg et al. (1981) showed that various doses of the neuroleptic, cis-flupenthixol, attenuated and then blocked (at high doses) responding for lever-pressing while leaving nose-poking responding less effected. They conclude from this result that the neuroleptic primarily produces its effect on lever-pressing behavior through motor impairments. The logic here is that the presence of nose-poking at high drug doses demonstrates the existence of some reinforcement capability of ESB under the neuroleptic.

Although we would not disagree that neuroleptics may produce motor impairments, this study does not quite demonstrate that fact. Because nose-poking is a motorically simpler task that appears to require less ESB reward to sustain it than lever-pressing (Corbett et al., in press), any demonstration that nose-poking behavior preferentially survives neuroleptic blockade may reflect the ability of the nose-poke response to get by with less reinforcement than the lever-pressing task. To make matters worse, Corbett, Stellar, Stinus, Kelley, and Fouriezos (1983) replicated the study in abbreviated form after correcting what they saw as a few procedural errors. They found a much weaker main effect. Since, to some extent, the appeal of the study depends upon a large difference between the drug effects on these two behaviors, a smaller difference weakens the conclusions. Blunting either the ESB reward or the motor capabilities could have produced the Ettenberg, et al. (1981) result; thus one cannot tell from this result alone which effect occurred.

In summary, the ESB work with systemic injection of dopamine receptor blockers shows that interrupting dopamine function results in a reduction of ESB reward and may lead to motor impairments. Selective reward effects may exist in some animals if the neuroleptic dose is carefully titrated to be at intermediate levels (Stellar et al., 1983) and this may vary with the task. The use of tasks that require little reinforcement to sustain responding and/or the use of tasks in which large motor deficits are required to disrupt responding will likely maximize the chances of observing a "selective" reward impairment. Although these task-to-task variations will probably continue to be a real but minor source of disagreement among studies, at least one can be careful about making claims. It would improve matters if the degree of sensitivity to motor disruption were measured with a physical obstacle (weighted lever, low dose of curare) before various paradigms are compared. For example, the lever-pressing extinction paradigm may only detect gross motor deficits, but the more physically demanding runway-based reward summation function paradigm may detect slight motor deficits.

Improving Selectivity through Drug Choice or Brain Injection

If one wanted to explore further the issue of obtaining more selective ESB reward effects, then at least two potential strategies exist: (a) to inject systemically but use drugs that are more selective for one type of dopamine receptor than another, and (b) to inject the drugs directly into selected brain regions. These two strategies are considered below. Also, in a different vein, but stimulated by data from brain injection studies, we then begin to discuss the nature of the "motor" impairment that might be produced by dopamine function disruption.

The classification of drugs according to their potencies in blocking the D1 and D2 dopamine receptor subtypes was discussed earlier. Gallistel and Davis (1983) took advantage of this literature to look at lateral hypothalamic ESB reward. They used the extinction method to measure selectively drug effects on ESB reward and tested a variety of drugs known to affect D1 and D2 receptors differently. Their results show a significant correlation between the affinity of the drugs for the D2 receptor and their ability to block ESB reward in this paradigm. The correlation was very poor for the D1 receptor. This implicates the D2 receptor in ESB reward.

As far as we are aware, the Gallistel and Davis (1983) work is the only study, to date, to approach the D1–D2 receptor question in lateral hypothalamic ESB with behaviorally selective measurement techniques. Liebman et al. (1982) and others have tested a variety of drugs on ESB self-stimulation behavior in the self-adjustment of duration paradigm (Liebman, 1983). However, as in the case of the Liebman et al. (1982) paper, the focus was more on discriminating norepinephrine from dopamine effects than on discriminating between dopamine receptor subtypes. Other papers have tested a variety of neuroleptic drugs on ESB self-stimulation (cf., Wise, 1982; Liebman, 1983; Phillips & Fibiger, 1978), but not from a viewpoint of dopamine receptor subtypes. One study (Ferrer, Sanguinetti, Vives, & Mora, 1983) explored the D1 versus D2 basis of frontal cortex self-stimulation and concluded that this system was D1. This is a different site from that stimulated by Gallistel and Davis (1983), which may explain the difference in the implicated receptor subtype. However, other differences exist. Gallistel and Davis tested more neuroleptics than did Ferrer, et al. (9 as opposed to 3), although Ferrer, et al. did test dopamine agonists as well. Ferrer, et al. also employed simple rate of response as their behavioral measure, which is a measure contaminated by performance factors. They did test open field activity in an attempt to reveal any motor side-effects, but one must be careful of this control since it involves behavior of a different type than lever-pressing. These considerations reflect again the complexity of testing ESB reward effects. Clearly, more studies are needed.

Brain injections offer a second way to increase the specificity of drug action, but the method also raises complications such as the problem of determining how far the injected substance has spread. In his review of this methodology, Routtenberg (1972) suggests a figure of about 1 mm or more, depending on the substance, whether it is delivered in crystalline or liquid form, according to the rate and amount delivered, etc. A number of studies have been done using this brain-injection method with neuroleptics (Mogenson, Takigawa, Robertson, & Wu, 1979; Mora, Sanguinetti, Rolls, & Shaw, 1975; Neill, Peay, & Gold, 1978; Phillips & Fibiger, 1978; Robertson & Mogenson, 1978; Neill et al., 1982; Stellar et al., 1983). Several of these types of studies have attempted to control for motor side-effects. For example, the crossed-injection method has been employed in which neuroleptics are injected into the brain (e.g., the caudate nucleus) on the ipsilateral versus the contralateral side of the brain with respect to the unilateral electrode, and simple rate of response is measured (Broekkamp & VanRossum, 1975; Clavier & Fibiger, 1977). In these two studies, the suppression of ESB self-stimulation was equal with injection on either side of the brain, leading the authors to conclude that the neuroleptic injection was having its depressing effect on behavior by inducing a motor deficit. Another study (Phillips, Carter, & Fibiger, 1979) found that self-stimulation rate decreased more with the ipsilateral injection than with the contralateral injection. This result prompted the authors to conclude that some motor effect of the brain injection had occurred, but that some reward effect occurred as well.

The conclusions for these three crossed-injection method studies were predicated on the belief that the dopamine systems were activated unilaterally by the electrode and that no or very few crossed projections of these systems existed. Therefore, if the contralateral injection decreased rate, it must be doing so through a decrement in general response capability. The larger ipsilateral effect observed in the Phillips et al. (1979) study suggests that something else above and beyond the motor effect was producing the response decrement seen here. Unfortunately, there are several problems with this type of study. First, we now know that the ascending projections of the dopamine systems do cross to some extent (Swanson, 1982; Fass & Butcher, 1981). Second, in the light of the descending path hypothesis concerning the neurons underlying hypothalamic self-stimulation (chapter 6), it seems less secure to expect that hypothalamic ESB results in strictly unilateral activation. Indeed, contralateral descending projections from the lateral hypothalamus to the substantia nigra have been reported (Gerfen et al., 1982). Finally, even if the previous two points were not true, one would still have to worry about a unilateral dopamine impairment resulting in a unilateral sensory inattention deficit (Marshall & Teitelbaum, 1974) and the possibility that such a deficit might be more effective when placed ipsilateral to the ESB reward electrode than when placed contralateral to the ESB reward electrode. The fact that the effects of ESB may be strikingly unilateral was shown by Beagley and Holley (1977), who demonstrated that the control of feeding behavior elicited by ESB was from contralaterally but not ipsilaterally presented visual stimuli.

Studies done on brain injection of neuroleptics into the nucleus accumbens (e.g., Mogenson et al., 1979; Phillips & Fibiger, 1978; Mora et al., 1975) show a decrease in ESB self-stimulation behavior after injection. Unfortunately, these three papers used rate of response as the behavioral measure, so that reward effects and motor effects cannot be distinguished by the self-stimulation measure alone (Mora et al. did measure motor function in another way). There are two exceptions in which rate-independent measures were employed. One study involved the use of the reward summation function technique and found preliminary evidence for both a reward shift and a motor impairment from accumbens injection of neuroleptic (Stellar et al., 1983). This finding is a bit disappointing in the sense that one might have hoped for a pure reward effect since dopamine blockade or destruction of the accumbens is not so strongly associated with motor function, as is the case with the caudate. The accumbens has often been associated with the limbic system (Chronister & DeFrance, 1981) and receives a much stronger anatomical projection from the limbic ventral tegmental area than from the substantia nigra (Figures 7.3A & B). However, such a finding also serves to underscore the intimate connections between limbic and motor function that were discussed previously in this chapter under the concept of "handshaking" (See Figure 7.4.) Along this line, we encourage the reader to remember that self-stimulation behavior can be obtained from the substantia nigra itself (Corbett & Wise, 1980; Gerfen et al., 1982). As mentioned before, the question of how separate or continuous are the ventral tegmental area and the substantia nigra is a difficult one.

Another paper that investigated the effect of accumbens injections was the study by Neill et al. (1982). This study employed the set–reset or the autotitration paradigm (see earlier discussion and chapter 5) to look at the effects of peripheral versus brain injections of a neuroleptic (haloperidol) and a dopamine agonist (amphetamine). The peripheral injections resulted in the expected findings of an increased reset threshold under haloperidol treatment—indicating a decreased ESB reward value—and a decreased reset threshold under amphetamine treatment, indicating an increased ESB reward value. Again, the logic here is that more resets indicate that the rat prefers to self-stimulate at higher ESB currents, which are nearer to the maximum ESB current obtainable. Presumably, this high current preference signifies the animal's attempts to offset a reduced ESB reward value that was produced by the drug. The authors now compared these results of systemic treatment to a brain injection of the same drugs. Paradoxically, the accumbens injections resulted in an opposite picture—that is, haloperidol decreased and amphetamine increased reset threshold. The significance of this is somewhat complicated by a concern with the paradigm itself (Fouriezos & Nawiesniak 1982; chapter 5), but setting this aside, the interpretation of the authors is particularly interesting in light of our struggle in this chapter with the separation of motor from reward effects in ESB studies.

What Neill et al. (1982) suggest to explain the above paradox is that the accumbens injections of haloperidol may decrease the effort that the rat is willing to put into the task. Since pressing the reset lever in this paradigm means leaving the self-stimulation lever, crossing around a 10-cm partition, and returning to the self-stimulation lever, an effort is involved in resetting that is above that involved with simply staying at the first lever, self-stimulating, and accepting a lower ESB current for a longer period. Therefore, if the animal's willingness to exert itself were decreased by haloperidol placed in the accumbens, then by this logic, one might expect a decrease in reset behavior. Unfortunately, this paradigm does not measure reward or motor effects; it only arranges that they produce opposite effects on reset behavior, and haloperidol in the accumbens could be either increasing reward or decreasing effort. However, in light of the other brain injection studies discussed, the hypothesis of ESB reward augmentation by neuroleptic administration seems a remote possibility.

Although other explanations of reduced resetting might be offered (e.g., response perseveration) to account for the above results, the decreased effort hypothesis is interesting in that it also could bear on other experimental results. For example, consider the failure to reach asymptote seen in the reward summation function experiment (Stellar et al., 1983) described above, which employed the physically demanding runway task. It should be noted that in this runway-based, reward summation function paradigm, reducing the pretrial ESB priming reduces the performance asymptote achieved, and thus appears as a motoric or performance deficit (Edmonds & Gallistel, 1974). However, increasing or decreasing priming ESB is widely accepted (Reid et al., 1973) as increasing or decreasing the animals's *motivation* for more ESB reward (Gallistel et al., 1974). Since it is hard to imagine how reducing pretrial ESB causes a motor impairment, the "effort" concept looks attractive and is quite close to the motivational construct given to priming ESB. The concept of effort that is raised here cannot be defended on the basis of a single experiment (Neill et al., 1982). We shall leave further discussion of this issue to a later section of this chapter.

Food Reward and the Effects of Dopamine Blockade

The logic and practice of studies of food reward and ESB reward are parallel. Indeed, many times techniques have been exchanged between these areas, with the exception of the ESB parametric psychophysical experiments, which are difficult or impossible to do with food. This parallel is certainly seen with the extinction method, in which the extinction pattern of responding is just as easily detectable with food or with ESB as the reinforcer. In a number of studies from Wise's laboratory, pimozide has been shown to produce an extinction of operant responding for food, water, or saccharine reward (Wise, Spindler, and Legault, 1978; Gerber, Sing, & Wise, 1981). These studies are reviewed in detail in a recent article (Wise, 1982), and so are not discussed in as much detail here. However, some salient points are worth making.

First, in the Wise et al. (1978) study, the rats ate food when it was presented to them even though they had extinguished lever-pressing for it. Generally, this is taken as evidence for the position that dopamine blockade does reduce the reinforcing properties of food and does not simply produce satiation or sickness that would render food unattractive and thereby cause operant responding for food to cease. However, from another viewpoint, this split between the operant response of obtaining food and the consummatory response of actually eating it is troublesome. In almost all theories of appetitive or operant behavior, it is the opportunity to execute the consummatory response that it rewarding (see chapter 2). Potential operant reinforcers may be judged, at least preliminarily, on the presence of a consummatory response. For example, if the rat does not want to eat, drink, or mate with the stimulus, the rat will not do operant work to produce its presence.

To explain the findings of Wise et al. (1978), one could claim that the reinforcement threshold for eating is lower than that for operant responding. Alternatively, one could claim that the motoric demands of eating are less than those of lever-pressing, or that the eating response is more of an elicited or reflexive behavior and is under different control than emitted operant responses. Indeed, latency to initiate eating of food in the home cage appears to be increased by pimozide, although once initiated, eating proceeds normally (Tombaugh, Tombaugh, & Anisman, 1979). In point of fact, we do not really know very much about the control (stimulus or motor) of these two different behaviors, especially as affected by drugs. For example, Teitelbaum et al. (1983) claim that locomotion and postural support constitute two subsystems of behavioral organization and that a point exists in recovery after profound dopamine and/or lateral hypothalamic destruction when the locomotion subsystem of behavior cannot function, but the posture and support subsystem remains viable. An animal in such a state of recovery will support itself and brace against a lateral push from the experimenter but is akinetic. In this context, one could imagine an animal that could show lower level consummatory behavior but not operant responding. The characterization of such an animal's deficit goes well beyond the simple conceptions of reward versus motor effects of drug administration.

As a second point about the extinction studies, a number of experiments have closely looked at the similarity between extinction induced by a neuroleptic, such as pimozide, and natural extinction derived from a withholding of reinforcement (Beninger, 1982; Mason, Beninger, Fibiger, & Phillips, 1980). The fact that responding under pimozide starts out at a high level is good evidence for the absence of a gross motor deficit such as in severe Parkinson's disease, but the story becomes more complex from there. Studies have compared natural and pimozide-induced extinction and found them different. For example, if partial reinforcement is given in training, then prolonged responding is seen in natural extinction (Skinner, 1938). This prolongation of extinction with partial reinforcement training should be seen under pimozide testing, but it is not. Under these circumstances, the extinction seen is very rapid (Tombaugh, Anisman, & Tombaugh, 1982; Gray & Wise, 1980). Indeed, Tombaugh, Ritch, & Shepard (1980) suggest that the parallel between pimozide and nonreinforcement treatments in inducing extinction may be peculiar to the continuous reinforcement schedule of testing.

The above discussion is hard to explain and forces Wise (1982) to postulate that, in addition to blunting primary reinforcers like food, pimozide also blunts cues or secondary reinforcers that are conditioned to the primary reinforcement. In Wise's article, this is referred to as the incentive motivational properties of reinforcers, and partial reinforcement schedules are postulated to depend heavily upon secondary reinforcement-induced incentive motivation in a way that continuous reinforcement schedules are not. Such speculation requires experimental justification, but it should be noted that a motivational construct has again surfaced. On a different but related topic, pimozide seems to be without effect on association learning itself. Tombaugh et al. (1980) have shown that the *accuracy* of a food-reinforced conditioned discrimination is unimpaired by pimozide. The same is true for aversively motivated discrimination (Corradini, Tombaugh, & Anisman, 1984), but both of these studies provide evidence for a suppression of behavioral responding by pimozide.

The comparison of natural and pimozide-induced extinction may be interpreted to suggest that pimozide does more than just blunt reinforcement or create simple, consistent motor effects. That is, dopamine blockade may make the animal's responses more costly in the following sense. When an animal executes a skeletal muscular act under neuroleptic treatment, it first finds the response more difficult to initiate and/or maintain than normally. This difficulty does not block responding or even seriously impair it. Indeed, it is hypothesized that the animal is still able to generate behavior in the normal range, but this requires greater effort. Because this effect is unexpected by the animal, one might claim that behavior under pimozide could start out at a normal level, with the animal putting more effort into the task, but then the animal will recalculate the cost/benefit equation associated with responding, and behavior will slow and may cease. It is interesting to note that in an old study when the lever-pressing task was made more difficult by weighting down the lever, *faster* extinction was seen (Mowrer & Jones, 1943; Solomon, 1948). The double extinction experiment (as in Gallistel, Boytim, Gomita, & Klebanoff, 1982) has never been done with a weighted lever. Perhaps this type of "motor deficit" is more subtle than the barbiturate and picrotoxin (seizure-producing) controls that have been tested in this double extinction paradigm and which this paradigm has been shown to discriminate from reward discontinuation (Gallistel, Boytim, Gomita, & Klebanoff, 1982). Additionally, it should be remembered that dopamine-lesioned animals can be activated by strong stimuli (Marshall et al., 1976). Therefore, activation coming from stimulus cues associated with the prior receipt of ESB reward may help to overcome the motor inactivation seen in animals following dopamine blockade.

Other evidence supporting the role of dopamine in natural reward comes from looking at acquisition-blocking effects of neuroleptics, or spontaneous recovery following extinction. These and other phenomenon are well-discussed in the Wise (1982) article and commentary. One different major piece of evidence that was not included in that review because of its more recent publication is the work of Heyman (1983) and associates (Heyman, Kinzie, & Seiden, 1983). Heyman (1983) used a variation on the basic matching-law procedure (Herrnstein, 1974; deVilliers, 1977) that was made to apply to a single lever situation. This was discussed in chapter 5 under the category of response-strength methods and earlier discussed in this chapter in regard to a study by

Hamilton and Stellar (1983). Here, food reward was offered on a number of variable interval schedules, and the resulting rates of lever pressing were plotted against the reinforcement obtained. As discussed in detail in chapter 5 (see figure 5.8), an equation derived from the matching law can be fit to the data by adjusting two parameters. The changes in these parameters from baseline to drug test conditions give information on the motor capacity and the strength of the reinforcement. In this equation, the motoric parameter essentially sets the asymptote of the curve, and the reinforcement parameter sets the amount of reinforcement required to get half-maximal responding. As represented in Figure 7.5, pimozide produces decrements in the asymptotic behavior reached and an increase in the number of reinforcements required to sustain half-maximal responding (Heyman, 1983). Thus, pimozide appears to produce both motor and reward effects in this paradigm where both are

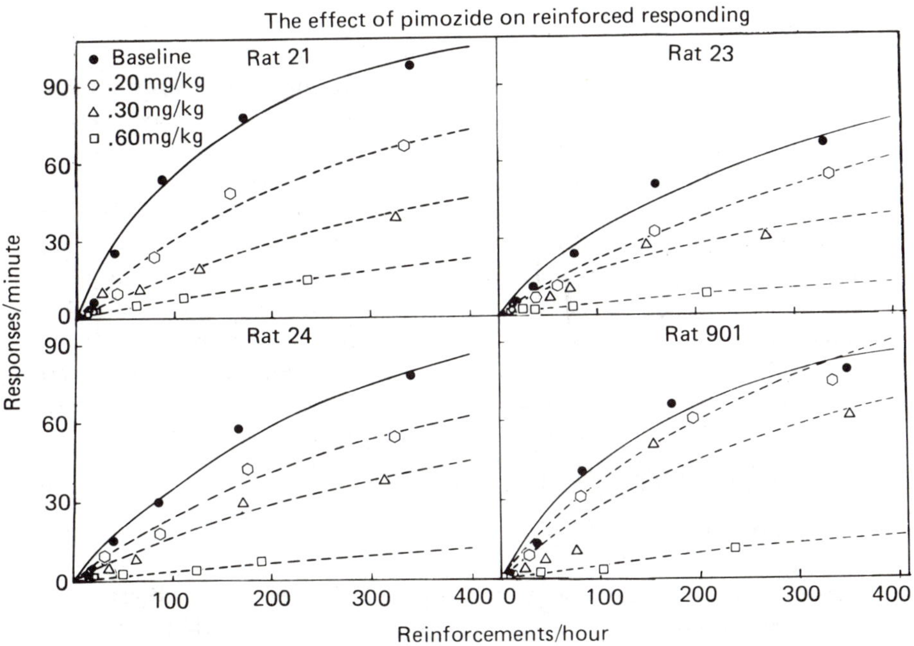

Figure 7.5 Data showing response rate of lever-pressing for a food reward on a variable interval (VI) schedule, where VI schedule varied from trial to trial. Density of obtained reinforcement is shown on the x-axis. Pimozide depressed rats, responding in a dose dependent manner, suppressing the asymptotic response level seen in the computer-generated curves of best fit. These curves were also shown to have a slower growth rate to their asymptotes. These observations suggest, respectively, a diminished behavioral capacity (motor deficit) and a decreased reinforcing quality of the food. (Heyman, 1983.) Reprinted by permission.

measured simultaneously. Amphetamine had largely the opposite effect (Heyman, 1983; Bradshaw, Ruddle, & Szabadi, 1981), increasing reinforcement efficiency, but inconsistently affecting motor capability. The advantages of this method are that motor and reward phenomena are measured quantitatively. In our opinion, this research provides major support for the idea that dopamine manipulation can produce both motor and reward effects.

In an elegant paradigm of conditioned reinforcement, Robbins (1976, 1978) has shown from another angle that dopamine may be involved in the reward processes. In this procedure, a thirsty rat is trained to lever-press for water reward on an intermittent schedule of reinforcement. A light or other neutral stimulus is presented just before the delivery of reinforcement, and so becomes conditioned to reinforcement delivery. In a second phase of the procedure, two levers are presented, and pressing one of them leads to the delivery of the previously conditioned light stimulus. Pressing the other lever gives nothing. Amount of responding on each of the two levers is measured, and the difference between them is taken as an indication of the ability of the conditioned stimulus (the light) to reinforce responding. Dopamine agonists, like amphetamine, administered in the second phase of the experiment, increased responding on the lever leading to the conditioned stimulus, but not on the other lever. The same basic paradigm was used with the same results when the primary reward in the first phase was ESB reward (Robbins & Koob, 1978). The water-conditioned reinforcer effects also seem dependent upon the integrity of the dopamine systems, since 6-OHDA lesions of the caudate or accumbens abolished the dopamine-agonist-induced increase in selective responding in the second phase (Robbins & Everitt, 1982). The results were somewhat complex in that accumbens lesions produced perseverative responding, while the caudate lesions produced indiscriminate responding on the two levers.

Lesion Studies

Lesions of the dopamine systems up to and over 95% depletion have been produced by the neurotoxin, 6-OHDA, which is taken up by catecholamine-containing neurons and selectively kills them. This action can be made even more specific by appropriate drug pretreatments that block uptake mechanisms in norepinephrine systems, thereby sparing them. These 6-OHDA lesions have been shown to greatly reduce or eliminate self-stimulation behavior (Breese, Howard, & Leahy, 1971; Cooper, Cott, & Breese, 1974; Phillips & Fibiger, 1976; Phillips et al., 1979), but having improved the selectivity of 6-OHDA's action, one is still left to face the complex problem of attributing the reduced performance to reward or motor effects. Another important complexity is the fact that recovery occurs in these subjects. We will not discuss recovery here but see Marshall (1984) for a review.

Phillips & Fibiger (1976) attempted to get at the motor vs reward question by using bilateral ESB sites in the caudate and an ipsilateral or contralateral lesion site in the substantia nigra. They found that ipsilateral lesions were far more effective in suppressing self-stimulation behavior than were contralateral sites. Ipsilateral lesions permanently reduced self-stimulation to less than 10% of its pre-lesion levels; whereas, contralateral lesions reduced responding, but this behavior recovered to 72% of pre-lesion levels within 4 weeks. This led to the conclusion that the ipsilateral lesion effect went beyond a motor effect, perhaps to decrease the effectiveness of ESB in generating reward. However, this effect was seen with *caudate* ESB electrodes. Working with bilaterally placed hypothalamic ESB electrodes, a unilateral substantia nigra injection was found to have comparable effects on ipsilateral and contralateral self-stimulation (Ornstein & Huston, 1975; Carey, 1982), and a motor effect explanation would account for the data from this site. Thus, the substantia nigra may play a role in the reward of caudate ESB, but it appears not to play much of a role in the reward from lateral hypothalamic ESB.

The above data fit with the regional metabolic activation data collected by 2-DG studies of lateral hypothalamic ESB, which show little activation in the substantia nigra while showing heavy activation in the ventral tegmental area. However, one should not easily rule out a role for the substantia nigra in lateral hypothalamic ESB self-stimulation. Another 2-DG study has shown that ventral tegmental area ESB can lead to profound uptake of the 2-DG in the substantia nigra (Porrino et al., 1984). Thus, the nigra may well be activated, perhaps at least to play a role in motor arousal. This last speculation is in line with the handshaking hypothesis of Nauta discussed earlier (Figure 7.4).

The findings of Ornstein and Huston (1975), discussed above, were extended to ESB sites in the substantia nigra itself by Clavier and Fibiger (1977), and this study reveals much about the complexity of the contralateral–ipsilateral method discussed above. Clavier and Fibiger lesioned the terminal fields of the nigrostriatal projection in the caudate and found an equal suppressive effect of ipsilateral and contralateral lesions on self-stimulation responding. Again, this leads one to consider a motor deficit explanation of the decreased ESB responding. A twist in their study (Clavier and Fibiger, 1977) was the finding that ipsilateral but not the contralateral lesions were very effective in abolishing the self-stimulation rate-enhancing effects of systemic amphetamine treatment. This led to the conclusion that perhaps the contralateral deficits are mostly motor and the ipsilateral deficits are mostly of the reward type. To make matters worse, as stated before, ipsilateral sensory inattention deficits may occur so that the presumed reward effect may actually be a performance-decreasing sensory-motor effect that is reversed by amphetamine. This clouds the reward versus motor interpretation of the contralateral control procedure. Also, as previously discussed here and in chapter 6, we now know the dopamine systems to be partially crossed, not wholly ipsilateral, as was thought at the time this research was conducted. All that can be said here is that this research is not inconsistent with the previous conclusions of the dopamine-blocking studies that dopamine is involved with both the reward and motor components of self-stimulation behavior.

Drug Self-Administration and Place Preference

Perhaps the most convincing examples of dopamine's potential for generating reward effects are the studies on self-administration of dopamine-stimulating drugs. In the self-administration paradigm, each reinforced lever-press triggers an intravenous injection of drug. Rats will self-administer the dopamine-stimulating drugs, amphetamine and cocaine (Pickens & Harris, 1968; Yokel & Pickens, 1973; Yokel & Wise, 1976; Risner & Jones, 1976; deWit & Wise, 1978). This self-administration can be blocked by systemic injection of neuroleptics (Yokel & Wise, 1976; deWit & Wise, 1978; Ettenberg et al., 1982) or by lesions of the dopaminergic terminals in the nucleus accumbens (Lyness, Friedle, & Moore, 1979; Roberts, Koob, Klonoff, & Fibiger, 1980). The basic pattern of responding following neuroleptic injection is to first elevate the rate of lever-pressing for self-administration. If the neuroleptic dose levels are low to moderate, the elevation of self-administration rate will be stable for a long time as the animal attempts to maintain the effective level of dopamine stimulation in the face of a partial blockade of the dopamine receptors. If the neuroleptic dose levels are high, then the elevation of responding is temporary and the rat ceases to respond, in an extinction pattern (Pickens, Meisch, & Thompson, 1978). This elevation of responding is opposite to that expected if the neuroleptic simply produced a gross motor deficit. Humans also will self-administer amphetamine over saline in laboratory experiments and report an increase in positive feelings. In humans, reported euphoric properties of amphetamine are reduced when the subjects are given neuroleptic pretreatments (Gunne, Anggard, & Jonsson, 1972). This whole area of self-administration research is reviewed in more detail in other sources (Wise, 1980; Kelley & Stinus, 1984).

Other evidence comes from place preference paradigms. Here, subjects are allowed to go to one of two distinctly different sides of a chamber, and their preference for one side over another is noted by the amount of time they spend in each side. The animal is then confined to one side of the chamber and given a drug suspected of having reward properties. This continues for a number of trials, often over several days. The animal is then tested in the chamber in a drug-free state, and alterations in its original preference are taken as evidence for the rewarding properties of the drug. If the drug was rewarding and the conditioning was successful, then the animal should strongly prefer the side in which the drug had been previously received. This paradigm does not allow for the measurement of motor effects of the drug, but since the animal is tested drug-free, one cannot argue that motor effects explain the results. In this paradigm, a number of drugs that promote dopamine function were shown to produce reward effects. Amphetamine, cocaine, and other compounds systemically given produce strong place preferences (Phillips & LePiane, 1980; Bozarth & Wise, 1981). These effects are antagonized by neuroleptics (Bozarth & Wise, 1981). Cocaine administration directly into the frontal cortex and the accumbens has also been shown to be rewarding (Goeders & Smith, 1983), indicating potential sites of action of the systemic effects.

Opiates

In addition to self-stimulation and work with drugs that directly mimic or stimulate dopamine function, other compounds have been shown to produce reward effects in both the self-administration and the place preference paradigms. For example, as is well known, the brain contains a number of opiate receptors that are found in anatomical association with the dopamine systems (Snyder & Childers, 1977; Kelley & Stinus, 1984). Morphine and heroin activate some of the opiate receptors and have been shown to produce a place preference whether administered systemically (Deneau, Yanagita, & Seevers, 1969; Woods & Schuster, 1968; Rossi & Reid, 1976; Sherman, Pickman, Rice, Liebeskind, & Holman, 1980; Bozarth & Wise, 1981) or into the ventral tegmental area (Phillips & LePiane, 1980; Bozarth, 1983). Place preference was also induced by ventral tegmental area administration of D-ala-met-enkephalin, an analogue of the naturally occurring opiate, enkephalin (Phillips & LePiane, 1982). These opiates are also readily self-administered intravenously (Ettenberg et al., 1982) or directly into the ventral tegmental area (Bozarth and Wise, 1981). Furthermore, the opiate reward effects appear to depend upon the integrity of the dopamine systems in that place preference for heroin is blocked by pimozide (Bozarth & Wise, 1981, 1983). Finally, intravenous administration of heroin (Gerber, Bozarth, & Wise, 1981) and ventral tegmental administration of morphine (Broekkamp et al., 1976) increase the rate of lateral hypothalamic self-stimulation. This finding is similar to the effects of drugs that promote dopamine release, such as cocaine or amphetamine (Leith & Barrett, 1981). For a more exhaustive review of the literature on opiate-induced reward effects see Bozarth (1983), Bozarth & Wise (1982), and Kelley and Stinus (1984).

The above hypothesis, that opiate reward works through a dopamine mechanism (Wise, 1980; Bozarth, 1983) is not without challenge. For example, while intravenous heroin self-administration can be blocked by the opiate antagonist, naloxone, to produce the expected increase in responding associated with a loss of reward effects, the dopamine antagonist, cis-flupenthixol, does not produce this effect. Rather, cis-flupenthixol only reduces responding for heroin (Ettenberg et al., 1982), which is not the pattern one expects from a selective reward block. However, one must remember that determining the reward versus nonreward (motor) effects of opiates on behavior is likely to be no less procedurally difficult or subtle than it is in studying dopamine. For example, in the Ettenberg et al. (1982) experiment described above, heroin may have produced such a strong *dopamine* reward that the cis-flupenthixol, at lower doses, might not have been effective in completely blocking it. At higher doses, the cis-flupenthixol might introduce motor effects that could prevent any increase in responding (to compensate for a decreased reward), and thus confound the issue of reward measurement. For further discussion of this possibility, see Bozarth and Wise (1983).

Some Models of Dopamine Function: Reward, Behavioral Activation, Effort

The discussions in this chapter suggest a somewhat general involvement of the effects of dopamine activation in various reward processes. In 1980, Wise published a model of this hypothesized central role of dopamine in reward function; it is shown in Figure 7.6 (Wise, 1980). In this figure, dopamine cells in the ventral tegmental area and perhaps the substantia nigra are seen as receiving inputs from a number of sources and then projecting this activation into the forebrain in the form of dopamine release. Rewarding ESB pulses from the lateral hypothalamus

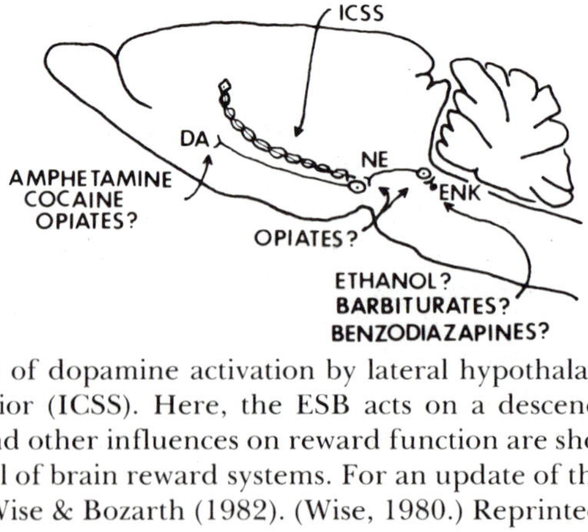

Figure 7.6 Model of dopamine activation by lateral hypothalamic ESB in self-stimulation behavior (ICSS). Here, the ESB acts on a descending myelinated system. Opiates and other influences on reward function are shown as proposed by Wise in a model of brain reward systems. For an update of the role of opiates and ethanol, see Wise & Bozarth (1982). (Wise, 1980.) Reprinted by permission.

are seen to act on myelinated cells in the lateral hypothalamus which then descend into the dopamine cell regions. Opiates and other rewards are thought to find other routes to the dopamine cell group. Thus, dopamine systems are postulated in this model to be a *final common path for reward effects* from a variety of sources, and release of dopamine in the terminal fields of the forebrain is a critical event in the elaboration of reward effects. Blockade of dopamine leads to a complete or nearly complete loss of reward (Wise, 1980). Figure 7.6 is an historically significant figure for its attempt at synthesis, though Wise and Bozarth (1982, 1984) have refined and updated its claims to some degree. This figure is the first diagram of the descending path hypothesis, though part of the work on which it rests comes from other groups (e.g. Shizgal, Bielajew, Corbett, et al. 1980).

Wise has moved back from this position slightly in his 1982 version of the hypothesis of reward to say that a *blunting* rather than a blocking of reward occurs following dopamine receptor blockade. However, the basic role of dopamine remains unchanged. Figure 7.6 and the attendant general theoretical position (Wise, 1980, 1982) represents a clear reward-function view of dopamine's role in behavior. For example, in defense of the anhedonia hypothesis against a pure motoric hypothesis of dopamine function, Wise suggests that a good deal (but perhaps not all) of the explanation of why dopamine-depleted rats do not move might be that they lack the "desire" to move because nothing is attractive enough or rewarding enough to get them to move—that is, they are anhedonic (Wise, 1982). Used in this way, the anhedonia hypothesis extends beyond a role in the elaboration of reward and into what seems a motivational function perhaps like incentive motivation (Bindra & Palfi, 1967; Bindra, 1968). Indeed, it may have been this motivational property of the term *anhedonia* that appealed to Wise in formulating this hypothesis. Again, the reader is referred to the Wise (1982) paper and its open peer commentary to get a feeling for the diversity of opinions on the dopamine blockade and anhedonia question.

A second model of dopamine function involves *behavioral activation*, a concept derived from the observation that dopamine agonist administration promotes increased general behavioral activity (Kelley, Stinus, & Iversen, 1980). Behaviors measured are typically locomotion, rearing, grooming, or other forms of simple unconditioned behaviors. Most heavily studied is perhaps open field locomotion and activity, taken as the total number of breaks of a photocell beam in a timed session. This concept of behavioral activation is very close to the concept of arousal, which has long been part of theories of motivated behavior in psychology and ethology (see chapter 2). It is also reflected in the shorthand clinical description of amphetamine and some other dopamine agonists as having "psychomotor" properties. Though all concepts of arousal share common ground, the concept of behavioral activation does have some important differences with the type of motor arousal underlying stereotypy, as discussed at the beginning of this chapter. The most important difference is that behavioral activation may depend upon the nucleus accumbens rather than the caudate, as shown by the fact that open field locomotion, induced by amphetamine, survives lesions of the caudate. Additionally, direct injection of dopamine agonists into the accumbens produces open field locomotion. The open field locomotion can also be produced by manipulation of the ventral tegmental area, which projects to the accumbens and depends on the integrity of the accumbens for the behaviorally activating effect. For a review of this literature, see Kelley and Stinus (1984).

Another model of dopamine function as related to ESB self-stimulation is shown in Figure 7.7, which is taken from the work of Neill et al. (1982). They postulate that dopaminergic activation in the accumbens increases the amount of effort that a subject will put into a given task. This is a general change in the animal's state that is not tightly time-locked to a particular ESB stimulus. The time-locked reward effects of the ESB that mediate operant reinforcement are postulated to bypass the dopamine cells and involve some other unspecified brain system, perhaps the nondopamine cells of the ventral tegmental area. Since dopamine-agonist administration directly into the accumbens can be rewarding (Hoebel et al., 1982), these authors have also postulated a related "mood" factor of

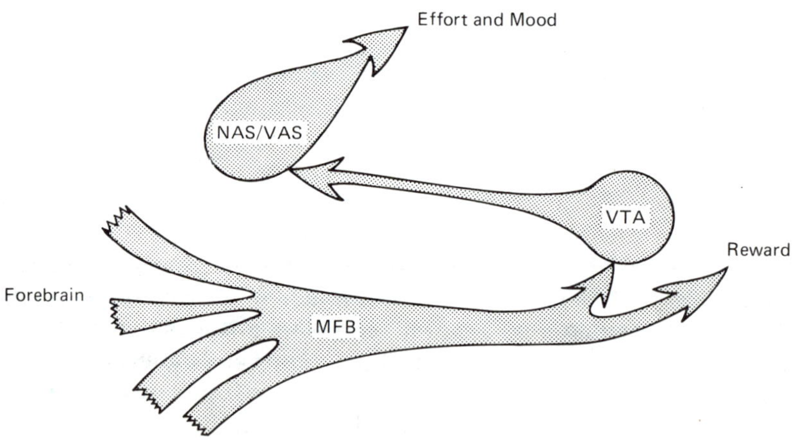

Figure 7.7 "Effort" and "mood" changes are hypothesized to be the primary consequences of dopamine release triggered by rewarding lateral hypothalamic ESB at the medial forebrain bundle (MFB). The actual phasic reinforcement effect of the ESB is hypothesized to depend on nondopaminergic neurons, perhaps bypassing the ventral tegmental area (VTA). NAS/VAS represents the nucleus accumbens and ventral anterior striatum. (Neill et al., 1982.) Reprinted by permission.

dopamine function in the accumbens. Thus, animals with high dopamine levels in the accumbens would experience some reward effects (the "mood" factor) and be willing to put more effort into a task (the "effort" factor). Some evidence for this was discussed earlier in relation to the study by Neill et al. (1982).

Although one observation is not much support for a model of this scope, other evidence may be obtainable. For example, the idea mentioned previously, that dopamine blockade increases the cost of responding, is similar to the decreased effort idea and may look to the same data base for support. Also, we have observed informally that a rat self-stimulating for ESB reward does not always appear to press the reward lever with the same force. This occurs despite the fact that the lever mechanism always requires the same force of pressing to activate the contacts. We have seen increases in non-obligatory response force at high ESB reward currents or pulse frequencies, and interestingly, under pharmacological treatments that increase dopamine function. With careful investigation to disassociate response force from other aspects of responding that affect reward delivery—for instance, response rate—non-obligatory force might be used as a measure of effort.

Although it is often dangerous to use new terms, especially such as "mood" or "effort" since they can cloud the issue by having imprecise definitions, this model of dopamine function points out the general kind of explanations that may be needed to better describe the role(s) of dopamine in behavioral function. Behavioral activation, effort, and the concept of cost-of-responding due to a subtle motor impairment are all related in that they are neither clear reward effects nor clear gross motor deficits that were described in the first two sections of this chapter. This is important since much of the work reviewed in this chapter takes this dichotomy between reward and motor function as the framework for research and thinking. Kelley and Stinus (1984) may provide a guide for our thinking when they suggest that the dopamine projection from the ventral tegmental area to the nucleus accumbens may be involved in both setting the value of external stimuli (reward effects, reinforcement) and to "*generate the state of motivational arousal necessary to guide appropriate responses*. . ." [italics added] (Kelley & Stinus, 1984, p. 41).

For us, the words "motivational arousal" as written by Kelley and Stinus (1984) capture the point of the above discussion. This is not a new idea, certainly, but it is surprising the extent to which current behavioral measurement methodologies and theories neglect explanations that fall between gross motor and reward function. An animal under neuroleptic treatment and showing an extinction response might be decreasing in its motivation as time progresses as well as learning to expect less reward. Neuroleptic blunting of motivation might explain the faster-than-expected extinction in partial reinforcement schedules and the asymptotic behavior decreases seen in the runway-based reward summation function.

Exploring the potential separation between reward, motivational, and motoric effects is an important challenge of the future. We need still better behavioral methods, finer neuroanatomy and neurochemistry (see Dunnett & Björkland, 1983) than we have produced to date. Then we can face the ultimate challenge of showing how reward, motivational, and motoric effects interact through dopamine and other systems, or how new concepts altogether are needed. In this effort, two related anatomical structures stand out and deserve special attention. These structures are the ventral tegmental area and the nucleus accumbens; they are discussed briefly below.

The Ventral Tegmental Area and the Nucleus Accumbens

The ventral tegmental area is that portion of the midbrain dopamine system that is most heavily implicated in ESB self-stimulation by the 2DG studies and the anatomical linkage studies discussed in the previous chapter. It possesses dopamine and non-dopamine cells that can be distinguished electrophysiologically. Lateral hypothalamic stimulation pulses alter the firing in almost all of the dopamine neurons (Maeda & Mogenson, 1981) although not all cells are activated. If the dopamine cells of the ventral tegmental area function as the second stage of relevant activated neurons following rewarding ESB delivered to the hypothalamus, then it should be possible to directly manipulate the neurons of the ventral tegmental area and alter the way that hypothalamic ESB generates reward and/or motivational arousal. For example, Figure 7.8 shows a diagram of some of the various neurotransmitter inputs to the ventral tegmental area. This figure is taken from the previously discussed paper of Kelley, Stinus, and Iverson (1980), and it is based upon their own work on brain injections of opiates into the ventral tegmental area and upon the work of others. It is important since it gives us an angle of attack on the problem of identifying the second stage of ESB reward-relevant circuitry if this second stage is indeed dopaminergic.

According to Figure 7.8, injection of opiates into the ventral tegmental area will cause a loss of inhibition upon these cells. This loss of inhibition was postulated to underlie the increase in behavioral activation reported by Kelley et al. (1980) and may underlie the direct reward effects of opiate injection into this region (Bozarth & Wise, 1983). Suppose now that one could deliver action potentials to the ventral tegmental area. It would be reasonable to assume that these action potentials would be more efficient at firing the ventral tegmental cells if some inhibitory inputs had been shut down. If hypothalamic ESB fires descending hypothalamic neurons (chapter 6), which then fire ventral tegmental cells, hypothalamic ESB should be more efficient in generating reward or behavioral activation effects after ventral tegmental opiate injection. This may have

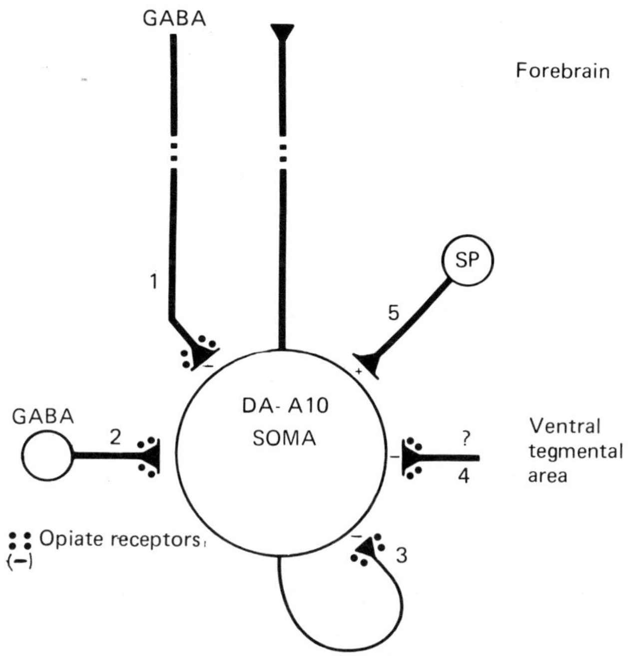

Figure 7.8 Suggested inputs to the dopamine-containing ventral tegmental area cell bodies (DA A10 soma), showing the way opiate receptors might inactivate various sources of inhibition. GABA and SP represent gamma-amino-buteric acid and substance P, respectively. (Kelley et al., 1980.) Reprinted by permission.

been shown by Broekkamp et al. (1976) who have reported an increase in rate of responding for ESB following ventral tegmental area injection of morphine. Also Gerber, Bozarth, and Wise (1981) reported that low doses of heroin (10 to 100 μg/kg) given intravenously facilitated response rate for lateral hypothalamic ESB reward. Unfortunately, both of these studies used rate of response as the behavioral measure, so that ESB reward effects cannot be said to be selectively increased, since elevations in behavioral activation could explain the results. This is a perfect opportunity to apply the quantitative behavioral methodologies that measure both performance and reward effects to assess the improvement of self-stimulation behavior by opiates.

In Figure 7.8, other neurotransmitter inputs are depicted besides the opiates. The same logic can be applied to these that was applied to the opiate studies. Neurophysiological unweighting of the dopamine neurons might occur if the dopamine autoreceptor were stimulated with apomorphine, or if picrotoxin were injected to block the GABA input (see Figure 7.8). Coupled with the quantitative methodologies for ESB reward measurement, such studies would give information not only on the pharmacology of the ventral tegmental area, but also on the role of the ventral tegmental area in ESB reward.

The nucleus accumbens deserves special attention since it is one of the major termination zones of the ventral tegmental area (Figure 7.3). It is an increasingly interesting area because of the limbic nature of its connections despite its location in the basal ganglia, a classic motor structure. The nucleus accumbens and the neighboring ventral anterior striatum receive a heavy projection from the amygdala, whereas the rest of the caudate gets a major projection from the cortex (Kelley et al., 1982). Dopamine-depleting lesions in the accumbens and neighboring structures reduce spontaneous activity and investigative behavior (Iverson & Koob, 1977; Koob, Riley, Smith, & Robbins, 1978; Fink & Smith, 1980). This parallels the effects of ventral tegmental area lesions (LeMoal et al., 1977), although partial lesions here can result in hyperactivity (Koob, Stinus, & LeMoal, 1981). Accumbens lesions block the self-administration of cocaine reward (Kelley & Stinus, 1984), and neuroleptics administered here attenuate ESB reward (Stellar et al., 1983; Mogenson et al., 1979; Mora et al., 1975). On the stimulant side, the accumbens is a site for ESB self-stimulation and a site for rewarding injection of dopamine agonists such as amphetamine (Hoebel et al., 1982). It is certainly a promising area for future research. However, this does not necessarily mean that the dopamine projections to the accumbens are part of the specific second stage of ESB reward. Using rate-intensity functions, Strecker, Roberts, & Koob (1982) found that after a partial depletion of dopamine in the accumbens, non-specific activation by apomorphine facilitated ESB reward. Strecker, et al. conclude that some nonspecific permissive role of dopamine in ESB reward is more likely. In this way dopamine function in the accumbens would parallel dopamine function in the motor system. These concepts were discussed under the gate or amplifier notion in chapter 6. Whatever the specific formulation, the accumbens seems to be an important site to look for the kinds of reward-motor interaction discussed here. For more information see Kelley & Stinus (1984) and Chronister & DeFrance (1981).

Whatever Happened to Norepinephrine?

Although a detailed history of the rise and fall of the norepinephrine hypothesis of ESB and other rewards is beyond the bounds of interest here, it is illuminating to consider a few points. Probably the "high" point of the hypothesis that norepinephrine brain systems, particularly those lying in the locus coeruleus, were important in reward came in 1975 with the publication of Stein's "Norepinephrine Reward Pathways: Role in Self-stimulation, Memory Consolidation, and Schizophrenia" (Stein, 1975). The major support for this reward hypothesis came from two sources. The first is anatomical. For example, it seemed that the locus coeruleus was a good place to locate electrodes in order to get self-stimulation behavior. Furthermore, the dorsal noradrenergic bundle, the primary ascending outflow of the locus coeruleus, was also a self-stimulation site (Stein, 1975). Finally, the lateral hypothalamus, frontal cortex, and other self-stimulation sites all contain norepinephrine, as does most of the brain (Moore & Bloom, 1978). The second line of evidence was pharmacological. Here, it was shown that norepinephrine-depleting drugs, such as disulfiram, decreased self-stimulation behavior. Treatment in the ventricles with norepinephrine was shown to reinstate self-stimulation responding after these depletions (Stein, 1975). Thus, the theory looked fairly good and some were setting about the business of applying this knowledge to schizophrenia and other problems, as shown above by the title of Stein's article.

The same two lines of evidence that erected the norepinephrine hypothesis of reward, also brought it down. On the anatomical side, it was shown with careful moveable electrode mapping studies that the locus coeruleus was *not* a site of self-stimulation (Corbett & Wise, 1979). Rather, the true site lies to the side and a bit ventral to the locus coeruleus. In addition, a careful study was conducted in which self-stimulation electrodes were placed unilaterally in the locus coeruleus, the dorsal noradrenergic bundle, and the lateral hypothalamus (Corbett, Skelton, & Wise, 1977). Each site was verified for self-stimulation behavior, and the dorsal noradrenergic bundle self-stimulation site was lesioned electrolytically. This should have cut the outflow of the locus coeruleus and compromised self-stimulation in either or both of the remaining two sites; however, it did not do this. Self-stimulation of the locus coeruleus remained intact, and self-stimulation of the lateral hypothalamus actually improved non-significantly following the lesion (Corbett et al., 1977). This occurred despite well placed lesions, as determined histochemically. The other line of evidence was pharmacological. Using more selective blockers and depletors that spared dopamine and serotonin, massive disruptions of the norepinephrine neurotransmission were produced with little effect on self-stimulation behavior. Furthermore, self-administration of cocaine is not blocked with norepinephrine blockers as it is with dopamine blockers. These and other developments were reviewed in detail by Fibiger (1978).

Conclusions

The mistaken attribution of norepinephrine as the reward substrate for ESB self-stimulation was brought about by the limitations of the physiological and pharmacological methods available at the time. Progress in such methods will naturally lead to improvements in understanding.

However, another source of error came from the over-simplification of the problem of measuring ESB reward effects and separating them from other contaminating effects. We are more sensitive to this problem today, but the issue remains. Are we over-simplifying again with a new neurotransmitter (dopamine) and at a slightly more advanced stage of behavioral measurement? The answer to this question is likely to be *yes*. We have suggested here that perhaps a new construct of motivational arousal (or effort) might be considered as a supplement to the reward–motor distinction. It is ironic that this "new" concept of motivational arousal is really an old concept, as is evidenced in chapters 2 and 3 in this book. It is also far from clear that this is enough or is a right fix to the current theories, which often see the problem in terms of simple motor–reward distinctions. Finally, while dopamine is being considered as a second stage of activation after a rewarding ESB pulse, we might do well to consider also the low-pass filter problem discussed in chapter 6 to keep us from too easily believing our own theories. Perhaps dopamine does not act as a second stage at all, but rather facilitates conduction of the ESB reward signal traveling along another pathway. In this way, dopamine's role in the limbic system might parallel its role in the motor system, as a modulator.

The behavior and the physiology are full of surprises. For example, it has been recently shown that cholecystokinin (CCK) exists in dopamine cell terminals and is co-released with dopamine (Hokfelt et al., 1980). Since neuroleptics block the dopamine cells they also increase the firing rate of the dopamine cells as the natural feedback mechanisms try to keep dopamine neurotransmission constant. Thus, more CCK will probably be released under these conditions, flooding the basal forebrain. Could some of the behavioral effects of neuroleptics really be mediated by CCK release? Since CCK injected systemically (Smith & Gibbs, 1979; Smith, 1983) and CCK injected into the ventricles (Della-Fera & Baile, 1979; E. Stellar, unpublished data) inhibit food intake, the point is an interesting one with regard to the effects of dopamine blockade on operant responding for food reward. It is certain that as our understanding of structure and function progress, new subtleties will be revealed, and that our present understanding of dopamine function is far from complete.

8
Overview

In this concluding chapter, we briefly review some of the behavioral characteristics of ESB reward as they relate to motivational issues, and then try to extract from the foregoing chapters generalizations and concepts that will be useful for future research on brain mechanisms of motivation and reward. After the review of behavioral issues in ESB reward, approach–withdrawal behavior and the concept of levels of brain function are discussed as they relate to motivation and the hierarchical organization of the nervous system. Then, we take up additional issues in the study of motivated behavior where there has been much debate in the past on how to construct appropriate conceptions of the underlying physiology. As a consequence, the pendulum has swung historically from one extreme to another in the quest for a theory of the controlling mechanisms: from emphasis on peripheral to emphasis on central controls, from a concept of specific drives to general arousal theory, from brain localization to a concept of hierarchical neural systems, from innate to acquired mechanisms. Much has been learned in the course of these swings, and each time a bit of enduring truth is left behind to be picked up and reinforced on the next swing. We are still in the early stages of the process.

Behavioral Phenomena Associated with ESB

In this first section of the chapter, we return to a consideration of some of the behavioral phenomena produced by ESB, and some lesion effect in the lateral hypothalamus. As stated previously (see chapter 5), the first major area of effort in the history of ESB study was explaining the many behavioral phenomena associated with ESB. Researchers wondered whether ESB at one site induced a comparable or different reward from ESB at another site. They asked how ESB self-stimulation behavior was affected by such motivational factors as natural hunger or by pretrial stimulation termed "priming." Today, researchers still wonder about these things, but they generally do not work on them. Often, self-stimulation behavior as a whole is not studied, but rather, a curve shift or a threshold shift is studied to try to isolate a portion of the behavioral effects, particularly the *reward* of the ESB. The purpose of this work is usually to characterize the underlying substrate, to study the effects of a lesion, or to measure the impact of a drug.

This change in interest appears to us to be a result of the realization of how difficult were the original behavioral questions and of how powerful the modern psychophysical and neurobiological tools are in answering questions of the underlying neural structure. Yet it is certainly the hope of many of us who work in this area that a firmer understanding of the relevant neural structure will shed some light on the early behavioral questions in new and powerful ways. The following discussion of ESB is selective in view of the fact that there are other good reviews of this literature (Rolls, 1976; Mogenson & Cieo, 1977; Olds, 1977; Gallistel, 1983).

Priming

Priming refers to the ability of rewarding ESB in the lateral hypothalamus to increase the vigor of performance of the next operant response for more of the same ESB. The term *priming* reminds one of the priming of a pump and refers to the belief that it is a motivational or craving process that gets the behavior started and that keeps it going. Originally, this concept was advanced by Deutsch (1960), Howarth and Deutsch (1962), and Gallistel (1967) to explain the rapidity with which rats would give up responding for ESB once the lever or other manipulandum was disconnected from the stimulator, as compared to the same experiment done with food or water reward. The rapid extinction was disconcerting because the strong preference for ESB over food, even to the point of starvation (Routtenberg & Lindy, 1965), suggests that ESB is a considerably stronger reward than food. Priming theorists explained that food rewards operated in the presence of a food-deprivation-induced motivational state, hunger. On the other hand, the motivational state underlying ESB reward was partially created by the ESB itself, and since there was no primary need for deprivation, this state decayed with time. Howarth and Deutsch (1962) demonstrated that, in an ESB extinction situation, simply retracting the lever to allow time for decay of the priming after-effect produced as much decrement in responding as if the lever had been present during extinction and the animal allowed to make unreinforced responses. Thus, we are left to conclude that it is not the animal's experience with nonreward that matters here, but simply the decay of the after-effect. Later, in more convincing and simpler experiments, Gallistel (1967, 1969a) showed that pretrial priming in a runway produced elevated responding for ESB reward and that this elevation in responding decreased or decayed with time since the last prime (Figure 8.1). Larger amounts of priming produced longer decay patterns in this experiment (cf., Gallistel, 1973). This decay is not seen for reward effects of ESB, which, like conventional rewards, are remembered from trial to trial and even from day to day.

The study of priming reached its peak by the early 1970s. A multi-author paper (Reid et al., 1973) showed priming to be a widespread effect that could be obtained in a number of laboratories with appropriate attention to the ESB parameters and testing methods. Priming could be obtained with pretrial ESB applied at any electrode site within the lateral hypothalamus, and the animal could be reinforced on any other electrode in this region (Gallistel, 1969b). This site-independence is all the more interesting when it is considered that effects of hunger and thirst states on ESB self-stimulation have been shown to be site-specific (Gallistel &

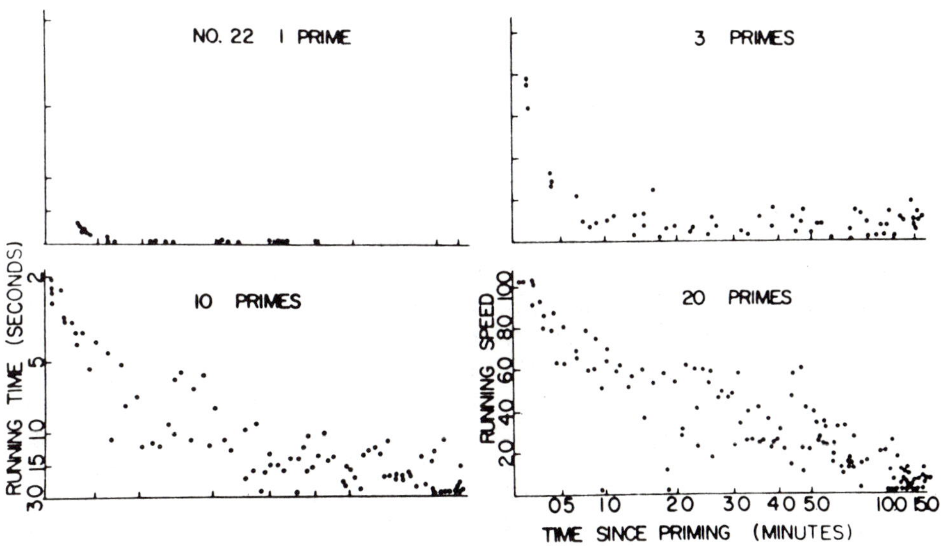

Figure 8.1 Running speed in a runway plotted against the time since the last pretrial priming ESB. As the amount of the priming increases on the different panels, the decay of vigor of runway performance grows longer. Note that, at no time in this experiment was the ESB reward for running the runway altered. (Gallistel, 1969a). Reprinted by permission.

Beagely, 1971). In comparing the vigor of behavior shown to two ESB rewards, Gallistel (1969a) demonstrated a paradox that could only be resolved by an understanding of priming effects. Here, rats could be made to run a runway faster to the *lower* of two ESB rewards if that lower reward were preceded by a sufficiently higher level of pretrial priming. This was true despite the fact that "T" maze testing showed that the rats did prefer the higher reward (Gallistel, 1969a). Only by postulating a stronger motivational craving (i.e., the priming effect) for the lower reward, could one explain these data.

One of the last papers attempting to establish the priming phenomenon showed that increases in runway running behavior, following an increment in the level of pretrial priming, were seen *immediately* in the first trial of testing (Gallistel et al., 1974). This contrasted with the temporal pattern of changes in running speed seen after the ESB reward was changed. Here, increasing the ESB reward obtained by running the runway produced no change in the animal's behavior on the first trial, since the animal had not yet sampled the new reward level. Later trials revealed a gradual upward adjustment of running speed in a classic learning curve that reflects the animal's growing experience with the new level of ESB reward (Gallistel et al., 1974). Thus, reward effects are thought to be memory-based and therefore time-independent, while priming effects are time-dependent and thus decay. In this same series, another paper (Edmonds & Gallistel, 1974) included a demonstration that pretrial priming increases raised the asymptotic level of responding on a reward summation function, but did not shift the locus of rise. According to our earlier analysis (chapter 5), this indicates that the priming did not alter the pulse effectiveness of the ESB in generating reward, but rather, acted as a performance variable to increase responding.

The above evidence constitutes a solid demonstration of the existence of the priming effect. At one time, still better evidence was thought to exist in support of a priming–reward distinction. Early studies of refractory period estimation showed a difference in the refractory period estimates for priming and reward effects of ESB (cf., Gallistel, 1973). However, Yeomans (1975) later demonstrated that all of these early studies were done without sufficient regard for the scaling problems of ESB refractory period estimation. When the studies were replicated with improved measurement techniques (see chapter 5), the reward–priming distinction did not appear (Gallistel et al., 1981). Subsequent writings (Gallistel, 1983) are left with the behavioral evidence presented in the preceding paragraphs. This support is sufficient to establish priming as an effect that must be considered when conducting ESB reward measurement experiments.

New support for a physiological distinction between reward and priming effects may come from the observation that priming temporarily restores lever-press behavior in a neuroleptic-treated rat undergoing extinction (Wasserman et al., 1982). From this, one could conclude that priming is independent of dopamine. However, since dopamine is likely to be involved in both reward effects of ESB and in motor activation and/or motivational arousal processes (see chapter 7), priming stimulation may simply release enough dopamine to produce arousal effects to temporarily overcome the neuroleptic blockade. This may be analogous to the classic response of akinetic Parkinson patients to stressful stimuli—that is, they move during the stimulation and collapse after the stimulation stops. Thus, one need not conclude that priming is independent of dopamine, and therefore physiologically different from reward effects of ESB; however, more research is needed. Regardless of the ultimate status of our knowledge about the neural substrate for the priming effect, we know it is a behavioral phenomenon that must be considered when measuring ESB reward (chapter 5), and it remains an interesting theoretical issue in speculations about the relationship of ESB self-stimulation to natural reward.

Relation of ESB to Natural Reward

The relationship of natural reward to ESB reward has long been of interest to researchers in this area. One question concerns the unique temporal relations of ESB reward versus that of other rewards. For example, food reward obtained by the typical operant response of pressing a lever must then be followed by a second behavior of moving over to the food dispenser and ingesting the pellet. This is really a two-component response. On the other hand, ESB reward obtained by pressing a lever is delivered at the moment the lever-press is detected by the equipment. In a clever series of experiments, the temporal arrangement was made equal. First, a rat was fitted with a tube that ran into the animal's mouth. Chocolate milk could be delivered through that tube as soon as the rat pressed the lever, thus mimicking the instantaneous delivery of a typical ESB reward (Panksepp & Trowell, 1967). This made acquisition just as fast under natural reward as under ESB reward. In a second experiment, rats were trained to press a lever for ESB reward, but before they actually could collect their reward, they had to lick a dry water spout. This mimicked the temporal arrangement of a typical natural reward delivery situation (Gibson, Reid, Sakai, & Porter, 1965). Under these conditions, ESB had the same temporal properties in acquisition and extinction as natural food and water rewards. Thus, ESB and natural reward may not be fundamentally different as long as temporal arrangements of reinforcement delivery are made the same. Yet one might still expect some differences.

One difference is the reliance of most natural rewards on a motivational state such as hunger or thirst. In ESB self-stimulation, no steady motivational state is present. In fact, if such a state is induced by deprivation of food or water, rats will show increases in ESB self-stimulation rate and vigor of performance (Hoebel, 1975). The basis for this increase is probably not increases in the size of reward properties of ESB, since all of the increase in runway running behavior produced by food deprivation appears on the first trial during which the animal is tested when hungry (Stellar & Gallistel, 1975). If ESB reward were increased, then the animal would not know of this increase until after the first trial, at least. In this respect, the deprivation has been observed by these authors to act similarly to pretrial priming stimulation. However, Stellar and Gallistel (1975) warn against making an inference that priming stimulation works simply by activating a temporary hunger state in the animal, since pretrial priming was shown to disrupt runway running for food or to disrupt the simple ingestion of food, even if it is highly palatable (Stellar & Heard, 1976; Cox, Kakolewski, & Valenstein, 1969).

Although the motivational state deriving from deprivation of food or water does not produce increases in the reward properties of lateral hypothalamic ESB, motivational states are known for their directing as well as their energizing properties. Gallistel and Beagely (1971) have demonstrated that changing the deprivation state from food deprivation to water deprivation can lead to shifts in preference of one lateral hypothalamic ESB site over another. This suggests that the ESB reward has some of the properties of a natural food or water stimulus. Although it is hard to know what these properties might be, it is well-established by electrophysiology that lateral hypothalamic neurons are driven by the sight of food or stimuli that are paired with food, but only if the animal is deprived (Rolls, 1982).

Evoked Motivational Effects

The difficulties in interpreting ESB effects in terms of natural motivational states are shown by the work of Valenstein and his associates. This work is predicated upon the observation that ESB of the lateral hypothalamus often leads to elicited feeding or drinking behavior when food or water are present (Margules & Olds, 1962; Cox, Kakloweski, & Valenstein, 1969; Hoebel, 1975). This phenomenon is termed "stimulus-bound feeding or drinking," and the implicit conclusion from this observation is that natural hunger or thirst was aroused by stimulation of a feeding or a drinking circuit and that the animal acted accordingly. Valenstein et al. (1968) showed that this was likely to be an over-simplification by demonstrating that a rat that ate, but did not drink, in response to ESB could be made to drink by "training." Training consisted of removing the food from the chamber, leaving the water, and regularly delivering ESB. With the dominant drive's goal object (e.g., the food) missing, the rats began to show drinking behavior. The food was then reintroduced in a final test session, and it was found that the proportion of time spent eating rather than drinking in response to ESB did not go back to that seen initially. Instead, the rat spent a great deal more time than expected showing drinking behavior.

The researchers concluded (Valenstein, Cox, & Kakolewski, 1968, 1970) that the effects of ESB could not have been to activate a fixed hunger circuit in the hypothalamus. A rat supposedly made hungry by ESB might also drink water if only water was present, and one could conclude that the animal was, to some lesser extent, also thirsty. However, such a rat would certainly have switched back to eating in the final test, when food was reintroduced, if the dominant motivation elicited by ESB was indeed hunger. Instead, Valenstein et al. (1969) argue that somehow we have a misconception when we think of this consummatory response as reflecting hunger elicited by ESB. Rather, they suggest that we think of the ESB as activating some arousal function that causes the animal to seek to execute a consummatory act. Choice of the particular consummatory act (e.g., feeding, drinking, gnawing) may be determined by which response is prepotent in the animal's behavioral repertoire. Thus, the elicited response may be more characteristic of the individual animal and its past experience than of the site of ESB (Valenstein et al., 1970). Indeed, some animals never show a consummatory response to ESB.

In 1972, Teitelbaum argued that the notion of fixed hypothalamic circuits for hunger and thirst could be salvaged by making the reasonable postulation that if mixed circuits for hunger and thirst existed, then they would likely be linked by mutual inhibition. Then, taking the model of mutual inhibition in the retina and other sensory systems that lead to perceptual contrast enhancement (Békésy, 1967), he argued that the underlying differences in activation of hunger and thirst systems could be small, but appear large behaviorally because of contrast enhancement. Small differences in baseline activity in the system, which could be induced by the training procedure, would then lead to large shifts in behavior. This argument is buttressed by the finding that very small stimulation electrodes were able to achieve much more specificity of initially elicited behavior than larger electrodes (Olds, Allan & Briese, 1971). Unfortunately, the Olds group did not try training their subjects the way Valenstein's group did.

A strong counter-argument to the Teitelbaum (1972) explanation was offered by making lesions through the ESB electrode (Bachus & Valenstein, 1979). These lesions destroyed the activated tissue and resulted in an increase in stimulating current needed to bring back elicited behavior. This was expected because higher currents are needed to activate tissue that is distant from the electrode tip. However, the lesions did not alter the *type* of ESB-evoked consummatory behavior that was seen in these animals. The lesion should have so reorganized the way that ESB impacts on the lateral hypothalamic tissue that the type of behavior seen in post-lesion testing would bear no special relationship to the pre-lesion behavior, but it did. They conclude that the type of behavior seen is not dependent on fixed circuits, but rather is a general manifestation of arousal. The response depends on the rat itself, on its conditioning history, and is labeled "prepotent" (Valenstein et al. 1969; Valenstein, 1975) perhaps to distance the concept from the fixed-circuit notion. The notion that the type of elicited behavior seen is dependent upon the rat rather than the specific neural circuits is reinforced by the finding that good predictions about which animals of a group will show schedule-induced polydipsia can be made if one knows which animals show elicited feeding behavior in response to ESB (Mittleman & Valenstein, 1984).

In this analysis, one must remember that a lateral hypothalamic electrode will have many effects on behavior. For example, in addition to any motivational characteristics, the stimulation is likely to have reward properties that could partially explain the training effect, discussed above, by appealing to superstitious conditioning. To make matters worse, those reward properties always occur whenever elicited eating is observed (Margules & Olds, 1962), and may be enhanced by the act of eating. It has been shown that the ESB current threshold to elicit lever-pressing can be made even lower if food is presented along with the lever so that eating can occur as well as pressing (Coons and Cruce, 1968).

To go back to an even more basic issue, rewarding ESB effects are strongly connected to the lateral hypothalamus, where ESB elicits feeding effects. However, early psychological theories describe the hunger (and other) motivational state(s) as aversive and would predict that a *reward* electrode should be in the neural system concerned with satiety. The nearest one can come to a hypothalamic satiety system is in the medial hypothalamus, where ESB is overwhelmingly aversive (Hoebel, 1975). All this suggests that we may need some additional ways of looking at changes in responding that are evoked by hypothalamic stimulation. One example of this is given in the next section.

Approach–Withdrawal Function

One of the other ways we might look at hypothalamic function is by taking a more general approach. For example, it has been shown (Stellar et al. 1979) that lateral hypothalamic stimulation leads to changes in a variety of approach and withdrawal behaviors as assessed by neurological tests. As an example of approach behaviors, it can be shown that orienting toward a touch to the snout or an attractive odor is enhanced by low levels of lateral hypothalamic ESB. Lower concentrations of a sweet-tasting sugar solution (but not water) are accepted by rats receiving this ESB, and some of these animals showed stimulus-elicited consummatory behavior (Stellar et al., 1979). A variety of other approach-type behaviors are activated by lateral hypothalamic stimulation. These include the stimulus-elicited eating, discussed above, predatory attack (Wassman & Flynn, 1962; Panksepp, 1971c), object carrying (Phillips, Cox, Kakolewski, & Valenstein, 1969), and exploration behaviors (Christopher & Butter, 1968). Finally, as discussed often in this book, rats will seek out and work for the brain stimulation itself.

On the other hand, lateral hypothalamic stimulation was shown to have a suppressive effect on several pain-motivated withdrawal behaviors. Escape and avoidance behaviors are suppressed (Rose, 1974; Stellar et al., 1979), and rats do not discriminate between hypothalamic stimulation plus footshock and hypothalamic stimulation alone (Cox & Valenstein, 1965). During lateral hypothalamic stimulation, rats fail to respond to strong ammonia-soaked swabs, which cause trigeminal pain in the olfactory membranes and they also show attenuated startle to intense auditory stimuli (Stellar, 1976). Unlike the effect of central gray stimulation (cf., Leibeskind & Paul, 1977), this hypothalamic "analgesia" does not extend to reflexes, as shown in Figure 8.2. The same animals that show suppression of shock-induced escape behavior will show only attenuation of a simpler flinch response and may show no effect at all on a quite simple single limb withdrawal test (Stellar, 1976; see Figure 8.2). Thus, one should be careful about using the term *analgesia* in this case since it does not apply to reflexes.

Stimulation of the ventromedial hypothalamus and lesion of the lateral hypothalamus produce exaggeration of withdrawal behaviors and suppression of approach (Stellar et al., 1979). This is not surprising in

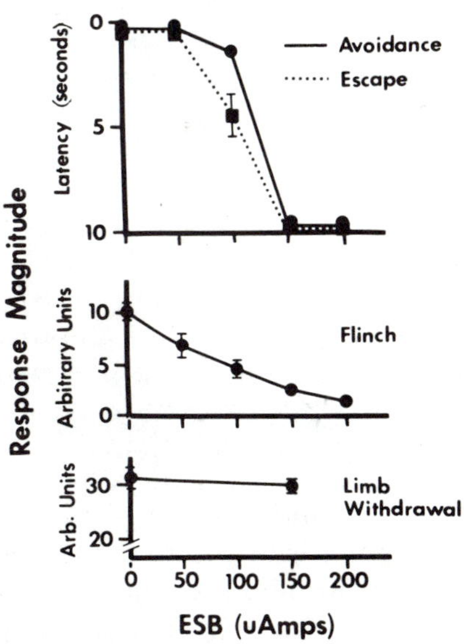

Figure 8.2 Data on the effects of rewarding lateral hypothalamic ESB on response suppression in several footshock tests. (Top) Escape latency in a jump-out box with 8 cm high walls. (Middle) Magnitude of the flinch response. (Bottom) Size of a simple withdrawal of the hind foot. Footshock current is 1.0 M amps (RMS). The latter two tests employed a brief (0.1 s) footshock. Note, as the response becomes progressively simpler (i.e., going from escape to flinch to hind foot withdrawal), the suppressive or "analgesic" effects of the ESB decrease.

the case of ventromedial hypothalamic stimulation because this stimulation is aversive (Olds & Olds, 1963; Stellar et al., 1979), but in the case of lesions of the lateral hypothalamus, most researchers had focused on the loss of the approach behavior of feeding as the important symptom. Yet, following this lesion, rats show withdrawal from almost every stimulus when they are able to show any behavior at all (Stellar et al., 1979). For example, introduction of bitter quinine into the mouth leads to a variety of behaviors designed to expel the substance (Norgren & Grill, 1982). This reaction is greatly exaggerated following a lateral hypothalamic lesion (Stellar et al., 1979). The combination of an arousal deficit (Marshall & Teitelbaum, 1974) and a bias toward withdrawal behaviors may explain why some animals show passive aphagia (they are hypoaroused) or active aphasia (they are withdrawal-biased), as seen by Schallert, Whishaw, De Ryck, & Teitelbaum (1978).

In this context, the question is whether the approach and withdrawal behaviors are natural ones beyond these hypothalamic effects and are therefore meaningful in a larger psychobiological context. One way to address this problem is to look at the research of others working outside this particular problem area. Long ago, Schneirla (1959, 1965) postulated that approach and withdrawal behaviors formed two natural classes of behavior that could be elicited by weak and strong stimuli, respectively. He constructed elaborate theories of development based upon these notions. Later, Glickman and Schiff (1967) postulated a relationship between approach reflexes and operant behavior. In this view, approach and withdrawal reflexes developed early in evolution to respond to stimuli that were either beneficial to survival (e.g., food) or harmful (e.g., pain), respectively. In their analysis, these reflexes and the associated stimuli then served as the bases for later evolutionary developments, giving rise to the brain systems that generate operant behavior. The natural result was that approach reflexes were linked to positive reinforcement stimuli. Although Glickman and Schiff are not alone in their view of the way reflex behavior in general might underlie operant behavior (see, Teitelbaum, 1977), this is one of the few papers to deal with the approach–withdrawal dichotomy in theory.

Early neurological work that predated this categorization of behavior came from the findings of Denny-Brown (1958). In a paper on apraxia, he demonstrated the existence of two classes of motor dysfunction that are associated with cortical lesions in humans. The first type is termed *approach apraxia* and is reflected as a release of a variety of tactually guided approach behaviors following certain lesions of the frontal lobe. These behaviors include a display of infantile rooting and sucking responses to light touch to the patient's cheek by the examiner's finger. Touch or pressure to the palm leads to grasping of the hand, and touch to the planter surface leads to grasping of the feet. At times, the hand grasp reaction may even be elicited visually or by tactile stimulation to the back of the hand, causing an orienting movement of the hand and arm, followed by a grasp (Denny-Brown, 1958). These reactions are often beyond the patient's control and may be strikingly unilateral. In illustration of this, it was observed that when such a frontal lobe patient grasped a door knob with the hand contralateral to the lesion, the patient could not let go and was forced to pry the fingers loose with the good hand. The second type of apraxia discussed by Denny-Brown (1958) was the avoidance (we would call it withdrawal) type. Here, patients with certain parietal lobe lesions were observed to retreat from tactile stimulation of the palm or face. This is opposite in sign to the syndrome of the frontal lobe.

Other neurological support comes from the study of the immediate behavioral changes following aspiration lesions of the caudate nucleus in cats (Villablanca, Marcus, & Olmstead, 1976). In this state, the cats exhibited strong orientation and approach behaviors toward tactile and auditory stimuli. For example, if the experimenter tapped on the table, the cat would run over and put its face up to the experimenter's hand. If the hand was then moved, the cat followed, giving the impression of being stuck to the examiner's hand. This type of behavior was not seen in these cats before lesion.

The above arguments establish the approach–withdrawal category as a useful way of looking at the effects of hypothalamic and perhaps other brain manipulations. The relevant question now is whether this model is at the correct level of generality for discussions of hypothalamic function. This question is impossible to answer with today's understanding of the way function emerges from structure, and these kinds of synthetic questions, in general, are the most difficult to address properly in psychobiology. As stated at the outset, the difficulty of this type of question is precisely what turned researchers to questions of structure. However, it is important to have a number of models available (i.e., hunger, approach–withdrawal, arousal) to keep our concepts from calcifying around one line of thought.

Hierarchical Organization

One way of thinking about motivation is not as a model of behavioral function. Rather, it is really a framework for looking at and organizing behavior from a structural perspective. This way of thinking is hierarchical and takes into account the multiple levels of brain representation of behavior. Hierarchical views of neural function have an old and rich tradition in neuroscience (Jackson, 1884; Sherrington, 1906; McLean, 1970). We have just looked at hierarchical organization or levels of function in Figure 8.2, where the "analgesic" effects of lateral hypothalamic brain stimulation were shown to be dependent upon the level of complexity of the response tested. Single limb withdrawal, a behavior that can be a spinally organized reflex, was not affected by the ESB, while simple escape, a behavior certainly requiring the brainstem (and very likely more rostral structures), was completely suppressed. Another example comes from the work on predatory attack and the biting reflex (Flynn et al., 1970), discussed in chapter 4. Here, the "motivational" state was seen to set up a reflex that was triggered by touch to the lip. The estrogenergic control of lordosis (Pfaff, 1980) and the organization of components of ingestive behavior in the decerebrate rat (Norgren & Grill, 1982) are further examples (also discussed in chapter 4). The problem with all of these studies is that, although they deal with reflex components of motivational states, they do not solve the problem of showing how motivated behavior might emerge from the hierarchical organization. Only rarely has this issue been raised and even more rarely has it been directly confronted as a research problem.

The work and recent writings of Gallistel and of Teitelbaum and his associates examine the issue of levels of function or hierarchical organization (Gallistel, 1980; Teitelbaum, 1977; Teitelbaum, 1982; Teitelbaum et al., 1983). Teitelbaum et al. (1983) investigated lower level control systems, or what they call "motor subsystems" in the organization of motivated behavior. Motor subsystems are functional units of motor organization that are more complex (at a higher hierarchical level) than reflexes, but simpler (at a lower hierarchical level) than motivated behaviors. For example, following lateral hypothalamic lesions, rats are akinetic; however, the motor subsystem responsible for posture and support may remain functional. In these cases, a rat will resist a push from the experimenter by postural bracing (see Figure 7.2) and appears stubbornly rooted to the spot. Such a rat can also be placed in unusual postures (e.g., head down with hind feet up on a brick) and will remain there for a long time. This is termed *catalepsy*. However, if the rat is pushed to displace its center of gravity so that it would fall over, it will move to reestablish a supportive posture. If dropped upside down onto a soft cushion, the rat will right itself in mid-air. If placed upside down on a flat surface, the rat will also right itself. Thus, movement does occur in these supposedly akinetic preparations, but does not do so outside the purposes of the posture and support subsystem.

One interesting side story has been the finding that temperature influences the posture and support subsystem. Cooling makes the animal more rigid and cataleptic in its posture and will ultimately induce shivering, while warming relaxes the posture and can even allow the experimenter to place the rat on its side without engaging the posture and support subsystem. These effects occur in lateral hypothalamically lesioned and in neonatal rats, both of which may have this subsystem operating in relative isolation from the higher level and more sophisticated behavioral controls of the normal adult animal (Teitelbaum et al., 1983). Teitelbaum et al. (1983) suggest that perhaps in evolution, thermal control mechanisms took advantage of the posture and support subsystem to serve temperature regulation. This is something one might not suspect and would never have discovered if the posture and support subsystems had not been experimentally isolated from other subsystems and from higher behavioral control.

The control of head and body movement represents another motor subsystem in the Teitelbaum et al. (1983) scheme. Here it is observed that, after lateral hypothalamic lesions, rats are akinetic but recover movement gradually. First, they move their heads from side to side in a lateral scanning movement. These scans grow in size with recovery until the animal can nearly turn, but the hind feet do not move unless the front feet literally drag them into a stepping movement as part of a lateral scan that has become a turn. Such animals at this stage of recovery can only pivot on the position of their hind feet. When forward locomotion recovers (a different system), the animal can move but is easily trapped in a cul-de-sac. Lateral scanning movements will not be able to get the rat out of the cul-de-sac if it is narrow, and the rat is trapped. With still more recovery, a vertical scanning movement occurs that enables the rat to lift its head and forequarters upward, but only if the nose and whiskers are in contact with the wall. These rats never rear in the middle of an open field. The vertical scan allows the animal to rise on its hind feet and turn laterally to escape the trap. Putting a top on the cul-de-sac traps the rat again, since the retropulsion movements required to back up do not recover for some time. In this way full movement can be seen to be a complex concatenation of components, including the ones mentioned above, that are smoothly and beautifully integrated into sophisticated behavioral acts by higher hierarchical systems.

At some level of the hierarchy, motivation appears. It is difficult to say exactly where this occurs. Gallistel (1983) suggests it is at the hypothalamic level, with its ability to potentiate and depotentiate (inhibit) lower level mechanisms. Teitelbaum (1982) also thinks that the hypothalamus might be a crucial place, for very large lateral hypothalamic lesions come close to producing what he calls the "zero condition" for motivated behaviors in which the animal shows little spontaneous behavior. He hopes that by a detailed analysis of the motor subsystems he isolates, as recovery proceeds from these large lateral hypothalamic lesions, he can synthesize motivated behavior from the components. This act of synthesis and its linkage to structure may be the hardest of all tasks in psychobiology. It may be especially hard in the case of the hypothalamus, which is perforated by many fiber systems (see Figure 6.1), and so may yield many disconnections between remote structures when it is lesioned.

Peripheral and Central-Neural Controls

Turning now to more general aspects of motivation, we address first the question of peripheral versus central control. Here, the issue should not be which is the controlling variable, but rather the relative contributions of each and how they interact. As pointed out in chapter 4, we are probably dealing with many reiterated peripheral to central-neural to peripheral loops in which the peripheral stimuli influence the central mechanisms, and the outputs of the central-neural mechanisms cause peripheral changes. These peripheral changes feed back to the brain, metabolically, hormonally, and over afferent neural pathways. Thus, sweet taste elicits a cephalic insulin release through a brainstem mechanism, and insulin speeds up entry of glucose into cells and of lipids into adipocytes; the glucose, among other things, changes the peripheral metabolic signals from the liver that reach the brain over the vagus nerve (see Friedman, 1980). At the same time, the sweet taste activates cells in the lateral hypothalamus, and lateral hypothalamic cells control gastric motility and secretion, which themselves have consequences for the brain. Also, the insulin may release serotonin and thus lead to general quiescence, satiation, and sleep. All of these events contribute to the final common pathways from the brain that lead to the appetitive and consummatory phases of motivation and its satiation.

A good example of the problem of peripheral–central-neural interaction, and a new opportunity to shed light on it, comes from the evidence that peptides like cholecystokinin (CCK) and angiotensin are synthesized in the brain as well as the periphery. We know that peripherally administered CCK (intraperitoneal injection) loses its effect as a satiety factor in the rat if the vagus nerve is cut subdiaphragmatically (Smith, Jerome, Cushin, Eterno, & Simansky, 1981). Yet CCK injected into the ventricles of sheep inhibits feeding (Della-Fera and Baile, 1979), and more dramatically, intraventricular injection of antibody to CCK increases feeding (Della-Fera, Baile, Schneider, & Grinker, 1981). Maddison (1977) found that intraventricular CCK reduced operant responding for food in rats, and our laboratory (E.S.) has recently seen suppression of both appetitive and consummatory aspects of feeding with pulse intracerebroventricular injection of CCK-8 (0.08 μg/kg) into the anterior cerebral ventricles of the rat. What we don't know is how peripheral and central CCK effects interact. Because of the blood–brain barrier, CCK does not enter the brain from the periphery as far as we know. Could peripheral signals over the vagus trigger central-neutral CCK activity? Could some third factor trigger both peripheral and central CCK simultaneously? That the area postrema might be a locus for central-peripheral interaction is suggested by the recent finding that lesions in the vicinity of this circumventricular organ, which lies outside the blood–brain barrier in the caudal IVth ventricle, eliminate peripheral CCKs's effect of reducing food intake (Van der Kooy, 1984). The importance of this caudal region of the medulla is underscored in the recent report that injection of nanogram quantities of CCK into the IVth ventricle suppresses food intake in rats (Ritter & Ladenheim).

In the case of angiotensin, we know that peripheral angiotensin binds to the subfornical organ (SFO) in the anterior IIIrd ventricle and that the SFO is also one of the circumventricular organs that lie outside the blood–brain barrier. At present, however, we don't know how or where centrally synthesized angiotensin acts or how its synthesis and release may be coordinated with the synthesis and release of peripheral angiotensin.

General Arousal Versus Specific Activation

Much debate has also centered on the question of whether motivation represents a general arousal and inhibition of behavior or whether it is a specific arousal of drives and the activation of particular motor patterns (see Stricker, 1983). Obviously, it is both. In all cases, the arousal and satiation of motivated behavior have general behavioral consequences, leading to changes in gross bodily activity, searching, and general excitement, on the one hand, and quiescence and refractoriness on the other. But in each case, the behavior involved and the patterns of stimulation arousing it are highly specific. Feeding, drinking, mating, and thermoregulatory behavior are all preceded by increased restlessness and general activity, but they are made up of very different appetitive and consummatory response patterns and are triggered by very different stimulus conditions. So again, it is a question of how the general and specific activation fit together in the underlying brain mechanism, for motivated behaviors not only have general arousal in common, but they all yield reward and affect. We know that the limbic system is involved, with the hypothalamus playing a major role. Self-stimulation studies tell us that one reward system may descend caudally through the medial forebrain bundle, perhaps to the ventral tegmental area, and then may ascend rostrally to involve the nucleus accumbens. We also know that dopamine-containing neurons are involved in both self-stimulation and food reward, but there is still debate on exactly how they are involved.

Localization of Function and Hierarchical Organization

The question of localization of function arises in the attempt to understand the brain mechanisms involved in motivated behavior, especially when small lesions are made or with discrete stimulation and single unit recording. The temptation is to draw conclusions about the functions of the localized neurons that have been recorded, stimulated, or damaged. With large lesions or transactions of the neuraxis, the emphasis is upon what the remaining part of the brain can do by itself. Teitelbaum (1982) has suggested that these two approaches bear a relationship to each other that is like a figure–ground relationship in perception. It is difficult to see (or do) both at once. However, the two approaches actually complement each other nicely if we remember that we are dealing with brain systems that extend, in some hierarchical order, up and down the neuraxis. Transections tell us about levels of function that remain, and localized lesions tell us about focal points within the brain systems where fibers of passage converge (e.g., MFB) or where integrative functions are performed, bringing together information from the internal environment and afferent neural input (e.g., preoptic and anterior hypothalamus in temperature regulation).

Localization may be indicated by selective binding of hormones (e.g., estrogen in the medial preoptic, anterior and ventromedial hypothalamus); the effects of discrete lesions, especially those that affect only cell bodies (e.g,, kainic acid); and selective response to humoral factors at the lowest thresholds, particularly at physiological levels (e.g., angiotensin on the SFO). Sometimes, however, lesions or stimulations only localize fibers of passage of widespread brain systems at accessible points of anatomical convergence rather than physiological integrating mechanisms. Nevertheless, the functioning of such extensive systems can be revealed by electrical stimulation in multiple loci (e.g., ESB in the MFB, VTA, and nucleus accumbens); through anatomical tracing methods, as in the tracing of the output of the SFO; and through recording following antidromic stimulation, as Rolls (1982) has shown.

Neural hierarchies are revealed by transections that demonstrate the functional capabilities and deficits at various levels of the neuraxis in response to sensory input or internal environment changes. As Teitelbaum has pointed out, partial transections (e.g, large LH lesions) are particularly suited to showing the neural hierarchies involved because the course of post-lesion recovery of function spreads the hierarchical order out in time. Thus, structures higher in the hierarchy recover later than lower structures, so that early deficits are attributed to their absence, and later recovery to the return of their function. Particularly striking is reinstatement of earlier, lesion-produced deficits by selective suppression of the rat's cortex with KC1, so that the hyperirritability of prior septal lesions or the lateral hypothalamic syndrome are made to return in recovered animals (Teitelbaum & Cytawa, 1965).

Nature–Nurture and the Role of Experience

We have probably outgrown the nature–nurture controversy in the study of motivated behavior. Much is "hard-wired," but modification of behavior in experience is the rule, especially in birds and mammals. Thus, imprinting is innate, but what gets imprinted depends on specific experience during a critical period in development. As Hoffman and Solomon (1974) and Starr (1978) have also shown, the intensity of following and distress-calling is modified, in the short run, by nonassociative experience, such as the duration and frequency of exposure to the mother duck, according to the opponent process paradigm. Lack of the effectiveness of experience, as in the blowfly or the decerebrate rat, greatly reduces the range of motivated behavior possible. Reward and reinforcement operate minimally, if at all, in these cases, so that it is not possible to use the operant measures of motivation that have proven so fruitful in the study of intact and even diencephalic (Huston, 1982) vertebrates.

Motivation and Phylogeny

As pointed out earlier, there is a lesson in phylogeny for our understanding of the innate and acquired biological controls of the brain mechanisms involved in motivated behavior and reward. First of all, as we examine the existing, specialized representatives of the process of evolution, we see the emergence of motivated behavior from simpler, stimulus-bound approach and avoidance behaviors (e.g., taxes). As the autonomic system develops, we see the emergence of affective display. As learning becomes more possible, incentives, reward, and reinforcement play a bigger role in the expression and control of motivated behavior. In the vertebrate series, there seems to be decreasing dependence on internal environment factors and more dependence on sensory stimulation, learning, and the cerebral cortex, as the study of mating behavior suggests, (Beach, 1947; cf., Dethier & Stellar, 1961). Finally, in humans, there is the emergence of hedonic experience, which can be verbally reported in a direct and objective manner (e.g., magnitude estimation) and which can only be inferred in animals.

Motivation and Ontogeny

A similar lesson can be derived from that other great experiment of nature, ontogenetic development. Teitelbaum (1977) has pointed out that, in the development of a mammal like a rat, there is encephalization of hunger and probably of other kinds of motivation. In this process, structures higher in the neuraxis come to play more of a role as they develop. Lesions of the lateral hypothalamus, for example, cut off the influence of these more rostral structures, but with recovery of function, their influence reappears and the deficits are reduced. As Teitelbaum says "recovery recapitulates ontogeny," thus reinforcing the notion of the encephalization of motivation.

Development of motivated behavior is anticipatory. Thus, as prepubEral injection of sex hormones in the rat has shown (Beach, 1942c), the immature rat has all the brain mechanisms for mating behavior long before it normally would use them. Similarily, Ellis and Epstein (1981), Blass et al. (1979), Hall (1979), and others have traced the development of ingestive behavior in the rat and have found the controls of adult eating and drinking present in the pre-weaning rat. Again, the brain mechanisms are developed precociously, for the sucking rat responds to intraventricular angiotensin with drinking and to intraventricular norepinephrine with eating long before the adult ingestive patterns would normally occur.

Conclusions

In this early stage of scientific study of brain mechanisms of motivation and reward, our accomplishment has been to develop a map of the structures and the physiological mechanisms involved and a set of general principles whereby they function in the control of behavior:

1. We have identified loci or structures in the brain that can be experimentally manipulated to make a big difference in the arousal and satiation of motivated behaviors and in the operation of reward and reinforcement.
2. We know those structures are widespread in the limbic system and represent excitatory and inhibitory systems that bias the animal to approach or withdrawal.
3. These systems are organized in hierarchical fashion, with multiple integrators at all levels of the neuraxis, but with major integrating functions at the level of the hypothalamus where inputs are received from sensory systems, the internal environment, and structures higher and lower in the neuraxis.
4. The integrators below the hypothalamus in the neuraxis, in the brain stem and spinal cord, also are responsive to multiple inputs and they control significant parts of the responses involved in motivated behavior.
5. The hypothalamus and other structures lining the ventricles received information from the internal environment through seven known circumventricular organs that lie outside the blood–brain barrier. The hypothalamus also exerts control over the internal environment through its influence on the pituitary and through its connections with the brainstem (the dorsal vagus complex, for example). These connections allow it to participate in neural control over autonomic functions and metabolism. By potentiating and depotentiating response mechanisms lower in the neuraxis, the hypothalamus and me-

dial forebrain bundle, in particular, exert control over motivated behavior.
6. The ascending monoaminergic pathways containing different neurotransmitters and connecting widely with forebrain structures, have introduced a whole new dimension in the understanding of the mechanisms underlying motivation and reward. Not only do they play a major role in the arousal of behavior, but much of their control is on motor mechanisms crucial in the patterning of responses.
7. Since learning and experience play such important roles in motivation and reward, one important task that lies ahead of us is to determine how they influence the complex systems with which we are now dealing.

Finally, we conclude that ESB and self-stimulation stand out as a model experimental system for dealing with many of the issues about motivation and reward listed above. Thanks to the use of psychophysical methods, the behavior can now lead to quantitative rather than only qualitative inferences about the underlying substrate or about changes in that substrate as it is manipulated with lesions or drugs. Often, the quantitative methods have built into them ways of dealing with motoric or other performance-altering effects of drugs or lesions. In some cases (e.g., tradeoff functions), the performance effects are factored out of the reward measure. In other cases (e.g., the reward summation function) the performance effects are measured as a second variable in addition to reward effects. Importantly, the quantitative approach also greatly aids the search for and electrophysiological identification of ESB reward-relevant cells by providing a concept of what must be the properties of the underlying substrate. Here, 2-DG methods can also give good clues as to where to start looking.

The goal of all this, of course, is to identify the neural circuits involved in ESB reward and motivational effects. In the lateral hypothalamus much progress has been made. In chapter 6, it was pointed out that a large proportion of the ESB reward-relevant fibers were likely to be medium- to small-size myelinated fibers that ran in a rostral to caudal direction through the medial forebrain bundle. To many of us who have watched the field of ESB research struggle with this complex phenomenon, the progress seems remarkable, and the best may be yet to come, as present research holds the goal of specific cellular identification of these elements. The second-order neurons in this system may be the dopamine cells discussed in chapter 7, and here, the nucleus accumbens may figure prominently. However, these conclusions must be made tentatively, since dopamine's role in behavior is far from clear. With the identification of a portion of the ESB reward substrate, the time may then be ripe for a return to the more functional questions of the relations between ESB self-stimulation and other motivated behaviors, and for a deeper understanding of the physiology of reward processes in all mammals, including humans.

Future Outlook

An even more important matter lies ahead of us now that we know some of the major features of the brain circuits involved in motivation and reward. Certainly, we can anticipate that further details of these neural circuits will be worked out, especially with the development of new technology. What is not yet clear is how we will move from behavior through the neural circuitry to the cellular and molecular mechanisms involved. For example, in the case of feeding and drinking, how do peptides like cholecystokinin and angiotensin exert their effects on the relevant neurons? What happens to the synthesis and release of such neurochemicals in normal fluctuations of hunger and thirst? How do pharmacological agents change these properties? How can these processes be understood in molecular terms? What influence do afferent neural impulses have on cholecystokinin and angiotensin release and activity? How do genetic mechanisms cast the die? These are the types of questions that Jacques Loeb would have liked to to have asked when he stated in 1918 that his purpose was to understand behavior in physical and chemical terms. These are the types of questions we need to learn how to frame better and how to pursue more intensively if we are to bring the investigation of motivation and reward into the forefront of progress in behavioral neuroscience, where it belongs.

References

Accornero, N., Bini, G., Lenzi, G.L., & Manfredi, M. (1977). Selective activation of peripheral nerve fibre groups of different diameter by triangular shaped stimulation pulses. *Journal of Physiology, 273*, 539–560.

Adolph, E.F. (1943). *Physiological regulations.* Lancaster, PA: Jaques Cottell Press.

Allport, F.H. (1924). *Social psychology.* Boston: Houghton-Mifflin.

Allport, G.W. (1937). *Personality: A psychological interpretation.* New York: Holt.

Antin, J., Gibbs, J., Holt, J., Young, R.C., & Smith, G.P. (1975). Cholecystokinin elicits the complete behavioral sequence of satiety in rats. *Journal of Comparative and Physiological Psychology, 89*, 784–790.

Asdourian, D., Stutz, R.M., & Rocklin, K.W. (1966). Effects of thalamic and limbic system lesions on self-stimulation behavior. *Journal of Comparative and Physiological Psychology, 61*, 468–472.

Ashmead, D.H., Reilly, B.M., & Lipsitt, L.P. (1980). Neonates-heart rate, sucking rhythm, and sucking amplitude as a function of sweet taste. *Journal of Experimental Child Psychology, 29*, 264–268.

Atrens, D., Ljunberg, T., & Ungerstedt, U. (1976). Modulation of reward and aversion processes in the rat diencephalon by neuroleptics: differential effects of clozapine and haloperidol. *Psychopharmacology, 49*, 97–100.

Bachus, S., & Valenstein, E.S. (1979). Individual behavioral responses to hypothalamic stimulation persist despite destruction of tissue surrounding electrode tip. *Neuroscience Abstracts, 5*, 229.

Ball, G.G. (1974). Vagotomy: effect of electrically elicited eating and self-stimulation in the lateral hypothalamus. *Science, 184*, 484–485.

Bard, P. (1928). A diencephalic mechanism for the expression of rage with special reference to the sympathetic nervous system. *American Journal of Physiology, 84*, 490–515.

Bard, P. (1934a) The neuro-humoral basis of emotional reactions. In C. Murchison (Ed.), *A handbook of general experimental psychology* (pp. 264–311). Worcester: Clark University Press.

Bard, P. (1934b). On emotional expression after decortication with some remarks on theoretical views. *Psychological Review, 41*, 309–329.

Bard, P. (1940). The hypothalamus and sexual behavior. *Research Publication of the Association of Nervous and Mental Disease, 20*, 551–579.

Bard, P., & Mountcastle, V.B. (1947). Some forebrain mechanisms involved in expression of rage with special reference to the suppression of angry behavior. *Research Publication of the Association of Nervous and Mental Disease, 27*, 362–404.

Beach, F.A. (1942a). Analysis of factors involved in the arousal, maintenance, and manifestation of sexual excitement in male animals. *Psychosomatic Medicine, 4*, 173–198.

Beach, F.A. (1942b). Analysis of the stimuli adequate to elicit mating behavior in the sexually unexperienced male rat. *Journal of Comparative Psychololgy, 33*, 163–207.

Beach, F.A. (1942c). Sexual behavior of prepuberal male and female rats tested with gonadal hormones. *Journal of Comparative and Physiological Psychology, 34*, 285–292.

Beach, F.A. (1942d). Central nervous mechanisms involved in the reproductive behavior of vertebrates. *Psychological Bulletin, 39*, 200–206.

Beach, F.A. (1947). Evolutionary changes in the physiological control of mating behavior in mammals. *Psychological Review, 54*, 297–315.

Beach, F.A. (1955). The descent of instinct. *Psychological Review, 62*, 401–410.

Beagley, W.K., & Holley, T.L. (1977). Hypothalamic stimulation facilitates contralateral visual control of a learned response. *Science, 196*, 321–322.

Beckstead, R.M. (1979). An autoradiographic examination of cortical and subcortical projections of the mediodorsal-projection (prefrontal) cortex in the rat. *Journal of Comparative Neurology, 184*, 43–62.

Beckstead, R.M., Domesick, V., & Nauta, W.J.H. (1979). Efferent connections of the substantia nigra and ventral tegmental area in the rat. *Brain Research, 175*, 191–217.

Beebe-Center, J.G. (1932). *The psychology of pleasantness and unpleasantness.* New York: D. van Nostrand.

Beebe-Center, J.G., Black, P., Hoffman, A.O., & Wade, M. (1948). Relative per diem consumption as a measure of preference in the rat. *Journal of Comparative and Physiological Psychology, 41*, 239–251.

Békésy, G.V. (1967). *Sensory inhibition.* Princeton: Princeton University Press.

Beninger, R. J. (1982). A comparison of the effects of pimozide and nonreinforcement on discriminated operant responding in rats. *Pharmacology, Biochemistry, and Behavior, 16*, 667–669.

Beninger, R.J., & Freedman, N.L. (1982). The use of two operants to examine the nature of pimozide-induced decreases in responding for brain stimulation. *Physiological Psychology, 10*, 409–412.

Bernard, C. (1957). *An introduction to the study of experimental medicine.* New York: Dover Publications, Reprint. (Original work published 1865.)

Bernstein, I.L. (1978). Learned taste aversions in children receiving chemotherapy. *Science, 200*, 1302–1303.

Bernstein, I.L., & Goehler, L.E. (1983). Vagotomy produces learned food aversions in the rat. *Behavioral Neuroscience, 97*, 585–594.

Bernstein, I.L., & Webster, M.M. (1980). Learned taste aversions in humans. *Physiology and Behavior, 25*, 363–366.

Bernstein, I.L., Zimmerman, J.C., Czeisler, C.A., & Weitzman, E.D. (1981). Meal patterns in "free-running " humans. *Physiology and Behavior, 27*, 621–623.

Berridge, K.C., Grill, H.J. (1983). Alternating ingestive and aversive consummatory responses suggest a two dimensional analysis of palatability in rats. *Behavioral Neuroscience, 97*, 563–573.

Bertino, M., Beauchamp, G.K., Riskey, D.R. & Engelman, K. (1981). Taste perception in three individuals on a low sodium diet. *Appetite, 2*, 67–73.

Bielajew, C. (1983a). *Psychophysical inference of the direction of normal conduction in the substrate for medial forebrain bundle stimulation.* Unpublished doctoral dissertation, Concordia University, Montreal, Canada.

Bielajew, C. (1983b). Technical comment. *Science, 222*, 1252.

Bielajew, C., Jordon, C., Fermi-Enright, J., & Shizgal, P. (1981). Refractory periods and anatomical linkage of the substrates for lateral hypothalamic and periaqueductal gray self-stimulation. *Physiology & Behavior, 27*, 95–104.

Bielajew, C., & Shizgal, P. (1980). Dissociation of the substrates for medial forebrain bundle self-stimulation and stimulation-escape using a two electrode stimulation technique. *Physiology & Behavior, 25*, 707–712.

Bielajew, C., & Shizgal, P. (1982). Behaviorally derived measures of conduction velocity in the substrate for rewarding medial forebrain bundle stimulation. *Brain Research, 237*, 107–119.

Bielajew, C., Walker, S., & Fouriezos, G. (1983). Refractoriness of reward-relevant neurons in the nucleus accumbens and adjacent structures. *Neuroscience Abstracts, 9*, 976.

Bindra. D. (1968). Neuropsychological interpretation of the effects of drive and incentive-motivation on general activity and instrumental behavior. *Psychological Review, 75*, 1–22.

Bindra, D., & Palfai, T. (1967). Nature of positive and negative incentive-motivational effects on general activity. *Journal of Comparative and Physiological Psychology, 63*, 288–297.

Bishop, M.P., Elder, S.T., & Heath, R.G. (1964). Attempted control of operant behavior in man with intracranial self-stimulation. In R.G Heath (Ed.), *The role of pleasure in behavior.* (pp.55–81). New York: Harper and Row.

Blass, E.M., & Epstein, A.N. (1971). A lateral preoptic osmosensitive zone for thirst in the rat. *Journal of Comparative and Physiological Psychology, 76*, 378–394.

Blass, E.M., & Fitzsimons, J.T. (1970). Additivity of effect and interaction of a cellular and an extracellular stimulus of drinking. *Journal of Comparative and Physiological Psychology, 70*, 200–205.

Blass, E.M., Hall, W.G., & Teicher, M.H. (1979). The ontogeny of sucking and ingestive behaviors. In J. M. Sprague & A.N. Epstein (Eds.), *Progress in psychobiology and physiological psychology*: (Vol. 8 pp. 243–299). New York: Academic.

Blundell, J.E. (1984). Systems and interactions: an approach to the pharmacology of eating and hunger. In A.J. Stunkard & E. Stellar (Eds.), *Eating and its disorders* (pp. 39–65). New York: Raven.

Booth, D.A. (1972). Conditioned satiety in the rat. *Journal of Comparative and Physiological Psychology, 81*, 457–471.

Boring, E.G. (1929). *A history of experimental psychology.*. New York: Appleton Century.

Boring, E.G. (1942). *Sensation and perception in the history of experimental psychology.* New York: Appleton Century.

Boyd, E.S., & Gardner, L.C. (1967). Effect of some brain lesions on intracranial self-stimulation in the rat. *American Journal of Physiology, 213*, 1044–1052.

Bozarth, M.A. (1983). Opiate reward mechanisms mapped by intracranial self-administration. In J.E. Smith & J.D. Lane (EDs.), *The neurobiology of opiate reward processes* (pp. 331–359) New York: Elsevier.

Bozarth, M.A., & Wise, R.A. (1981). Heroin reward is dependent on a dopaminergic substrate. *Life Sciences, 29*, 1881–1886.

Bozarth, M.A., & Wise, R.A. (1982). Actions of drugs of abuse on brain reward systems: an update with specific attention to opiates. *Pharmacacology, Biochemistry, and Behavior, 17*, 239–243.

Bozarth, M.A., & Wise, R.A. (1983). Neural substrates of opiate reinforcement. *Progress in neuro-pharmacology and biological psychiatry, 7*, 569–575.

Bradshaw, C.M., Ruddle, H.V., & Szabadi, E. (1981). Relationshp between response rate and reinforcement frequency in variable-interval schedules. III. The effect of d-amphetamine. *Journal of the Experimental Analysis of Behavior, 36*, 29–39.

Breese, G.R., Howard, J.L., & Leahy, J.P. (1971). Effect of 6-hydroxydopamine on electrical self-stimulation of brain. *British Journal of Pharmacology, 43*, 255–257.

Brobeck, J.R. (1946). Mechanisms of the development obesity in animals with hypothalamic lesions. *Physiological Reviews, 26*, 541–599.

Broca, P. (1878). Anatomie comparie des circonvolutions cerebrales. Le grand lobe limbique et la scissure limbique dun la serie des mammiferes. *Rhoue Antropologie, 1*, 385–498.

Broekkamp, C.L., Phillips, A.G., & Cools, A.R. (1979). Facilitation of self-stimulation behavior following intracerebral microinjection of opioids into the ventral tegemental area. *Phamacology, Biochemistry, and Behavior, 11*, 289–295.

Broekkamp, C.L., VanDenBoggard, J.H., Heijnen, H.J., Rops, R.H., Cools, A.R., & VanRossum, J.M. (1976). Separation of inhibiting and stimulating effects of morphine on self-stimulation behavior by intracerebral microinjections. *European Journal of Pharmacology, 36*, 443–446.

Broekkamp, C., & VanRossum, J. (1975). The effect of microinjections of morphine and halperidol into the neostriatum and nucleus accumbens on self-stimulation behavior. *Archives of International Pharmacology, 217*, 110–117.

Brown, J.S. (1979). Motivation. In E. Hearst (Ed.) *The first century of experimental psychology* (pp. 231–272).Hillsdale, NJ: Erlbaum.

Bunney, B. (1983). Neuroleptics: electrophysiological pharmacology. In J.T. Coyle & S.J. Enna (Eds.), *Neuroleptics: Neurochemical, behavioral, and clinical perspectives* (pp. 157–181). New York: Raven.

Butler, R.A. (1953). Discrimination learning by rhesus monkeys to visual-exploration motivation. *Journal of Comparative and Physiological Psychology, 46*, 95–98.

Cabanac, M. (1971). Physiological role of pleasure. *Science, 173*, 1103–1107.

Cabanac, M. (1979). Sensory pleasure. *The Quarterly Review of Biology, 54*, 1–29.

Cabanac, M., Massonnet, B., & Belaiche, R. (1972). Preferred skin temperature as a function of internal and mean skin temperature. *Journal of Applied Physiology, 33*, 699–703.

Cabanac, M., Minaire, Y. & Adair, E.R. (1968). Influence of internal factors on the pleasantness of a gustative sweet sensation. *Communications in Behavioral Biology, 1*, 77–82.

Cannon, W.B. (1927). The James-Lange theory of emotion: A critical examination and alternative theory. *Americal Journal of Psychology, 39*, 106–124.

Cannon, W.B. (1932). *The wisdom of the body*. New York: Norton.

Carey, R.J. (1982). Effect of unilateral 6-OHDA lesions of the substantia nigra on lateral hypothalamic self-stimulation. In B.G. Hoebel & D. Novin (Eds.), *The neural basis of feeding and reward.* (pp. 249–304). Brunswick, ME: Haer Institute.

Cassens, G.P., Actor, C., Kling, M., & Schildkraut, J.J. (1981). Amphetamine withdrawal effects of threshold of intracranial reinforcement. *Psychopharmacology, 73*, 318–322.

Cassens, G.P., & Mills, A.W. (1973). Lithium and amphetamine: Opposite effects on threshold of intracranial reinforcement. Psychopharmacology, 30, 283–290.

Chambers, W.W., Seigel, M.S., Liu, J.C., & Liu, C.N. (1974). Thermaregulatory responses of decerebrate and spinal cats. *Experimental Neurology, 42*, 282–299.

Christopher, M. & Butter, C.M. (1968). Consummatory behaviors and locomotion exploration evoked from self-stimulation sites in rats. *Journal of Comparative and Physiological Psychology, 66*, 335–339.

Chronister, R.B., & DeFrance, J.F. (1981). Nucleus accumbens in historical perspective. In: R. Chronister & J. DeFrance (Eds.), *The neurobiology of the nucleus accumbens* (pp. 1–6). Brunswick, ME: Haer Institute.

Clavier, R.M., & Fibiger, H.C. (1977). On the role of ascending catecholaminergic projections in intracranial self-stimulation of the substantia nigra. *Brain Research, 131*, 271–281.

Clavier, R.M., & Gerfen, C. (1979). Self-stimulation of the sulcal prefrontal cortex in the rat: direct evidence for ascending dopaminergic mediation. *Neuroscience Letters, 12*, 183–187.

Cofer, N.C., & Appley, M.H. (1964). *Motivation: Theory and research.* New York: Wiley.

Colle, L.M. (1984). *Dopamine terminal ablations attenuate lateral hypothalamic reward.*

Paper presented at Canadian Psychological Association meetings. Ottawa, Canada.

Coons, E.E., & Cruce, J.A.F. (1968). Lateral hypothalamus: Food and current intensity in maintaining self-stimulation of hunger. *Science, 159*, 1117–1119.

Cooper, B.R., Cott, J.M., & Breese, G.R. (1974). Effects of catecholamine-depleting drugs and amphetaine on self-stimulation of brain following various 6- hydroxydopamine treatments. *Psychopharmacologia, 37*, 235–248.

Cooper, J.R., Bloom, F.E., & Roth, R.H. (1982). *The Biochemical basis of neuropharmacology*. New York: Oxford University Press.

Corbett, D., Laferriere, A., & Milner, P. (1982). Elimination of medial prefrontal cortex self-stimulation following transection of efferents to the sulcal cortex in the rat. *Physiology and Behavior, 29*, 425–431.

Corbett, D., Laferriere, A., & Milner, P. (1982b). Plasticity of the medial prefrontal cortex: facilitation of self-stimulation by prior electrical stimulation. *Physiology and Behavior, 28*, 531–534.

Corbett, D., Silva, L., & Stellar, J.R., (in press). An investigation of the factors affecting development of frontal cortex self-stimulation. *Physiology and Behavior.*

Corbett, D., Skelton. R.W., & Wise, R.A. (1977). Dorsal bundle lesions fail to disrupt self-stimulation from the region of the locus coeruleus. *Brain Research, 133*, 37–44.

Corbett, D., & Stellar, J.R. (1983). Neurological reactivity during medial prefrontal cortex stimulation: Effects of self-stimulation experience, *Physiology and Behavior, 31*, 771–776.

Corbett, D., Stellar, J., Stinus, L., Kelley, A., & Fouriezos, G. (1983). Time course of a-flupenthixol action explains "response artifacts" of neuroleptic action on brain stimulation reward. *Science, 222*, 1251–1252.

Corbett, D., & Wise, R. (1979). Intracranial self-stimulation in relation to the ascending noradrenergic fiber systems of the pontine tegmentum and caudal midbrain: a moveable electrode mapping study. *Brain Research, 177*, 423–436.

Corbett, D., & Wise, R. (1980). Intracranial self-stimulation in relation to the ascending dopamine systems of the midbrain: a moveable electrode mapping study. *Brain Research, 185*, 1–15.

Corbit, J.D. (1973). Voluntary control of hypothalamic temperature. *Journal of Comparative and Physiological Psychology, 83*, 394–411.

Corbit, J.D., & Ernits, T. (1974). Specific preference for hypothalamic cooling. *Journal of Comparative and Physiological Psychology, 86*, 24–27.

Corbit, J.D., & Stellar, E. (1964). Palatability, food intake, and obesity in normal and hyperphagic rats. *Journal of Comparative and Physiological Psychology, 58*, 63–67.

Corradini, A., Tombaugh, T., & Anisman, H. (1984). Effects of pimozide on escape and discrimination performance in a water-escape task. *Behavior Neuroscience, 98*, 96–106.

Cox, V., Kakolewski, J., & Valenstein, E. (1969). Inhibition of eating and drinking following hypothalamic stimulation in the rat. *Journal of Comparative and Physiological Psychology, 68*, 530–535.

Cox, V., & Valenstein, E.S. (1965). Attenuation of aversive properties of peripheral shock by hypothalamic stimulation. *Science, 149*, 323–325.

Craig, W. (1918). Appetites and aversions as constituents of instincts. *Biological Bulletin, 34*, 91–107.

Creese, I., Sibley, D.R., Hamblin, M.W., & Leff, S.E. (1983). The classification of dopamine receptors: relationship to radioligand binding. In M. Cowan, E. Shooter, C. Stevens, & R. Thompson (Eds.), *Annual Review of Neuroscience, 6*, 43–72.

Crook, C.K., & Lipsitt, L.P. (1976). Neonatal nutritive sucking: effects of taste stimulation upon sucking rhythm and heart rate. *Child Development, 47*, 518–522.

Crow, T.J. (1972). Catecholamine-containing neurons and electrical self-stimulation: a review of some data. *Psychological Medicine, 2*, 414–421.

Culberton, J., Kling, J., & Berkeley, M. (1966). Extinction responding following ICSS and food reinforcement. *Psychonomic Science, 5*, 127–128.

Cytawa, J., & Teitelbaum, P. (1967). Spreading depression and recovery of subcortical functions. *Acta Biologiae Experimentalis, 27*, 345–353.

Dahlstrom, A., & Fuxe, K. (1964). Evidence for the existence of monoamine-containing neurons in the central nervous system. I. Demonstration of monamines in the cell bodies of brain stem neurons. *Acta Physiologica Scandinavica, 62* (Suppl.), 1–55.

Darwin, C. (1873). *The expression of the emotions in man and animals.* New York: D. Appelton and Company.

Della-Fera, M.A., & Baile, C.A. (1979). Cholecystokinin octapeptide: Continuous picomole injections into the cerebral ventricles of sheep suppress feeding. *Science, 206*, 471–473.

Della-Fera, M.A., Baile, C.A., Schneider, B.S., & Grinker, J.A. (1981). Cholecystokinin antibody injected in cerebral ventricles stimulates feeding in sheep. *Science, 212*, 687–689.

Dempsey, E.W., & Rioch. D.M. (1939). The localization in the brain stem of the oestrous responses of the female guinea pig. *Journal of Neurophysiology, 2*, 9–18.

Deneau, G., Yanagita, T., & Seevers, M. (1969). Self-adminstration of psychoactive substances by the monkey: a measure of psychological dependence. *Psychopharmacology, 16*, 30–48.

Denny-Browm, T. (1958). The nature of apraxia. *Journal of Nervous and Mental Disease, 126*, 9–32.

Desor, J., Maller, O., & Turner, R. (1973). Taste in acceptance of sugars by human infants. *Journal of Comparative and Physiological Psychology, 84*, 456–501.

Dethier, V.G. (1957). Communcation by insects: Physiology of dancing. *Science, 125*, 331–336.

Dethier, V.G. (1976). *The hungry fly.* Cambridge, MA: Harvard University Press.

Dethier, V.G. (1982). The contribution of insects to the study of motivation. In. A.R. Morrison, & P.L. Strick, (Eds.), *Changing concepts of the nervous system.* (pp. 445–455). New York: Academic.

Dethier, V. G., & Stellar, E.(1961). *Animal Behavior*. Englewood Cliffs, NJ: Prentice Hall.

Deutsch, J.A. (1960). *The structural basis of behavior*. Chicago: Chicago University Press.

Deutsch, J.A. (1964). Behavioral measurement of the neural refractory period and its application to intracranial self-stimulation. *Journal of Comparative and Physiological Psychology, 58*, 1–9.

Deutsch, J.A., & Howarth, C.I. (1963). Some tests of a theory of intracranial self-stimulation. *Psychological Review, 70*, 444–460.

deVilliers, P. (1977). Choice in concurrent schedules and a quantitative formulation of the law of effect. In W. Honig & J. Staddon (Eds.), *Handbook of operant behavior* (pp. 233–287). Englewood Cliffs, NJ: Prentice Hall.

Dewey, J. (1886). *Psychology*. New York: Harper and Row.

deWit, H., & Wise, R.A. (1978). Blockade of cocaine reinforcement in rats with the dopamine receptor blocker pimozide but not with the noradrenergic blockers phentolamine or phenoxybenzamine. *Canadian Journal of Psychology, 31*, 195–203.

Domesick, V.B. (1981). Further observations on the anatomy of nucleus accumbens and caudatoputamen in the rat: Similarities and contrasts. In R.B. Chronister and J.F. DeFrance (Eds.), *The neurobiology of the nucleus accumbens*. (pp. 7–38). Brunswick, ME: Haer Institute.

Douglin, D.C., & Glassman, R.B. (1979). Gradual increase in self-stimulation response rates: Effect of electrode loci. *Physiological Psychology, 7*, 135–138.

Drewnowski, A., & Greenwood, M.R.C. (1983). Cream and sugar: Human preferences for high-fat foods. *Physiology and Behavior, 30*, 629–633.

Dunnett, S.B., & Björkland, A. (1983). Exploring dopamine function with nigral transplants. *IBBO News, 3*, 17–21.

Dunnett, S.B., Björklund, A., & Stenevi, U. (1983). Transplant-induced recovery from brain lesions: a review of the nigrostriatal model. In R.B. Wallace & G.P. Das (Eds.), *Neural transplantation research* (pp. 191–216). New York: Springer-Verlag.

Edmonds, D.E., & Gallistel, C.R. (1974). Parametric analysis of brain stimulation reward in the rat. III. Effect of performance variables on the reward summation function. *Journal of Comparative and Physiological Psychology, 87*, 876–884.

Edmonds, D.E., & Gallistel, C.R. (1977). Reward vs. performance in self-stimulation: Electrode-specific effects of methyl-p-tyrosin on reward in the rat. *Journal of Comparative and Physiological Psychology, 91*, 962–974.

Edwards, M., Wishik, J., & Sinnamon, H. (1979). Catecholaminergic and cholinergic agents and duration regulation of ICSS in the rat. *Pharmacology, Biochemistry, and Behavior, 10*, 723–731.

Ekman, P. (1982). *Emotion and the human face*. Cambridge: Cambridge University Press.

Ekman, P., Levenson, R.W., & Friesen, W.V. (1983). Autonomic nervous system activity distinguishes among emotions. *Science, 221*, 1208–1210.

Ellis, S., & Epstein, A.N. (1981). Feeding and drinking are aroused by chemical injection into infant brain. *Neuroscience Abstracts, 7*, 853.

Epstein, A.N. (1982a). Instinct and motivation as explanations for complex behavior. In D.W. Pfaff (Ed.), *The physiological mechanisms of motivation.* (pp. 25–58). New York: Springer-Verlag.

Epstein, A.N. (1982b). The physiology of thirst. In D.W. Pfaff (Ed.), *The physiological mechanisms of motivation.* (pp. 165–214). New York: Springer-Verlag.

Epstein, A.N. (1983). The neuropsychology of drinking behavior. In E. Satinoff & F. Teitelbaum (Eds.), *Handbook of behavioral neurobiology: Vol. 6. Motivation.* (pp. 367–423). New York: Plenum.

Epstein, A.N., Kissileff, H.R., & Stellar, E. (Eds.) (1973). *The neuropsychology of thirst.* Washington, DC: V.H. Winston and Sons.

Epstein, A.N. Zhang, D-M., Schultz, J., Rosenberg, M., Kupsha, P., Stellar, E. (1984). The failure of ventricular sodium to control sodium appetite in the rat. *Physiology and Behavior, 32*, 683–686.

Ernits, T., & Corbit, J.D. (1973). Taste as a dipsogenic stimulus. *Journal of Comparative and Physiological Psychology, 83*, 27–31.

Ettenberg, A., Cinsavich, S., & White, N. (1979). Performance effects with repeated-response measures during pimozide-produced dopamine receptor blockade. *Pharmacology, Biochemistry, and Behavior, 11*, 557–561.

Ettenberg, A., Koob, G., & Bloom, F. (1981). Response artifact in the measurement of neuroleptic-induced anhedonia. *Science, 213*, 357–359.

Ettenberg, A., Pettit, H., Bloom, F., & Koob, G. (1982). Heroin and cocaine intravenous self-administration in rats: mediation by separate neural systems. *Psychopharmacology, 78*, 204–209.

Ettenberg, A., & White, N. (1981). Pimozide attenuates conditioned taste preferences induced by self-stimulation in rats. *Pharmacology, Biochemistry, and Behavior, 15*, 915–919.

Falk, J.L. (1971). The nature and determinants of adjunctive behavior. *Physiology and Behavior, 6*, 577–588.

Fallon, J.H. & Moore, R.V. (1978). Catecholamine innervation of the basal forebrain, IV. Topography of the dopamine projection to the basal forebrain and neostriatum. *Journal of Comparative Neurology, 180*, 545–580.

Fass, B., & Butcher, D.L. (1981). Evidence for a crossed nigrostriatal pathway in rats. *Neuroscience Letters, 22* 109—113.

Ferrer, J., Sanguinetti, A., Vives, F., & Mora, F. (1983). Effects of agonists and antagonists of D1 and D2 dopamine receptors on self-stimulation of the medial prefrontal cortex in the rat. *Pharmacology, Biochemistry, and Behavior, 19*, 211–217.

Fibiger, H.C. (1978). Drugs and reinforcement mechanisms: a critical review of the catecholamine theory. *Annual Review of Pharmacology and Toxicology, 18*, 37–56.

Fibiger, H.C., Carter, D. & Phillips, A. (1976). Decreased intracranial self-stimulation after neuroleptics or 6-hydroxydopamine: evidence for mediation by motor deficits rather than by reduced reward. *Psychopharmacology, 47*, 21–27.

Findly, J.D., Robinson, W.W., & Peregrino, L. (1972). Addiction to secobarbital and chlordiazepoxide in the rhesus monkey by means of a self-infusion preference procedure. *Psychopharmacology, 26*, 93–114.

Fink, J.S., & Smith, J.P. (1980). Mesolimbicocortical dopamine terminal fields are necessary for normal locomotor and investigatory exploration in rats. *Brain Research, 199*, 359–384.

Fluharty, S.J., & Epstein, A.N. (1983). Sodium appetite elicited by intracerebroventricular infusion of angiotensin II in the rat: II. Synergistic interaction with systemic mineralocorticoids. *Behavioral Neuroscience, 97*, 746–758.

Flynn, F.W., & Grill, H.J. (1983). Insulin elicits ingestion in decerebrate rats. *Science, 221*, 188–190.

Flynn, J.P., Vanegas, H., Foote, W., & Edwards, S. (1970). Neural mechanisms involved in a cat's attack on a rat. In R. Whalen, R.F. Thompson, M. Verseano, & N.M. Weinberger (Eds.), *The neural control of behavior* (pp. 135–173). New York: Academic.

Foerster, A.P. (1982). Spontaneous regeneration of cut axons in adult rat brain. *Journal of Comparative Neurology. 210*, 335–356.

Fouriezos, G. (1980, June). *Effective spread of current from a monopolar stimulating electrode*. Paper presented at meeting of Canadian Psychological Association. Calgary, Canada.

Fouriezos, G., Hanson, P., & Wise, R.A. (1978). Neuroleptic-induced attenuation of brain stimulation reward in rats. *Journal of Comparative and Physiological Psychology, 92*, 661–671.

Fouriezos, G., & Nawiesniak, E. (1982). Comparison of two methods of estimating thresholds of intracranial self-stimulation. *Neuroscience Abstracts, 8*, 624.

Fouriezos, G, & Wise, R.A. (1976). Pimozide-induced extinction of intracranial self-stimulation: response patterns rule out motor or performance deficits. *Brain Research, 103*, 377–380.

Franklin, K. (1978). Catecholamines and self-stimulation: Reward and performance effects dissociated. *Pharmacology, Biochemistry, and Behavior, 9*, 813–820.

Franklin, K., & McCoy, S.N. (1979). Pimozide-induced extinction in rats: Stimulus control of responding rules out motor deficit. *Pharmacology, Biochemistry, and Behavior, 11*, 71–75.

Fray, P. (1981). Concurrent VIVI schedules to assess the reinforcing strength of electrical brain stimulation. In O. Bradshaw, E. Szabadi, & C.F. Lowe (Eds.), *Quantification of steady-state operant behavior* (pp. 361–364). New York: Elsevier.

Fray, P., Dunnett, S., Iverson, S., Björklund, A., & Stenevi, U. (1983). Nigral transplants reinervating the dopamine-depleted neostriatum can sustain intracranial self-stimulation. *Science, 219*, 416–419.

Friedman, M.I. (1980). Hepatic-cerebral interactions in insulin-induced eating and gastric acid secretion. *Brain Research Bulletin, 5* (Suppl. 4), 63–68.

Friedman, M.I., & Stricker, E.M. (1976). The physiological psychology of hunger: a physiological perspective. *Physiological Review, 83*, 409–431.

Frisch, K. von. (1967). *The dance language and orientation of bees*. Cambridge MA: Harvard University Press.

Gallistel, C.R. (1967). Intracranial stimulation and natural reward: Differential effects of trial spacing. *Psychonomic Science, 9*, 167–168.

Gallistel, C.R. (1969a). The incentive of brain-stimulation reward. *Journal of Comparative and Physiological Psychology, 69*, 713–721.

Gallistel, C. R. (1969b). Self-stimulation: Failure of pretrial stimulation to affect rat's electrode preference. *Journal of Comparative and Physiological Psychology, 69*, 722–729.

Gallistel, C.R. (1973). Self-stimulation: The neurophysiology of reward and motivation. In J.A. Deutsch (Ed.), *The physiological basis of memory* (pp. 210–267). New York: Academic.

Gallistel, C.R. (1978). Self-stimulation in the rat: Quantitative characteristics of the reward pathway. *Journal of Comparative and Physiological Psychology, 92*, 977–998.

Gallistel, C. R. (1980a). *The organization of action: a new synthesis.* Hillsdale, NJ: Lawrence Erlbaum Associates.

Gallistel, C.R. (1980b). From muscles to motivation. *American Scientist, 68*, 398–409.

Gallistel, C.R. (1983). Self-stimulation. In J.A. Deutsch (Ed.), *The physiological basis of memory* (pp.269–349). New York: Academic.

Gallistel, C.R., & Beagely, G. (1971). Specificity of brain stimulation reward in the rat. *Journal of Comparative and Physiological Psychology, 76*, 199–205.

Gallistel, C.R., Boytim, M., Gomita, Y., & Klebanoff, L. (1982). Does pimozide block the reinforcing effect of brain stimulation? *Pharmacology, Biochemistry, and Behavior, 17*, 769–781.

Gallistel, C.R., & Davis, A.J. (1983). Affinity for the dopamine D2 receptor predicts neuroleptic potency in blocking the reinforcing effect of MFB stimulation. *Pharmacology, Biochemistry, and Behavior, 19*, 867–872.

Gallistel, C.R., Karreman, G., & Reivich, M. (1977). [14C] 2-deoxyglucose uptake marks systems activated by rewarding brain stimulation. *Brain Research Bulletin, 2*, 149–152.

Gallistel, C.R., Piner, C., Allen, T.O., Adler, N.T., Yadin, E., & Negin, M. (1982). Computer-assisted analysis of 2-DG autoradiographs. *Neuroscience and Biobehavior Review, 6*, 409–420.

Gallistel, C.R., Shizgal, P., & Yeomans, J. (1981). A portrait of the substrate for self-stimulation. *Psychological Review, 88*, 228–273.

Gallistel, C. R., Stellar, J.R., & Bubis, E. (1974). Parametric analysis of brain stimulation reward in the rat. I. The transient process and the memory-containing process. *Journal of Comparative and Physiological Psychology, 87*, 848–859.

Garcia, J., Kimmeldorf, D.J., & Koelling, R.A. (1955). Conditioned aversion to saccharine resulting from exposure to gamma radiation. *Science, 122*, 157–158.

Garcia, J., & Koelling, R.A. (1967). A comparison of aversions induced by X-rays, toxin, and drugs in the rat. *Radiation Research, 7*, 439–450.

Gerber, G.J., Bozarth, M.A., & Wise, R.A. (1981). Small-dose intravenous heroin facilitates hypothalamic self-stimulation without response suppression in rats. *Life Sciences, 28*, 557–562.

Gerber, G.J., Sing, J., & Wise, R.A. (1981). Pimozide attenuates lever pressing for water in rats. *Pharmacology, Biochemistry, and Behavior, 14*, 201–205.

Gerfen, C., Staines, W., Arbuthnott, G., & Fibiger, H.C. (1982). Crossed connections of the substantia nigra in the rat. *Journal of Comparative Neurology, 207*, 283–303.

Gerhardt, S., & Liebman, J. (1981). Differential effects of drug treatments on nose-poke and bar-press self-stimulation. *Pharmacology, Biochemistry, and Behavior, 15*, 767–771.

German, D.C., & Bowden, D.M. (1974). Catecholamine systems as the neural substrate for intracranial self-stimulation: a hypothesis. *Brain Research, 73*, 381–419.

German, D.C., Dalsass, M., & Kiser, R.S. (1980). Electrophysiological examination of the ventral tegmental (A10) area of the rat. *Brain Research, 181*, 191–197.

Gibson, W., Reid, L., Sakai, M. & Porter, P. (1965). Intracranial reinforcement compared with sugar-water reinforcement. *Science, 148*, 1307–1359.

Glick, S.D., Greenstein, S., & Waters, D.H. (1974). Lateral hypothalamic lesions and striatal dopamine levels. *Life Sciences, 14*, 747–750.

Glick, S.D., & Ross, D.A., (1981). Lateralization of function in the rat brain: Basic mechanisms may be operative in humans. *Trends in Neuroscience, 4*, 196–199.

Glickman, S.E., & Schiff, B.B. (1967). A biological theory of reinforcement. *Psychological Review, 74*, 81—109.

Goeders, N.E., & Smith, J.E. (1983). Cortical dopaminergic involvement in cocaine reinforcement. *Science, 221*, 773–775.

Gold, R.M. (1973). Hypothalamic obesity: the myth of the ventromedial nucleus. *Science, 182*, 488–490.

Goltz, F. (1892). Der Hund ohne Grosshirn. *Pflüger Archive gesamte Physiologie, 51*, 570–614.

Gomita, Y., & Gallistel, C.R. (1982). Effects of reinforcement blocking doses of pimozide on neural systems driven by rewarding stimulation of the MFB: A 14c-2-deoxyglucose analysis. *Pharmacology, Biochemistry, and Behavior, 17*, 841–845.

Grau, J.W., Hyson, R.L., Maier, S.F., Madden, J., & Barchas, J.D. (1981). Long-term stress-induced analgesia and activation of the opiate system. *Science, 213*, 1409–1411.

Gray, T., & Wise, F.A. (1980). Effects of pimozide on lever-pressing behavior maintained on an intermittent reinforcement schedule. *Pharmacology, Biochemistry, and Behavior, 12*, 931–935.

Greengard, P. (1976). Possible role for cyclic nucleotides and phosphorylated membrane proteins in postsynaptic actions of neurotransmitters. *Nature, 260*, 101–108.

Grijalva, G.V., Lindholm, E., & Novin, D. (1980). Physiological and morphological changes in the gastrointestinal tract induced by hypothalamic intervention: an overview. *Brain Research Bulletin, 5* (Suppl. 1), 19–31.

Grinker, J.A. (1977). Effects of metabolic state on taste parameters and intake: comparisons of human and animal obesity. In J.M. Weiffenbach (Ed.), *Taste and develoment: The genesis of sweet preference* (pp. 309–327). Bethesda, MD: DHEW Publication No. (NIH) 77–1068.

Grossman, S.P. (1984). Contemporary problems concerning our understanding of brain mechanisms that regulate food intake and body weight. In A.J.

Stunkard & E. Stellar (Eds), *Eating and its disorders* (pp. 5–13). New York: Raven.

Grossman, S.P., Dacey, D., Haloris, A.E., Collier, T., & Routtenberg, A. (1978). Aphagia and adipsia after preferential destruction of nerve cell bodies in the hypothalamus. *Science, 202*, 537–539.

Guieu, J.D., & Hardy, J.D. (1971). Integrative activity of preoptic units. I. Response to local and peripheral temperature changes. *Journal of Physiology* (Paris), *63*, 253–256.

Gunne, L.M., Anggard, E., & Jonsson, L.E. (1972). Clinical trials with amphetamine-blocking drugs. *Psychiatria, Neurologia, Neurochirogia* (Amsterdam), *75*, 225–226.

Gutman, N. (1953). Operant conditioning, extinction, and periodic reinforcement in relation to concentration of sucrose used as reinforcing agent. *Journal of Experimental Psychology, 46*, 213–224.

Guyenet, P.G., & Aghajanian, G.K. (1978). Antidromic identification of dopaminergic and other output neurons of the rat substantia nigra. *Brain Research, 130*, 69–84.

Hall, R.D., Bloom, F.E., & Olds, J. (1977). Neuronal and neurochemical substrates of reinforcement. *Neurosciences Research Program Bulletin, 15*, 133–314.

Hall, W.G. (1979). The ontogeny of feeding in rats. I. Ingestive and behavioral response to oral infusions. *Journal of Comparative and Physiological Psychology, 93*, 977–1000.

Hamilton, A.L., & Stellar, J.R. (1983). *A simple method for distinguishing factors which affect reward from those affecting motor performance in responding for electrical stimulation of the brain.* Paper presented at Eastern Psychological Association, Philadelphia, PA.

Hamilton, C.L. (1969). Problems of refeeding after starvation in the rat. *Annals of the New York Academy of Sciences, 157*, 1004–1017.

Han, P.W., & Frohman, L.A. (1970). Hyperinsulinemia in tube-fed hypophysectomized rats bearing hypothalamic lesions. *American Journal of Physiology, 219*, 1632–1636.

Hardy, J.D., & Guieu, J.D. (1971). Integrative activity of preoptic units. II. Hypothetical network. *Journal of Physiology* (Paris), *63*, 264–267.

Harlow, H.F., & Zimmerman, R.R., (1959). Affectional responses in the infant monkey. *Science, 130*, 421–432.

Harvey, J.A., & Hunt, H.F. (1965). Effect of septal lesions on thirst in the rat as indicated by water consumption and operant responding for water reward. *Journal of Comparative and Physiological Psychology, 59*, 49–56.

Hawkins, R.C. (1975). *Human temperature regulation and the perception of thermal comfort.* Unpublished doctoral dissertation, University of Pennsylvania.

Head, H., & Holmes, G. (1911). Sensory disturbances from cerebral lesion. *Brain, 34*, 102–254.

Heath, R.G. (1964a). Pleasure response of human subjects to direct stimulation of the brain. In R.G. Heath (Ed.), *The role of pleasure in behavior* (pp. 219–243). New York: Harper and Row.

Heath, R.G., (Ed.). (1964b). *The role of pleasure in behavior.* New York: Harper and Row.

Herrick C.J. (1918). *An introduction to neurology*. Philadelphia: W.B. Saunders.

Herrnstein, R.J. (1974). Formal properties of the matching law. *Journal of Experimental Analysis of Behavior, 21*, 159–164.

Hess, W.R. (1954). *Diencephalon: Autonomic and extrapyramidal functions*. New York: Grune and Stratton.

Hess, W.R. (1957). *The functional organization of the diencephalon*. New York: Grune and Stratton.

Hetherington, A.W., & Ranson, S.W. (1942). The spontaneous activity and food intake of rats with hypothalamic lesions. *American Journal of Physiology, 136*, 609–617.

Heyman, G. (1983). A parametric evaluation of the hedonic and motoric effects of drugs: pimozide and amphetamine. *Journal of Experimental Analysis of Behavior, 40*, 113–122.

Heyman, G., Kinzie, D., & Seiden, L.S. (1983). Pimozide and chlorpromizine reduce reinforcement efficacy and motor capacity in the rat. *Neuroscience Abstracts, 9*, 562.

Hodos, W., & Valenstein, E. (1962). An evaluation of response rate as a measure of rewarding intracranial stimulation. *Journal of Comparative and Physiological Psychology, 55*, 80–84.

Hoebel, B.G. (1975). Brain reward and aversion systems in the control of feeding and sexual behavior. In J. Cole & T. Sonderegger (Eds.), *Nebraska Symposium on Motivation, 1974* (pp. 49–112). Lincoln: University of Nebraska Press.

Hoebel, B.G. (1976). Brain stimulation reward and aversion in relation to behavior. In A. Wauquier & E.T. Rolls (Eds.), *Brain stimulation reward* (pp. 355–372). New York: Elsevier.

Hoebel, B.G. (1984). Neurotransmitters in the control of feeding and its rewards: monoamines, opiates, and brain-gut peptides, In A.J. Stunkard & E. Stellar (Eds.), *Eating and its disorders* (pp. 15–38). New York: Raven.

Hoebel, B.G., Hernadez, L., McLean, S., Stanley, B., Aulissi, E., Glimcher, P., & Margolin, D. (1982). Catecholamine, enkephalin, and neurotensin in feeding and reward. In B.G. Hoebel & D. Novin (Eds.), *The neural basis of feeding and reward* (pp. 465–478). Brunswick, ME: Haer Institute.

Hoebel, B.G., & Novin, D. (Eds.) (1982). *The neural basis of feeding and reward*. Brunswick, ME: Haer Institute.

Hoebel, B.G., & Teitelbaum, P. (1962). Hypothalamic control of feeding and self-stimulation. *Science, 135*, 375–377.

Hoffman, H.S., & Solomon, R.L. (1974). An opponent process theory of motivation: Some affective dynamics in imprinting. *Learning and Motivation, 5*, 149–164.

Hokfelt, T., Rehfeld, J.H., Skirboll, L., Ivenmark, B., Goldstein, M., & Markley, K. (1980). Evidence for the coexistance of dopamine and CCK in mesolimbic neurons. *Nature, 285*, 476–478.

Howarth, C.I., & Deutsch, J.A. (1962). Drive decay: The cause of fast "extinction" of habits learned for brain stimulation. *Science, 137*, 35–36.

Hull, C.L. (1943). *Principles of behavior*. New York: Appelton-Century-Crofts.

Huston, J.P. (1982). Searching for the neural mechanism of reinforcement (of "stamping-in"). In B.G. Hoebel & D. Novin (Eds.), *The neural basis of feeding and reward* (pp. 75–83). Brunswick, ME: Haer Institute.

Huston, J.P., & Borbely, A.A. (1973). Operant conditioning in forebrain ablated rats by use of rewarding hypothalamic stimulation. *Brain Research, 50*, 467–472.

Huston, J.P., & Borbely, A.A. (1974). The thalamic rat: General behavior, operant learning with rewarding hypothalamic stimulation, and effects of amphetamine. *Physiology and Behavior, 12*, 433–448.

Huston, J.P., & Mills, A.W. (1971). Threshold of reinforcing brain stimulation. *Communications in Behavioral Biology, 5*, 331–340.

Huston, J.P., Ornstein, K., & Lehner, R. (1978). Self-stimulation in the hypothalamus after ipsilateral disconnection from the brainstem and removal of the telencephalon. *Neuroscience Letters, 10* (Suppl. 1), 55.

Huston, J.P., Pritzel, M., & Buscher, W. (1981). Hypothalamic self-stimulation in rats with one hemisphere isolated anterior to the midbrain and the other hemisphere devoid of telencephalon. *Neuroscience Abstracts, 7*, 650.

Hustvedt, B.E., & Løvø, A. (1972). Correlation between hyperinsulinemia and hyperphagia in rats with ventromedial hypothalamic lesions. *Acta Physiologia Scandinavia, 84*, 29–33.

Hyde, T.M., & Miselis, R.R. (1983). Effects of area postrema/caudal medial nucleus of solitary tract lesions on food intake and body weight. *American Journal of Physiology, 244*, R577–R587.

Inoue, S., & Bray, G.A. (1980). Role of the autonomic nervous system in the development of ventromedial hypothalamic obesity. *Brain Research Bulletin, 5*, (Suppl. 4), 119–125.

Iversen, S.D., & Iversen, L.L. (1981). *Behavioral pharmacology*. New York: Oxford University Press.

Iversen, S.D., & Koob, G.F. (1977). Behavioral implications of dopaminergic neurons in the mesolimbic system. In E. Costa & G. Gessa (Eds.), *Advances in biochemical psychopharmacology*. (Vol. 16). New York: Raven.

Jackson, J.H. (1958). The Croonian lectures on evolution and dissolution of the nervous system. In J. Taylor (Ed.), *Selected Writings of John Hughlings Jackson*. London: Staples Press. (Reprinted from *British Medical Journal, 1884, 1*, 591–593, 660–663, 703–707.)

James, W. (1884). The physical basis of the emotions. *Psychological Review, 1*, 516–529.

James, W. (1890). *Principles of psychology*. New York, Henry Holt.

Janas, J., & Stellar, J. (1984). *Effects of transections of the medial forebrain bundle on self-stimulation reward*. Paper presented at Canadian Psychological Association. Ottowa, Canada.

Jennings, H.S. (1906). *Behavior of the lower organism*. New York: Columbia University Press.

Johanson, C.E., & Uhlenhuth, E.H. (1980). Drug preference and mood in humans: d-amphetamine. *Psychopharmacology, 71*, 274–279.

Jordan, H.A. (1969). Voluntary intragastric feeding: Oral and gastric contributions to food intake and hunger in man. *Journal of Comparative and Physiological Psychology, 68*, 498–506.

Jordan, H.A., Moses, H., MacFayden, B.V., & Dudrick, S.J. (1974). Hunger and satiety in humans during parenteral hyperalimentation. *Psychosomatic Medicine, 36*, 144–155.

Jordan, H.A., Stellar, E., & Duggan, S.Z. (1968). Voluntary intragastric feeding in man. *Communications in Behavioral Biology, 1*, 65–68.

Joyce, J. (1983). Multiple dopamine receptors and behavior. *Neuroscience and Biobehavioral Reviews, 7*, 227–256.

Kandel, E.R. (1979). Cellular insights into behavior and learning. *Harvey Lectures, 73*, 19–92.

Kapatos, G., & Gold, R.M. (1973). Evidence for ascending noradrenergic mediation of hypothalamic hyperphagia. *Pharmacology, Biochemistry, and Behavior, 1*, 81–87.

Katz, R.J. (1979). The temporal structure of reinforcement: An analysis of brain-stimulated reward. *Behavioral and Neural Biology, 26*, 416–430.

Kebabian, J. W., & Calne, D.B. (1979). Multiple receptors for dopamine. *Nature, 277*, 93–96.

Keesey, R.E., & Powley, T.L. (1973). Self-stimulation and body weight in rats with lateral hypothalamic lesions. *American Journal of Physiology, 224*, 970–978.

Kelley, A., Domesick, V., & Nauta, W.J.H. (1982). The amygdalostriatal projection in the rat: an anatomical study by anterograde and retrograde tracing methods. *Neuroscience, 7*, 615–650.

Kelley, A., & Stinus, L. (1984). Neuroanatomical and neurochemical substrates of affective behavior. In N.A. Fox & R.J. Davidson (Eds.), *Affective development: A psychobiological perspective* (pp. 1–75). Hillsdale, NJ: Erlbaum.

Kelley, A., Stinus, L., & Iversen, S.D. (1980). Interactions between d-ala-met-enkephalin, A10 dopaminergic neurons, and spontaneous behavior in the rat. *Behavioral Brain Research, 1*, 3–24.

Kennedy, C., DesRosiers, M., Jehle, J., Reivich, M., Sharpe, F., & Sckoloff, L. (1975). Mapping of functional neural pathways by autoradiographic survey of local metabolic rate with [14C] deoxyglucose. *Science, 187*, 850–852.

Kent, E.W., & Grossman, S.P. (1973). Elimination of learned behaviors after transections of fibers crossing the lateral border of the hypothalamus. *Physiology and Behavior, 10*, 953–963.

Kety, S.S. (1970). The biogenic amines in the central nervous system: Their possible roles in arousal, emotion, and learning. In F.O. Schmitt (Ed.), *The neurosciences: Second study program* (pp. 324–336). New York: Rockefeller University Press.

King, B.M., Carpenter, R.G., Stamoutsos, B.A., Frohman, L.A., & Grossman, S.P. (1978). Hyperphagia and obesity following ventromedial hypothalamic lesions in rats with subdiaphragmatic vagotomy. *Physiology and Behavior, 20*, 643–651.

Kissileff, H.R. (1970). Free feeding in normal and "recovered lateral" rats monitored by a pellet-detecting eatometer. *Physiology and Behavior, 5*, 163–174.

Kling, J.W., & Riggs, L.A. (1971). *Woodworth and Schlosberg's experimental psychology*. New York: Holt, Rinehart, & Winston.

Klüver, H., & Bucy, F.C. (1939). Preliminary analysis of functions of the temporal lobes in monkeys. *Archives of Neurological Psychiatry, 42,* 979–1000.

Kolb, B., Nonneman, A., & Singh, R. (1974). Double dissociation of spatial impairments and perseveration following selective prefrontal lesions in rats. *Journal of Comparative and Physiological Psychology, 87*, 772–780.

Koob, G.F., Riley, S.J., Smith, S.C., & Robbins, T.W. (1978). Effects of 6-hydroxydopamine lesions of the nucleus accumbens septi and olfactory tubercle on feeding, locomotor activity, and amphetamine anorexia in the rat. *Journal of Comparative and Physiological Psychology, 92*, 917–926.

Koob, G.F., Stinus, L. & LeMoal, M. (1981). Hyperactivity and hypoactivity produced by lesions to the mesolimbic dopamine system. *Behavioral Brain Research, 3*, 341–359.

Krieg, W. (1932). The hypothalamus of the albino rat. *Journal of Comparative Neurology, 55*, 19–89.

Kuffler, S., & Vaughn-Williams, E. (1953). Small-nerve junction potentials. The distribution of small motor nerves to frog skeletal muscle and the membrane characteristics of the fibers they innervate. *Journal of Physiology, 121*, 289.

Lange, C.G. (1885). *Om Sindshevaegelser.* Copenhagen: Kronar.

Langston, J., Ballard, P., Tetrud, J., & Irwin, I. (1983). Chronic parkinsonism in humans due to a product of meparidine-analog synthesis. *Science, 219*, 979–980.

Lashley, K.S. (1938). An experimental analysis of instinctive behavior. *Psychological Review, 45*, 445–471.

Lehrman, D.S., Wortis, R.P., & Brody, P. (1961). Gonadotropin secretion in response to external stimuli of varying duration in the ring dove (Streptopelia visoria). *Society for Experimental Biology nad Medicine, 106*, 298–300.

Leibowitz, S.F. (1978). Adrenergic stimulation of the paraventricular nucleus and its effects on ingestive behavior as a function of drug dose and time of injection in the light-dark cycle. *Brain Research Bulletin, 3*, 357–363.

Leibowitz, S.F. (1982). Hypothalamic catecholamine systems in relation to control of eating behavior and mechanisms of reward. In B.G. Hoebel & D. Novin (Eds.), *The neural basis of feeding and reward* (pp. 241–257). Brunswick, ME: Haer Institute.

Leith, N., & Barrett, R. (1981). Self-stimulation and amphetamine: tolerance to d and l isomers and cross tolerance to cocaine and methylphenidate. *Psychopharmacology, 74*, 23–28.

LeMagnen, J. (1971). Advances in studies on the physiological control and regulation of food intake. In E. Stellar & J.M. Sprague (Eds.), *Progress in physiological psychology* (pp. 204–261). New York: Academic.

LeMagnen, J. (1981). Metabolic basis for the dual periodicity of feeding in rats. *Behavioral Brain Sciences, 4*, 561–607.

LeMagnen, J. (1983). Body energy balance and food intake: a neuroendocrine regulatory mechanism. *Physiological Review, 63*, 314–386.

LeMoal, M., Stinus, L., Simon, H., Tassin, J.P., Thierry, A.M., Blanc, G., Glowinski, J., & Cardo, B. (1977). Behavorial effects of a lesion in the ventral mesencephalic tegmentum: evidence for involvement of A10 DA neurons. In E. Costa & G. Gessa (Eds.), *Advances in biochemical psychopharmacology,* (Vol. 16). New York: Raven.

Liebeskind, J.C., & Paul, L.A. (1977). Psychological and physiological mechanisms of pain. *Annual Review of Psychology, 28*, 41–60.

Liebman, J. (1983). Discriminating between reward and performance: a critical review of intracranial self-stimulation methodology. *Neuroscience and Biobehavioral Reviews, 7*, 45–72.

Liebman, J., Hall, N., & Prowse, J. (1982). Effects of various catecholamine receptor agonists, muscle relaxation and physical hindrance on shuttle box self-stimulation. *Pharmacology, Biochemistry, and Behavior, 16*, 789–790.

Lindsley, D.B. (1951). Emotion. In S.S. Stevens (Ed.), *Handbook of experimental psychology* (pp. 473–516). New York: Wiley.

Lindvall, O., & Björklund, A. (1974). The organization of the ascending catecholamine neuron systems in the rat brain as revealed by the glyoxylic acid fluorescence method. *Acta Physiologiae Scandinavia, 412* (Suppl.), 1–48.

Liu, J.C. (1979). Tonic inhibition of thermoregulation in the decerebrate monkey (Saimiri sciureus). *Experimental Neurolology, 64*, 632–648.

Loeb, J. (1918). *Forced movements, tropisms, and animal conduct.* New York: Lippincott.

Lorens, S.A. (1966). Effect of lesions in the central nervous system on lateral hypothalamic self-stimulation in the rat. *Journal of Comparative and Physiological Psychology, 62*, 256–262.

Lorens, S.A. (1976). Anatomical substrate of intracranial self-stimulation: Contribution of lesion studies. In A. Wauquier & E.T. Rolls (Eds.), *Brain-stimulation reward* (pp. 41–50). New York: Elsevier.

Lyness, W.H., Friedle, N.M., & Moore, K.E. (1979). Destruction of dopaminergic nerve terminals in nucleus accumbens: effect of d-amphetamine self-administration. *Pharmacology, Biochemistry, and Behavior, 11*, 553–556.

MacDonnell, M.F., & Flynn, J.P. (1966). Control of sensory fields by stimulation of hypothalamus. *Science, 152*, 1406–1408.

MacLean, P.D. (1949). Psychosomatic disease and the "visceral brain." *Psychosomatic Medicine, 11*, 338–353.

MacLean, P.D. (1970). The triune brain: Emotion and scientific facts. In F.O. Schmitt (Ed.), *The Neurosciences second study program* (pp. 336–349). New York: Rockefeller University Press.

Maddison, S. (1977). Intraperitoneal and intracranial cholecystokinin depress operant responding for food. *Physiology and Behavior, 19*, 819—824.

Maeda, H., & Mogenson, G. (1981). A comparison of the effects of electrical stimulation of the lateral and ventromedial hypothalamus on the activity of neurons in ventral tegmental area and substantia nigra. *Brain Research Bulletin, 7*, 283–291.

Margules, D.L., & Olds, J. (1962). Identical "feeding" and "rewarding" systems in the lateral hypothalamus of rats. *Science, 135*, 374–375.

Marshall, J.F. (1984). Brain function: neural adaptations and recovery from injury, *Annual Review of Psychology*, (pp. 277–308). Palo Alto, CA: Annual Review Inc.

Marshall, J.F. (1979). Somatosensory inattention after dopamine-depleting intracerebral 6-OHDA injections: spontaneous recovery and pharmacological control. *Brain Research, 177*, 311–324.

Marshall, J.F., Levitan, D., & Stricker, E.M. (1976). Activation-induced restoration of sensorimotor functions in rats with dopamine depleting lesions. *Journal of Comparative and Physiological Psychology, 90*, 536–546.

Marshall, J.F., Richardson, J.S., & Teitelbaum, P. (1974). Nigrostriatal bundle damage and the lateral hypothalamic syndrome. *Journal of Comparative and Physiological Psychology, 87*, 808–830.

Marshall, J.F., & Teitelbaum, P. (1974). Further analysis of sensory inattention following lateral hypothalamic damage in rats. *Journal of Comparative and Physiological Psychology, 86*, 375–395.

Mason, P.A., Milner, P.M., & Giftachristas, N. (1984). Temporal summation characteristics of brain stimulation as function of reward magnitude. *Canadian Psychology, 25*, 310 (Abstract).

Mason, S.F., Beninger, R.J., Fibiger, H.C., & Phillips, A.G. (1980). Pimozide-induced suppression of responding: evidence against a block of food reward. *Pharmacology, Biochemistry and Behavior, 12*, 917–923.

Matthews, G. (1977). Neural substrate for brain stimulation reward in the rat. Cathodal and anodal strength-duration properties. *Journal of Comparative and Physiological Psychology, 91*, 858–874.

Matthews, G. (1978). Strength-duration properties of single units driven by electrical stimulation of the lateral hypothalamus in rats. *Brain Research Bulletin, 3*, 171–174.

Mayer, A., (1900). Variations de la tension osmotique du sang chez les animoux prives de liquides. *Compte Rendu des Seances de la Societe le Biologie, 52*, 153–155.

McCleary, R.A. (1953). Taste and post-ingestion factors in specific hunger behavior. *Journal of Comparative and Physiological Psychology, 46*, 411–421.

McDougall, W. (1908). *An introduction to social psychology*. New York: Methuen.

Miliaressis, E., Rompré, P., & Durivage, A. (1982). Psychophysical method for mapping behavior substrates using a moveable electrode. *Brain Research Bulletin, 8*, 693–701.

Miller, N.E. (1959). Liberalization of basic S-R concepts; extensions to conflict behavior, motivation, and social learning. In S. Koch (Ed.), *Psychology: A study of a science* (Vol. II pp. 196–292). New York: McGraw-Hill.

Miller, N.E. (1961). Implication for theories of reinforcement. In D. Sheer (Ed.), *Electrical stimulation of the brain* (pp. 575–581). Austin: University of Texas Press.

Miller, N.E., Bailey, C.J., & Stevenson, J.A.F. (1950). "Decreased hunger" but increased food intake resulting from hypothalamic lesions. *Science, 112*, 256–259.

Millhouse, C.E. (1969). A Golgi study of the descending medial forebrain bundle. *Brain Research, 15*, 341–363.

Millhouse, C.E. (1979). A Golgi anatomy of the rodent hypothalamus. In P.J. Morgane & J. Panksepp (Eds.), *Handbook of the hypothalamus, Vol. 1: Anatomy of the hypothalamus* (pp. 221–265). New York: Dekker.

Miselis, R.R. (1981). The efferent projections of the subfornical organ of the rat: a circumventricular organ with a neural network subserving water balance. *Brain Research, 230,* 1–23.

Miselis, R.R., Shapiro, R., & Hand, P. (1979). Subfornical organ efferents to neural systems for control of body water. *Science, 205,* 1022–1025.

Misher, A., & Brooks. F.P. (1966). Electrical stimulation of hypothalamus and gastric secretion in the albino rat. *American Journal of Physiology, 211,* 403–406.

Mittleman, G., & Valenstein, E.S. (1984). Ingestive behavior evoked by hypothalamic stimulation and schedule-induced polydipsia are related. *Science, 224,* 415–417.

Mogenson, G., & Cioe, J. (1977). Central reinforcement: A bridge between brain function and behavior. In W. Honig & J. Staddon (Eds.), *Handbook of operant behavior* (pp. 570–595). Englewood Cliffs, NJ: Prentice Hall.

Mogenson, G., & Phillips, A. (1978). Brain-stimulation reward after twenty-five years. *Canadian Journal of Psychology, 32,* 54–57.

Mogenson, G., Takigawa, M., Robertson, A., & Wu, M. (1979). Self-stimulation of the nucleus accumbens and ventral tegmental area of Tsai attenuated by microinjections of spiroperidol into the nucleus accumbens. *Brain Research, 171,* 247–259.

Mook, D.G. (1963). Oral and post-ingestional determinants of the intake of various solutions in rats with esophageal fistulas. *Journal of Comparative and Physiological Psychology, 56,* 645–659.

Moore, R., & Bloom, F. (1978). Central catecholamine neuron systems: anatomy and physiology of the dopamine systems. *Annual Review of Neuroscience, 1,* 129–169.

Mora, F., Sanguinetti, A., Rolls, E.T., & Shaw, S.G. (1975). Differential effects on self-stimulation and motor behavior produced by microintracranial injections of a dopamine-receptor blocking agent. *Neuroscience Letters, 1,* 179–184.

Morgan, C.T. (1943). *Physiological psychology.* New York: McGraw-Hill.

Morgane, P.J. (1962). Disassociation of hypothalamic self-stimulation and primary feeding system. *Clinical Research, 10,* 185.

Morgane, P.J. (1979). Historical and modern concepts of hypothalamic organization and function. In P.J. Morgane & J. Panksepp (Eds.), *Handbook of the hypothalamus: Vol. I. Anatomy of the hypothalamus* (pp. 1–64). New York: Dekker.

Morgane, P.J., & Panksepp, J. (Eds.). (1979a). *Handbook of the hypothalamus: Vol. I. Anatomy of the hypothalamus.* New York: Dekker.

Morgane, P.J. & Panksepp, J. (Eds.), (1979b). *Handbook of the hypothalamus: Vol. II. Physiology of the hypothalamus.* New York: Dekker.

Morgane, P.J., & Panksepp, J. (Eds.). (1981). *Handbook of the hypothalamus: Vol. III. Behavioral studies of the hypothalamus.* (Parts A & B). New York: Dekker.

Morrison, A.R., & Strick, P.L. (Eds.), (1982). *Changing concepts of the nervous system.* New York: Academic.

Morruzi, G., & Magoun, H.W. (1949). Brainstem reticular formation and activation of the EEG. *Electroencephalography and Clinical Neurophysiology, 1*, 455–473.

Mowrer, O.H., & Jones, H.M. (1943). Extinction and behavioral variablility as functions of effortfulness of task. *Journal of Experimental Psychology, 33*, 369–386.

Munoz, C., Sprick, V., Huston, J.P. (1983). Lateral hypothalamic self-stimulation after lesions in the anterior or lateral hypothalamus. *Neuroscience Abstracts, 9*, 637.

Nachman, M. (1970). Learned taste and temperature aversions due to lithium chloride sickness after temporal delays. *Journal of Comparative and Physiological Psychology, 73*, 22–30.

Nauta, W.J.H. (1964). Some efferent connections of the prefrontal cortex in the monkey. In J.M. Warren, & K. Akert (Eds.), *The frontal granual cortex and behavior* (pp. 397–409). New York: McGraw-Hill.

Nauta, W.J.H., & Domesick, V. (1983). Neural associations of the limbic system. In Beckman (Ed.), *Neural substrates of behavior*. New York: Spectrum.

Nauta, W.J.H., & Haymaker, W. (1969). Hypothalamic nuclei and fiber connections. In W. Haymaker, E. Anderson, & W.J.H. Nauta (Eds.), *The hypothalamus* (pp. 136–209). Springfield, IL: Thomas.

Neeley, S.P., & Stellar, J.R. (1983). Reward and aversive effects of lateral hypothalamic stimulation in rats measured by a modified runway and reward summation technique. *Physiology and Behavior, 31*, 657–662.

Neill, D., Gaar, L., Clark, A., & Britt, M. (1982). "Rate-free" measures of self-stimulation and microinjections: evidence toward a new concept of dopamine and reward. In B.G. Hoebel & D. Novin (Eds.), *The neural basis of feeding and reward* (pp. 289–298). Brunswick, ME: Haer Institute.

Neill, D., Peay, L., & Gold. M. (1978). Identification of a subregion within rat neostriatum for the dopaminergic modulation of lateral hypothalamic self-stimulation. *Brain Research, 153*, 515–528.

Nicolaidis, S. (1968). Discriminatory responses of hypothalamic osmosensitive units to gustatory stimulation in cats. In C. Pfaffmann (Ed.), *Olfaction and taste* (Vol. III, pp. 569–573). New York: Rockefeller University Press.

Nicolaidis, S. (1980). Hypothalamic convergence of external and internal stimulation leading to early ingestive and metabolic responses. *Brain Research Bulletin, 5* (Suppl. 4), 97–101.

Nicolaidis, S. (1981). Lateral hypothalamic control of metabolic factors related to feeding. *Diabetologia, 20*, 426–434.

Nieuwenhuys, R., Geeraedts, L.M.G., & Veening, J.G. (1982). The medial forebrain bundle of the rat. I. General introduction. *Journal of Comparative Neurology, 206*, 49–81.

Norgren, R. (1977). Synopsis of gustatory neuroanatomy. In J. LeMagnen & P. McLeod (Eds.), *Olfaction and taste* (Vol. VI, pp. 225–232). Washington, DC: IRL Publishers.

Norgren, R., & Grill, H. (1982). Brainstem control of ingestive behavior. In D.W. Pfaff (Ed.), *The physiological mechanisms of motivation* (pp. 99–131). New York: Springer-Verlag.

Norgren, R., & Leonard, C.M. (1973). Ascending central gustatory pathways. *Journal of Comparative Neurology, 150*, 217–238.

Novin, D., & VanderWeele, D.A. (1977). Visceral involvement in feeding: there is more to regulation than the hypothalamus. In J.M. Sprague & A.N. Epstein (Eds.), *Progess in psychobiology and physiological psychology (Vol. 7*, pp. 193–241). New York: Academic.

Novin, D., Wyrwicka, W., & Bray, G.A. (Eds.), (1976). *Hunger: Basic mechanisms and clinical implications.* NewYork: Raven.

Olds, J. (1956). A preliminary mapping of electrical reinforcing effects in the rat brain. *Journal of Comparative and Physiological Psychology, 49*, 281–285.

Olds, J. (1958a.) Effects of hunger and male sex hormone on self-stimulation of the brain. *Journal of Comparative and Physiological Psychology, 51*, 320–324.

Olds, J. (1958b.) Satiation effects in self-stimulation of the brain. *Journal of Comparative and Physiological Psychology, 51*, 675–678.

Olds, J. (1958c). Self-stimulation of the brain: Its use to study local effects of hunger, sex, and drugs. *Science, 127*, 315–324.

Olds, J. (1961). Differential effects of drives and drugs on self-stimulation at different brain sites. In D. Sheer (Ed.), *Electrical simulation of the brain* (pp. 350–370). Austin: University of Texas Press.

Olds, J. (1977). *Drives and rewards: Behavioral studies of hypothalamic functions.* New York: Raven.

Olds, J., Allan, W.S., & Briese, E. (1971). Differentiation of hypothalamic drive and reward centers. *American Journal of Physiology, 22*, 368–375.

Olds, J., & Milner, P. (1954). Positive reinforcement produced by electrical stimulation of septal area and other regions of the rat brain. *Journal of Comparative and Physiological Psychology, 47*, 419–427.

Olds, M.E., & Olds, J. (1963). Approach-avoidance analysis of the rat diencephalon. *Journal of Comparative Neurology, 120*, 259–295.

Olds, M.E., & Olds, J. (1969). Effects of lesions in the medial forebrain bundle on self-stimulation behavior. *American Journal of Physiology, 217*, 1253–1264.

Oltmans, G.A., & Harvey, J.A. (1972). LH syndrome and brain catecholamine levels after lesions of the nigrostriatal bundle. *Physiology and Behavior, 8*, 69–78.

Oomura, Y., Shimiza, N., Miyahara, S., & Hattori, K. (1982). Chemosensitive neurons in the hypothalamus. Do they relate to feeding behavior. In B.G. Hoebel & D. Novin (Eds.), *The neural basis of feeding and reward* (pp. 551–556). Brunswick, ME: Haer Institute.

Ornstein, K., & Huston. J.P. (1975). Influence of 6-hydroxydopamine injections in the substantia nigra on lateral hypothalamic reinforcement. *Neuroscience Letters, 1*, 339–342.

Panksepp, J. (1971a). Is satiety mediated by the ventromedial hypothalamus? *Physiology and Behavior, 7*, 381–384.

Panksepp, J. (1971b). A re-examination of the role of the ventromedial hypothalamus in feeding behavior. *Physiology and Behavior, 7*, 385–394.

Panksepp, J. (1971c). Aggression elicited by electrical stimulation of the hypothalamus in albino rats. *Physiology and Behavior, 6*, 321–324.

Panksepp, J., & Trowill, J. (1967a). Intraoral self-injection. I. Effects of delay of reinforcement on resistance to extinction and implication for self-stimulation. *Psychonomic Science, 9*, 405–406.

Panksepp, J., & Trowill, J. (1967b). Intraoral self-injection. II. The stimulation of self-stimulation phenomenon with a conventional reward. *Psychonomic Science, 9*, 407–408.

Papez, J.W. (1937). A proposed mechanism of emotion. *Archives of Neurology and Psychiatry, 38*, 725–744.

Pavlov, I.P. (1927). *Conditioned reflexes: An investigation of the physiological activity of cerebral cortex.* New York: Oxford University Press.

Peck, J.W., & Novin, D. (1971). Evidence that osmoreceptors mediating drinking in rabbits are in the lateral preoptic area. *Journal of Comparative and Physiological Psychology, 74*, 134–147.

Penfield, W., & Rasmussen, T. (1950). *The cerebral cortex of man.* New York: Macmillian.

Pfaff, D.W. (1980). *Estrogens and brain function.* New York: Springer-Verlag.

Pfaff, D.W. (1982a). Neurobiological mechanisms of sexual behavior. In D.W. Pfaff (Ed.), *The physiological mechanisms of motivation* (pp. 287–317). New York: Springer-Verlag.

Pfaff, D.W. (Ed.), (1982b). *The physiological mechanisms of motivation.* New York: Springer-Verlag.

Pfaffmann, C. (1960). The pleasures of sensation. *Psychological Review, 67*, 253–268.

Pfaffmann, C. (1965). de Gustibus. *American Psychologist, 20*, 21–31.

Pfaffmann, C. (1980). Wundt's scheme of sensory affect in the light of research on gustatory preferences. *Psychological Research, 42*, 165–174.

Pfaffmann, C. (1982). Taste: a model of incentive motivation. In D.W. Pfaff (Ed.), *The physiological mechanisms of motivation* (pp. 61–97). New York: Springer-Verlag.

Phillips, A.G., Carter, D.A., & Fibiger, H.C. (1979). Dopaminergic substrates of intracranial self-stimulation in the caudate-putamen. *Brain Research, 104*, 221–232.

Phillips, A.G., Cox, V.C., Kakolewski, J.W., & Valenstein, E.S. (1969). Object carrying in rats: An approach to the behavior produced by stimulation. *Science, 166*, 903–905.

Phillips, A.G., & Fibiger, H.C. (1976). Long-term deficits in stimulation-induced behaviors and self-stimulation after 6-hydroxydopamine administration in rats. *Behavioral Biology, 16*, 127–143.

Phillips, A.G., & Fibiger, H.C. (1978). The role of dopamine in maintaining self-stimulation of the nucleus accumbens in the rat. *Canadian Journal of Psychology, 32*, 58–76.

Phillips, A.G., & LePiane, F.G. (1980). Reinforcing effects of morphine microinjection into the ventral tegmental area. *Pharmacology, Biochemistry, and Behavior, 12*, 965–968.

Phillips, A.G., & LePiane, F.G. (1982). Reward produced by microinjections of (d-ala), metenkephalinamide into the ventral tegmental area. *Behavioral Brain Research, 5*, 224–225.

Phillips, M.I. (1978). Angiotensin the brain. *Neuroendocrinology, 25*, 354–377.

Phillipson, O.T. (1979). Afferent projections to the ventral tegmental area of Tsai and interfasicular nucleus: A horseradish peroxidase study in the rat. *Journal of Comparative Neurology, 187*, 117–134.

Pickens, R., & Harris, W.C. (1968). Self-adminstration of d-amphetamine by rats. *Psychopharmacologia, 12*, 158–163.

Pickens, R., Meisch, R.A., & Thompson, T. (1978). Drug self-administration: an analysis of the reinforcing effects of drugs. In L. Iversen, S. Iversen, & S. Snyder (Eds.), *Handbook of Psychopharmacology* (Vol. 12. pp. 1–37). New York: Plenum.

Pickens, R., & Thompson, T. (1968). Cocaine-reinforced behavior in rats: Effects of reinforcement magnitude and fixed ratio size. *Journal of Pharmacology and Experimental Therapeutics, 161*, 122–129.

Pletscher, A. (1976). Biomedical and pharmacological aspects of Parkinson's syndrome: a short review. In W. Birdsmayer & O. Hornykiewicz (Eds.), *Advances in Parkinsonisms* (pp. 21–36). New York: Roche.

Pon, S., & Stellar, J. (1981). *Behavioral effects of unilateral hypothalamic lesions in hemiforebrain-ablated rats.* Paper presented at the Eastern Psychological Association, New York.

Porrino, L.J., Esposito, R.U., Seeger, T.F., Crane, A.M., Pert, A., & Sokoloff, L. (1984). Metabolic mapping of the brain during rewarding self-stimulation. *Science, 224*, 306–309.

Powley, T.L. (1977). The ventromedial hypothalamic syndrome, satiety and a cephalic phase hypothesis. *Psychological Review, 84*, 89–126.

Powley, T.L., & Opsahl, C.A. (1974). Ventromedial hypothalamic obesity abolished by subdiaphragmatic vagotomy. *American Journal of Physiology, 226*, 25–33.

Powley, T.L., & Opsahl, C.A. (1976). Autonomic components of the hypothalamic feeding syndromes. In D. Novin, W. Wyrwicka, & G.A. Bray (Eds.), *Hunger. Basic mechanisms and clinical implications.* (pp. 313–326). New York: Raven.

Pribram, K.H., & Kruger, L. (1954). Functions of the "olfactory brain." *Annals of the New York Academy of Sciences, 58*, 109—138.

Pycock, C.J. (1980). Turning behavior in animals. *Neuroscience, 5*, 461–514.

Ranson, S.W. (1939). Somnolence caused by hypothalamic lesions in the monkey. *Archives of Neurology and Psychiatry, 41*, 1–23.

Reid, L., Gibson, W., Glendhill, S., & Porter, P. (1964). Anticonvulsant drugs and self-stimulation behavior. *Journal of Comparative and Physiological Psychology, 57*, 353–356.

Reid, L., Hunsicker, J.P., Kent, E.W., Lindsay, J.G., & Gallistel, C.R. (1973). Incidence and magnitude of the "priming effect" in the self-stimulating rats. *Journal of Comparative and Physiological Psychology, 82*, 286–293.

Reynolds, G.S. (1968). *A primer of operant conditioning*. Glenview, IL: Scott, Foresman.

Richter, C.P. (1942–1943). Total self regulatory functions in animals and human beings. *Harvey Lectures Series, 38*, 63–103.

Risner, M.E., & Jones, B.E. (1976). Role of noradrenergic and dopaminergic processes in amphetamine self-administration. *Pharmacology, Biochemistry, and Behavior, 5*, 477–482.

Ritter, R.C. and Ladenheim, E.F. (1984) Fourth ventricle infusion of cholecystokinin suppresses feeding in rats. *Neuroscience Abstracts, 10*, 652.

Ritter, R.C., Slusser, P.F., & Stone, S. (1981). Glucoreceptors controlling feeding and blood glucose: location in hindbrain. *Science, 213*, 451–453.

Robbins, T.W. (1976). Relationship between reward-enhancing and stereotypical effects of psychomotor stimulant drugs. *Nature, 264*, 57–59.

Robbins, T.W. (1978). The acquisition of responding with conditioned reinforcement: effects of pipradrol, methylphenidate, d-amphetamine, and nomifensine. *Psychopharmacology, 58*, 79–87.

Robbins, T.W., & Everitt, B.J. (1982). Functional studies of the central catecholamines. In J.R. Smythies & R.J. Bradley (Eds.), *International review of neurobiology*, (pp. 303–366). New York: Academic.

Robbins, T.W., & Koob, G.F. (1978). Pipradrol enhances reinforcing properties of stimuli paired with brain stimulation. *Pharmacology, Biochemistry, and Behavior, 8*, 219–222.

Roberts, D.C., Koob, G.F., Klonoff, P., & Fibiger, H.C. (1980). Extinction and recovery of cocaine self-administration following 6-hydroxydopamine lesions of the nucleus accumbens. *Pharmacology, Biochemistry, and Behavior, 12*, 781–787.

Robertson, A., Laferriere, A., & Milner, P. (1982a). Development of brain stimulation reward in the medial prefrontal cortex: Facilitation by prior electrical stimulation of the sulcal prefrontal cortex. *Physiology and Behavior, 28*, 869–872.

Robertson, A., Laferriere, A., & Milner, P. (1982b). Treatment with anticonvulsant drugs retards the development of brain-stimulation reward in the prefrontal cortex, *Physiology and Behavior, 29*, 275–280.

Robertson, A., & Mogenson, G. (1978). Evidence for a role of dopamine in self-stimulation of the nucleus accumbens of the rat. *Canadian Journal of Psychology, 32*, 67–76.

Rohner, F., Dufour, A.O., Karakash, C., Marchand, Y.L., Ruf, K.B., & Jeannenand, B. (1977). Immediate effect of lesion of the ventromedial hypothalamic area upon glucose-induced insulin secretion in anaesthetized rat. *Diabetologia, 13*, 239–242.

Roll, S.K. (1970). Intracranial self-stimulation and wakefulness: effect of manipulating ambient brain catecholamines. *Science, 168*, 1370–1372.

Rolls, B.J., Rolls, E.T., & Rave, E.A. (1982). The influence of variety on human food selection and intake. In L.M. Barker, (Ed.), *The psychobiology of human food selection.* (pp. 101–122). Westport, CT: AVI.

Rolls, E.T. (1971a). Contrasting effects of hypothalamic and nucleus accumbens septi self-stimulation on the brain stem single unit activity and cortical arousal. *Brain Research, 31*, 275–285.

Rolls, E.T. (1971b). Absolute refractory period of neurons involved in MFB self-stimulation. *Physiology and Behavior, 7*, 311–315.

Rolls, E.T. (1974). The neural basis of brain-stimulation reward. *Progress in Neurobiology, 3*, 71–160.

Rolls, E.T. (1975). *The brain and reward.* Oxford: Pergamon.

Rolls, E.T. (1976). The neurophysiological basis of brain-stimulation. In A. Wauquier, & E.T. Rolls, (Eds.), *Brain-stimulation reward* (pp. 65–87). New York: Elsevier.

Rolls, E.T. (1977). Neural activity during natural and brain stimulation reward. In R.W. Hall, F.E. Bloom, & J. Olds, (Eds.), *Neuroscience research program bulletin* (pp. 231–240). Cambridge, MA: MIT Press.

Rolls, E.T. (1982). Feeding and reward. In B.G. Hoebel & D. Novin (Eds.), *The Neural basis of feeding and reward* (pp. 323–327) Brunswick, ME: Haer Institute.

Rolls, E.T., Kelly, P.H., & Shaw, S.G. (1974). Noradrenaline, dopamine, and brain-stimulation reward. *Pharmacology, Biochemistry, and Behavior, 2*, 735–740.

Rolls, E.T., & Rolls, B.J. (1982). Brain mechanisms involved in feeding. In L.M. Barker (Ed.), *Psychobiology of human food selection* (pp. 33–62). Westport, CT: AVI.

Rompré, P., Phillipe, L., & Miliaressis, E. (1983). A method providing reliable measurements of intracranial self-stimulation in spite of the presence of contingent motoric activity. *Neuroscience Abstracts, 9*, 976.

Rose, M. (1974). Pain-reducing properties of rewarding electrical brain stimulation in the rat. *Journal of Comparative and Physiological Psychology, 87*, 607–617.

Rosellini, R.A., & Lashley, R.L. (1982). An opponent process theory of motivation. VIII. Pellet preference and adjunctive behavior. *Learning and Motivation, 13*, 222–239.

Rosenblatt, J.S. (1965). The basis of synchrony in the behavioral interaction between the mother and her offspring in the laboratory rat. In B.H. Foss (Ed.), *Determinants of infant behavior* (Vol. 3, pp. 3–45). London: Meuthen.

Rossi, N., & Reid, L. (1976). Affective states associated with morphine injections. *Physiological Psychology, 4*, 269–274.

Roth, R. (1983). Neuroleptics: functional neurochemistry. In J. Coyle & S. Enna (Eds.), *Neuroleptics: Neurochemical, behavioral, and clinical perspectives* (pp. 119–156). New York: Raven.

Routtenberg, A. (1970). Forebrain pathways of reward in Rattus norvegicus. *Journal of Comparative and Physiological Psychology, 75*, 269–276.

Routtenberg, A. (1972). Intracranial chemical injection and behavior: a critical review. *Behavioral Biology, 7*, 601–641.

Routtenberg, A., (1976). Self-stimulation pathways: Origins and terminations—a three-stage technique. In A. Wauquier & E.T. Rolls (Eds.), *Brain-stimulation reward* (pp. 31–39). New York: Elsevier.

Routtenberg, A. (Ed.). (1980). *Biology of reinforcement: Facets of brain stimulation reward.* New York: Academic.

Rottenberg, A., & Lindy, J. (1965). Effects of the availability of rewarding septal and hypothalamic stimulation on bar pressing for food under conditions of deprivation. *Journal of Comparative and Physiological Psychology, 60*, 158–161.

Routtenberg, A., & Sloan, M. (1972). Self-stimulation in the frontal cortex in Rattus norvegicus. *Behavioral Biology, 7*, 567–572.

Russek. M. (1971). Hepatic receptors and the neurophysiological mechanisms controlling feeding behavior. In S. Ehrenpreis (Ed.), *Neuroscience research.* (pp. 213–282). New York: Academic.

Sacks, O. (1973). *Awakenings*. New York: E.P. Dutten.

Satinoff, E. (1983). A reevaluation of the concept of the homeostatic organization of temperature regulation. In E. Satinoff & P. Teitelbaum (Eds.), *Handbook of behavioral neurobiology: Vol. 6. Motivation.* (pp. 443–472). New York: Plenum.

Satinoff, E., & Rutstein, J. (1970). Behavioral thermoregulation in rats with anterior hypothalamic lesions. *Journal of Comparative and Physiological Psychology, 71*, 77–82.

Satinoff, E., & Shan, S. (1971). Loss of behavioral thermoregulation after lateral hypothalamic lesions in rats. *Journal of Comparative and Physiological Psychology, 77*, 302–312.

Satinoff, E., & Teitelbaum, P. (Eds.). (1983). *Handbook of behavioral neurobiology: Vol. 6. Motivation.* New York: Plenum.

Schaefer, G.J., & Holtzman, S.G. (1979). Free-operant and auto titration brain self-stimulation procedures in the rat: A comparison of drug effects. *Pharmacology, Biochemistry, and Behavior, 10*, 127–135.

Schaefer, G.J., & Michael, R.P. (1980). Acute effects of neuroleptics on brain self-stimulation thresholds in rats. *Psychopharmacology, 67*, 9–15.

Schallert, T., De Ryck, M., Whishaw, I.Q., Ramirez, V.D. & Teitelbaum, P. (1979). Excessive bracing reactions and their control by atropine and 1-dopa. *Experimental Neurology, 64*, 33–43.

Schallert, T., & Whishaw, I.Q. (1978). Two types of aphagia and two types of sensorimotor impairments after lateral hypothalamic lesions. Observations in normal weight, dieted, and fattened rats. *Journal of Comparative and Physiological Psychology, 92*, 720–741.

Schallert, T., Whishaw, I.Q., De Ryck, M. & Teitelbaum, P. (1978). The postures of catecholamine-depletion catelepsy: Their possible adaptive value in thermoregulation. *Physiology and Behavior, 21*, 817–820.

Schallert, T., Whishaw, I.Q., & Flannigan, K.P. (1977). Gastric pathology and feeding deficits induced by hypothalamic damage in rats. Effects of lesion type, size, and placement. *Journal of Comparative and Physiological Psychology, 91*, 598–610.

Schenk, S., & Shizgal, P. (1982). The substrates for lateral hypothalamic and medial prefrontal cortex self-stimulation have different refractory periods and show poor spatial summation. *Physiology and Behavior, 28*, 133–138.

Schneirla, T.C. (1959). An evolutionary and developmental theory of biphasic processes underlying approach and withdrawal. In M.R. Jones (Ed.), *The Nebraska symposium on motivation* (pp. 1–43). Lincoln, NE: University of Nebraska Press.

Schneirla, T.C. (1965). Aspects of stimulation and organization in approach/withdrawal processes underlying vertebrate behavioral development. In D. Lehrman, R. Hinde, & E. Shaw (Eds.), *Advances in the study of behavior* (pp. 1–74). New York: Academic.

Schreiner, L., & Kling, A., (1956). Rhinocephalon and behavior. *American Journal of Physiology, 184*, 486–490.

Sclafani, A., Aravich, P.F., & Landman, M. (1981). Vagotomy blocks hypothalamic hyperphagia in rats on a chow diet and sucrose solution, but not on a palatable mixed diet. *Journal of Compatative and Physiological Psychology, 95*, 720–734.

Sclafani, A., & Springer. D. (1976). Dietary obesity in adult rats. Similarities to hypothalamic and human obesity syndromes. *Physiology and Behavior, 17*, 461–471.

Sem-Jacobsen, O.W., & Torkildsen, A. (1960). Depth recording and electrical stimulation in the human brain (pp. 275–290). In E.R. Ramey & D.S. O'-Doherty (Eds.), *Electrical studies on the unanesthetized brain.* New York: Harper & Row.

Seward, J.P., Uyeda, A., & Olds, J. (1959). Resistance to extinction following cranial self-stimulation. *Journal of Comparative and Physiological Psychology, 52*, 294–299.

Sherman, J., Pickman, C., Rice, A., Leibeskind, J., & Holman, E. (1980). Rewarding and aversive effects of morphine: temporal and pharmacological properties. *Pharmacology, Biochemistry, and Behavior, 13*, 501–505.

Sherrington, C. (1906). The integrative action of the nervous system. New York: Scribners.

Shizgal, P., Bielajew, C., Corbett, D., Skelton, R., & Yeomans, J. (1980). Behavioral methods for inferring anatomical linkage between rewarding brain stimulation sites. *Journal of Comparative and Physiological Psychology, 94*, 227–237.

Shizgal, P., Bielajew, C., & Kiss, I. (1980). Anodal hyperpolarization block technique provides evidence for rostro-caudal conduction of reward signals in the medial forebrain bundle. *Neuroscience Abstracts, 6*, 422.

Shizgal, P., Kiss, I., & Bielajew, C. (1982). Psychophysical and electrophysiological studies of the substrate for brain stimulation reward. In B.G. Hoebel & D. Novin (Eds.), *The neural basis of feeding and reward* (pp. 419–429). Brunswick, ME: Haer Institute.

Shizgal, P., & Matthews, G. (1977). Electrical stimulation of the rat diencephalon: Differential effects of interrupted stimulation on on- and off-responding. *Brain Research, 29*, 319–333.

Shizgal, P., & Rompré, P. (1984). Electrophysiological characteristics of forebrain cells directly driven by medial forebrain bundle stimulation in the rat. *Neuroscience Abstracts, 10*, 310.

Silva, L.R., Vogel, J., & Corbett, D. (1982). Frontal cortex self-stimulation: Evidence for independent substrates within areas 32 and 24. *Neuroscience Abstracts, 9*, 625.

Simon, H., LeMoal, M., & Calas, A. (1979). Efferents and afferents of the ventral tegmental-A10 region studied after local injection of [3H] Leucine and horseradish perioxidase. *Brain Research, 178*, 17–40.

Skinner, B.F. (1938). *The behavior of organisms*. New York: Appleton-Century.

Smith, G.P. (1983). The place of gut peptides in the treatment of obesity. In P.B. Curtis-Prior (Ed.), *Biochemical pharmacology of obesity*. New York: Elsevier.

Smith, G.P., & Gibbs, J. (1979). Postrandial satiety. In J.M. Sprague & A.N. Epstein (Eds.), *Progress in psychobiology and physiological psychology*. (Vol. 8, pp. 179–242). New York: Academic.

Smith, G. P., Jerome, C., Cushin, B.J., Eterno, R., & Simansky, K.J. (1981). Abdominal vagotomy blocks the satiety effect of cholecystokinin in the rat. *Science, 213*, 1036–1037.

Smith, J.C. (1971). Radiation: Its detection and its effects on taste preferences. In. E. Stellar & J.M. Sprague (Eds.), *Progress in physiological psychology*. Vol. 4, pp. 53–118). New York: Academic.

Smith, J.C., Williams, D.P., & Jue, S.S. (1976). Rapid oral mixing of glucose and saccharin by rats. *Science, 191*, 304–305.

Smith, S.G., & Davis, W.M. (1973). Haloperidol effects on morphine self-administration: testing for pharmacological modification of the primary reinforcement mechanisms. *Psychological Record, 23*, 215–221.

Snyder, S.H. (1977). Opiate receptors and internal opiates. *Scientific American, 236*, 44–56.

Snyder, S.H., & Childers, S. (1979). Opiate receptors and opioid peptides. In M. Cowan, Z. Hall, & E. Kandel (Eds.), *Annual Review of Neuroscience, 2*, 35–64.

Sokoloff, D., Reivich, M., Kennedy, C., & DesRosiers, M. (1977). The 14C-deoxyglucose method for measurement of local cerebral glucose utilization. Theory, procedure, and normal values in the conscious and anesthetized albino rat. *Journal of Neurochemistry, 28*, 897–916.

Solomon, R.L. (1948). Effort and extinction: A confirmation. *Journal of Comparative and Physiological Psychology, 41*, 93–100.

Solomon, R.L. (1977). An opponent-process theory of motivation. V. Affective dynamics of eating. In L.M. Barker, M.R. Best, & M. Domjan (Eds.), *Learning mechanisms in food selection*. Houston: Baylor University Press.

Solomon, R.L. (1980). The opponent-process theory of acquired motivation . *American Psychologist, 35*, 691–712.

Solomon, R.L. (1982). The opponent process in acquired motivation. In D.W. Pfaff (Ed.), *The physiological mechanisms of motivation* (pp. 321–336). New York: Springer-Verlag.

Solomon, R.L., & Corbit, J.D. (1974). An opponent-process theory of motivation. I. Temporal dynamics of affect. *Psychological Review, 81*, 119–145.

Spencer, H. (1872). *The principles of psychology*. New York: Appelton-Century-Crofts.

Starr, M.D. (1978). An opponent process theory of motivation. VI. Time and intensity variables in the development of separation-induced distress calling in ducklings. *Journal of Experimental Psychology: Animal Behavior Processes, 4*, 338–355.

Stein, L. (1975). Norepinephrine reward pathways: Role in self-stimulation, memory consolidation, and schizophrenia. In. J. Cole, & T. Sonderegger

(Eds.), *Nebraska Symposium on Motivation, 1974* (pp. 113–159). Lincoln, NE: University of Nebraska Press.

Stein, L. (1980).The chemistry of reward. In A. Routtenberg, (Ed.), *Biology of reinforcement: Facets of brain stimulation reward* (pp. 109–130). New York: Academic.

Stein, L., & Ray. O. (1959). Self-regulation of brain stimulating current intensity in the rat. *Science, 130*, 570–572.

Stein, L., & Wise, C.D. (1967). Release of hypothalamic norepinephrine by rewarding electrical stimulation or amphetamine in the unanesthetized rat. *Federation Proceedings, 26*, 651. (Abstract).

Stein, L., & Wise, C.D. (1969). Release of norepinephrine from hypothalamus and amygdala by rewarding medial forebrain bundle stimulation and amphetamine. *Journal of Comparative and Physiological Psychology, 67*, 189–198.

Steiner, J.E. (1977). Facial expressions of the neonate infant indicating the hedonics of food-related chemical stimuli. In J.M. Weiffenbach, (Ed.), *Taste and Development: The genesis of sweet preference* (pp. 173–187). Bethesda, MD: DHEW Publication No. (NIH) 77-1068.

Steinfes, G., Heym, J., Strecker, R., & Jacobs, B. (1983). Behavioral correlates of dopamine unit activity in freely moving cats. *Brain Research, 258*, 217–228.

Steinfels, G., Strecker, R., Heym, J., & Jacobs, B. (1982). Correlates of dopamine unit activity with feeding and other behaviors in freely moving cats. In B.G. Hoebel & D. Novin (Eds.), *The neural basis of feeding and reward* (pp. 391–404). Brunswick, ME: Haer Institute.

Stellar, E. (1954). The physiology of motivation. *Psychological Review, 61*, 5–22.

Stellar, E. (1982). Brain mechanisms in hedonic processes. In. D.W. Pfaff (Ed.), *The physiological mechanisms of motivation* (pp. 377–407). New York: Springer-Verlag.

Stellar, E., & Hill, J.H. (1952). The rat's rate of drinking as a function of water deprivation. *Journal of Comparative and Physiological Psychology, 45*, 96–102.

Stellar, E., & Jordan, H.A. (1970). Perception of satiety. In D.A. Hamburg (Ed.), *Perception and its disorders* (pp. 298–317). Baltimore: Williams & Wilkin.

Stellar, E., & McCleary, R.A. (1952). Food preference as a function of the method of measurement. *American Psychologist: 7*, 256. (Abstract).

Stellar, J. R. (1976). *Approach-withdrawal analysis of the lateral and medial hypothalamus.* Unpublished doctoral dissertation, University of Pennsylvania.

Stellar, J.R., Brooks, F.H., & Mills, L.E. (1979). Approach and withdrawal analysis of the effects of hypothalamic stimulation and lesions in rats. *Journal of Comparative and Physiological Psychology, 93*, 446–466.

Stellar, J.R., & Gallistel, C.R. (1975). Runway performance of rats for brain-stimulation or food reward: Effects of hunger and priming. *Journal of Comparative and Physiological Psychology, 89*, 590–599.

Stellar, J. R., & Heard, K. (1976). Aftereffects of rewarding lateral hypothalamic brain stimulation and feeding behavior. *Physiology and Behavior, 17*, 865–867.

Stellar, J.R., Illes, J., & Mills, L.E., (1982). Role of ipsilateral forebrain in lateral hypothalamic stimulation reward in rats. *Physiology and Behavior, 29*, 1089–1097.

Stellar, J.R., Kelley, A., & Corbett, D. (1983). Effects of peripheral and central dopamine blockade on lateral hypothalamic self-stimulation: Evidence for both reward and motor deficits. *Pharmacology, Biochemistry, and Behavior, 18*, 433–442.

Stellar, J.R., & Neeley, S.P. (1982). Reward summation function measurements of lateral hypothalamic stimulation reward: Effects of anterior and posterior medial forebrain bundle lesions. In. B.G. Hobel & D. Novin, (Eds.), *The neural basis of feeding and reward* (pp. 431–443). Brunswick, ME: Haer Institute.

Stricker, E.M. (1983). Brain neurochemistry and the control of food intake. In E. Satinoff & P. Teitelbaum (Eds.), *Handbook of behavioral neurobiology: Vol. 6. Motivation* (pp. 329–366). New York: Plenum.

Stricker, E.M., Swerdloff, A.F., & Zigmond, M.J. (1976). Intrahypothalamic injections of kainic acid produces feeding and drinking deficits in rats. *Brain Research, 158*, 470–473.

Stricker, E.M., & Zigmond, M.J. (1976a). Brain catecholamines and the lateral hypothalamic syndrome. In D. Novin, W. Wyrwicka, & G. Bray (Eds.), *Hunger: Basic mechanisms and clincal implications* (pp. 19–32). New York: Raven.

Stricker, E.M., & Zigmond, M.J. (1976b). Recovery of function after damage to central catecholamine-containing neurons: A neurochemical model for the lateral hypothalamic syndrome. In J.M. Sprague, & A.N. Epstein, (Eds.), *Progress in psychobiology and physiological psychology* (Vol. 6, pp. 121–188). New York: Academic.

Stunkard, A., & Stellar, E. (Eds.). (1984). *Eating and its disorders*. New York: Raven.

Swanson, L.W. (1982). The projections of the ventral tegmental area and adjacent regions: A combined fluorescent retrograde tracer and immunofluorescence study in the rat. *Brain Research Bulletins, 9*, 321–353.

Teitelbaum, P. (1967). *Physiological psychology: Fundamental principles*. Englewood Cliffs, NJ: Prentice-Hall.

Teitelbaum, P. (1971). The encephalization of hunger. In E. Stellar & J.M. Spraque (Eds.), *Progress in physiology psychology* (Vol. 4, pp.319–350). New York: Academic

Teitelbaum, P. (1973). Discussion on the use of electrical stimulation to study hypothalamic structure and function. In A. Epstein, H. Kissileff, & E. Stellar (Eds.), *The neuropsychology of thirst: New findings and advances in concepts*. (pp. 143–154). New York: Winston & Sons.

Teitelbaum, P. (1977). Levels of integration of the operant. In W. Honig & J. Staddon (Eds.), *Handbook of operant behavior* (pp. 7—27). Englewood Cliffs, NJ: Prentice-Hall.

Teitelbaum, P. (1982). What is the "zero condition" for motivated behavior? In B.G. Hoebel & D. Novin (Eds.), *The neural basis of feeding and reward* (pp. 7–24). Brunswick, ME: Haer Institute.

Teitelbaum, P., & Cytawa, J. (1965). Spreading depression and recovery from lateral hypothalamic damage. *Science, 147*, 61–63.

Teitelbaum, P., & Epstein, A.N. (1963). The role of taste and smell in the regulation of food and water intake. In C. Pfaffmann (Ed.), *Olfaction and taste* (pp. 347–360). New York: Macmillan.

Teitelbaum, P., Schallert, T., & Whishaw, I.Q. (1983). Sources of spontaneity in motivated behavior. In E. Satinoff & P. Teitelbaum (Eds.), *Handbook of behavioral neurobiology: Vol. 6. Motivation* (pp. 23–65). New York: Plenum

Thorndike, E.L. (1898). Animal intelligence: An experimental study of the associative processes in animals. *Psychological Review Monograph Supplement, 2*, 1–109.

Thorndike, E.L. (1911). *Animal intelligence.* New York: Macmillan.

Tinbergen, N. (1951). *The study of instinct.* New York: Oxford University Press.

Titchener, E.B. (1896). *An outline of psychology.* New York: Macmillan.

Tolman, E.C. (1932). *Purposive behavior in animals and men.* New York: Appleton-Century-Crofts.

Tombaugh, T., Anisman, H., & Tombaugh, J. (1982). Extinction and dopamine receptor blockade after intermittent reinforcement training: failure to observe functional equivalence. *Psychopharmocology, 70*, 19–28.

Tombaugh, T., Ritch, M., & Shepard, D.T. (1980). Effects of pimozide on accuracy of performance and discrimination of correct responding on a simultaneous discrimination task in the rat. *Pharmacology, Biochemistry, and Behavior, 13*, 859–862.

Tombaugh, T., Tombaugh, J., & Anisman, H. (1979). Effects of dopamine receptor blockade on alimentary behaviors: home cage food consumption, magazine training, operant acquisition, and performance. *Psychopharmacology, 66*, 219–226.

Troland, L.T. (1928). *The fundamentals of human motivation.* New York: Nostrand.

Twitchell, T.E. (1970). Reflex mechanisms and the development of prehension. In K.J. Connolly (Ed.), *Mechanics of motor skill development* (pp. 25–45). New York: Academic.

Unemoto, M. (1968). Self-stimulation of the lateral hypothalamus after electrolytic injury of the medial forebrain bundle in the cat. *Brain Research, 11*, 325–335.

Ungerleider, L., & Coons, E.E. (1970). A behavioral measure of homosynaptic and heterosynaptic temporal summation in the self-stimulation of rats. *Science, 169*, 785–787.

Ungerstedt, U. (1971a). Stereotaxic mapping of the monoamine pathways in the rat brain. *Acta Physiologiae Scandinavia, 367* (Suppl.), 1–48.

Ungerstedt, U. (1971b). Striatal dopamine release after amphetamine or nerve degeneration revealed by rotational behavior. *Acta Physiologiae Scandinavia, 367* (Suppl.), 49–68.

Valenstein, E.S, (1964). Problems of measurement and interpretation with reinforcing brain stimulation. *Psychological Review, 71*, 415–437.

Valenstein, E.S. (1966). The anatomical locus of reinforcement. In E. Stellar & J.M. Sprague (Eds.), *Progress in physiological psychology* (Vol. 1, pp. 149–190). New York: Academic.

Valenstein, E.S. (1969). Behavior elicited by hypothalamic stimulation: A prepotency hypothesis. *Brain, Behavior, and Evolution, 2*, 295–316.

Valenstein, E.S. (1975). Brain stimulation and behavioral control. In J. Cole & T. Sonderegger (Eds.), *Nebraska symposium on motivation, 1974* (pp. 251–292). Lincoln, NE: University of Nebraska Press.

Valenstein, E., & Beer. B. (1964). Continuous opportunity for reinforcing brain stimulation. *Journal of Experimental Analysis of Behavior, 7*, 183–184.

Valenstein, E.S., Cox, V.C., & Kakolewski, J.W. (1967). Polydipsia elicited by the synergistic action of a saccharin and glucose solution. *Science, 157*, 552–554.

Valenstein, E.S., Cox, V.G., & Kakolewski, J.W. (1968). Modification of motivated behavior elicited by electrical stimulation of the hypothalamus. *Science, 159*, 1119–1121.

Valenstein, E.S, Cox, V.G., & Kakolewski, J.W. (1970). Reexamination of the role of the hypothalamus in motivation. *Psychological Review, 77*, 16–31.

Valenstein, E.S, & Valenstein, T. (1964). Interaction of positive and negative reinforcing systems. *Science, 145*, 1456–1458.

Van der Kooy, D. (1984). Area postrema: Site where cholecystokinin acts to decrease food intake. *Brain Research, 295*, 345–347.

Veening, J., Swanson, L., Maxwell, W., Nieuwenhuys, R., & Geeraedts, L. (1982). The medial forebrain bundle of the rat. II. An autoradiographic study of the major descending and ascending components. *Journal of Comparative Neurology, 206*, 82–108.

Velley, L., Chaminade, C., Roy, M.T., Kempf, E., & Cardo, B. (1983). Intrinsic neurons are involved in lateral hypothalamic self-stimulation. *Brain Research, 268*, 79–86.

Villablanca, J.R, Marcus, R.J., & Olmstead, C.E. (1976). Effects of caudate nuclei of frontal cortical ablations in cat. I. Neurology and gross behavior. *Experimental Neurology, 52*, 389–420.

Wald, G., & Jackson, P. (1944). Activity and nutritional deprivation. *Proceedings of the National Academy of Sciences, 30*, 255–263.

Waraczynski, M., & Stellar, J.R. (1984). *Choice method analysis of brain stimulation reward psychophysics.* Paper presented at Canadian Psychological Association meeting. Ottawa, Canada.

Warden, C.J. (1931). *Animal motivation studies: The albino rat.* New York: Columbia University Press.

Wasserman, E.M., Gomita, Y., & Gallistel, C.R. (1982). Pimozide blocks reinforcement but not priming from MFB stimulation in the rat. *Pharmacology, Biochemistry, and Behavior, 17*, 783–787.

Wassman, M.J., & Flynn, J. (1962). Directed attack elicited from the hypothalamus. *Archives of Neurology, 6*, 220–227.

Watson, J.B. (1919). *Psychology from the standpoint of a behaviorist.* New York: Lippincott.

Wauquier, A., & Rolls, E.T. (1976). *Brain-stimulation reward.* New York: Elsevier

Waxman, S.G. (1978). Variations in axonal morphology and their functional significance. In S.G. Waxman (Ed.), *Physiology and pathobiology of axons.* New York: Raven.

Weijnen, J.A.W.M., & Mendelson, J. (Eds.). (1977). *Drinking behavior*. New York: Plenum.

Weiss, K.R., Koch, U.T., Koester, J., Rosen, S.C., & Kupfermann, I. (1982). The role of arousal in modulating feeding behavior of Aplysia. Neural and behavioral studies. In B.G. Hoebel & D. Novin (Eds.), *The neural basis of feeding and reward* (pp. 25–57). Brunswick, ME: Haer Institute.

Wheatley, M.D. (1944). The hypothalamus and affective behavior in cats. *Archives of Neurological Psychiatry, 52*, 296–316.

Wiesner, B.P., & Shepard, N.M. (1933). *Maternal behavior in the rat*. Edinburgh: Oliver and Boyd

Wilcott, R.C. (1981). Medial and orbital cortex and the suppression of behavior in the rat. *Physiology and Behavior, 27*, 237–241.

Windle, W.F. (1981). *Stephen Walter Ranson: Ground-breaking neuroscientist*. Los Angeles: Brain Research Institute.

Wise, R.A. (1980). Action of drugs of abuse on brain reward systems. *Pharmacology, Biochemistry, and Behavior, 13*, 213–223.

Wise, R.A. (1981). Intracranial self-stimulation: Mapping against the lateral boundaries of the dopaminergic cells of the substantia nigra. *Brain Research, 213*, 190–194.

Wise, R.A. (1984). Neuroleptic and operant behavior: The anhedonia hypothesis. *Behavior and Brain Sciences, 5*, 39–87.

Wise, R.A. (1983). Technical comment. *Science, 222*, 1253.

Wise, R.A., & Bozarth, M. (1982). Action of drugs of abuse on brain reward systems: An update with specific attention to opiates. *Pharmacology, Biochemistry, and Behavior, 17*, 239–243.

Wise, R.A., & Bozarth, M. (1984). Brain reward circuitry: Four circuit elements "wired" in apparent series. *Brain Research Bulletin, 12*, 203–208.

Wise, R.A., Spindler, J., & Legault, L. (1978). Major attenuation of food reward with performance-sparing doses of pimozide in the rat. *Canadian Journal of Psychology, 32*, 77–85.

Woods, J., & Schuster, C. (1968). Reinforcement properties of morphine, cocaine, and SPA as a function of unit dose. *International Journal of Addiction, 3*, 231–237.

Woods, S.C., Lotter, E.C., McKay, L.D., & Porte, D. (1979). Chronic intracerebroventricular infusion of insulin reduces food intake and body weight of baboons. *Nature, 282*, 503–505.

Woodworth, R.S. (1918). *Dynamic psychology*. New York: Columbia University Press.

Worms, P., Broekkamp, C., & Lloyd, K. (1983). Behavioral effects of neuroleptics. In J. Coyle & S. Enna (Eds.), *Neuroleptics: Neurochemical, behavioral, and clinical perspectives* (pp. 93–117). New York: Raven.

Wundt, W. (1873–1874). *Grundzuge der physiologiechen Psychologie*. Leipzig: Engelmann.

Yadin, E., Guarini, V., & Gallistel, C.R. (1983). Unilaterally activated systems in rats self-stimulating at sites in the medial forebrain bundle, medial prefrontal cortex, or locus coeruleus. *Brain Research, 266*, 39–50.

Yeomans, J.S. (1975). Quantitative measurement of neural post-stimulation excitability with behavioral methods. *Physiology and Behavior, 15*, 593–602.

Yeomans, J.S. (1979). The absolute refractory periods of self-stimulation neurons. *Physiology and Behavior, 22*, 911–919.

Yeomans, J.S. (1982). The cells and axons mediating medial forebrain bundle reward. In B.G. Hoebel & D. Novin (Eds.), *The neural basis of feeding and reward* (pp. 405–417). Brunswick, ME: Haer Institute.

Yeomans, J., Gallistel, C.R., & Reivich, M. (1978). Autoradiographic mapping of brain regions activated during self-stimulation using 14C-2-deoxyglucose. *Neuroscience Abstracts, 4*, 230.

Yeomans, J.S., Matthews, G., Hawkins, R.D., Bellman, K., & Doppelt, H. (1979). Characterization of self-stimulation neurons by their local potential summation properties. *Physiology and Behavior, 22*, 921–929.

Yeomans, J.S., Prior, P., & Bateman, F.D. (1982). Current-distance relationship for neurons mediating circling behavior elicited by tectopontine tract stimulation. *Neuroscience Abstracts, 8*, 292.

Yim, C.Y., & Mogenson, G.J. (1980). Effect of iontophoretically applied dopamine on the response of nucleus accumbens neurons to electrical stimulation of the amygdala. *Neuroscience Abstracts, 6*, 447.

Yokel, R.A., & Pickens, R. (1973). Self-administration of optical isomers of amphetamine and methylamphetamine by rats. *Journal of Pharmacological and Experimental Theraputics, 187*, 27–33.

Yokel, R.A., & Pickens, R. (1974). Drug level of d- and l- amphetamine during intravenous self-administration. *Psychopharmacologia, 34*, 255–264.

Yokel, R.A., & Wise, R.A., (1976). Attenuation of intravenous reinforcement by central dopamine blockade in rats. *Psychopharmacology, 48*, 311–318.

Young, P.T., (1936). *Motivation of behavior: The fundamental determinants of human and animal activity.* New York: Wiley.

Young, P.T. (1941). The experimental analysis of appetite. *Psychological Bulletin, 38*, 129–164.

Young, P.T. (1945). Studies of food preferences, appetite, and dietary habit. V. Techniques for testing food preferences and the significance of results obtained with different methods. *Comparative Psychology Monographs, 19*, 1–58.

Young, P.T., & Greene, J. T. (1953). Quantity of food ingested as a measure of relative acceptability. *Journal of Comparative and Physiological Psychology, 46*, 288–294.

Zarevics, P., & Setler, P.E. (1979). Simultaneous rate-independent and rate-dependent assessment of intracranial self-stimulation: evidence for the direct involvement of dopamine in brain reinforcement mechanisms. *Brain Research, 169*, 499–512.

Zhang, D-M., Stellar, E., & Epstein, A.N. (1984). Together intracranial angiotensin and systemic mineralocorticoid produce avidity for salt in the rat. *Physiology and Behavior, 32*, 677–681.

Index